Table of Symptoms page 40

ALSO BY SUSAN M. LOVE, M.D.,
WITH KAREN LINDSEY

Dr. Susan Love's Breast Book

DR. SUSAN
LOVE'S
HORMONE
BOOK

DR. SUSAN LOVE'S HORMONE BOOK

Making Informed Choices About Menopause

SUSAN M. LOVE, M.D.,

WITH KAREN LINDSEY

RANDOM HOUSE

NEW YORK

Grateful acknowledgment is made to the following for permission to use
specified material:

John Boik: Table 10.1: "Natural Agents That Affect Hormone Bioavailability"
from *Cancer and Natural Medicine* by John Boik. Reprinted by permission.

*Key Porter Books, Dutton Signet, a division of Penguin Books USA Inc., and
Janine O'Leary Cobb:* Table 3.1: "Menopausal Ailments" from *Understanding
Menopause* by Janine O'Leary Cobb. Copyright © 1988 by Key Porter Books.
Copyright © 1993 by Janine O'Leary Cobb. Rights throughout the United
States are controlled by Dutton Signet, a division of Penguin Books USA Inc.
Reprinted by permission of Key Porter Books, Dutton Signet, a division of
Penguin Books USA Inc., and Janine O'Leary Cobb.

Rodale Press, Inc.: Table from article entitled "Get Your Isoflavones Here" by
Holly McCord, R.D., with Teresa Yeykal from *Prevention* magazine (August
1996). Copyright © 1996 by Rodale Press, Inc. Reprinted by permission of
Rodale Press, Inc. For subscription information, please call 1-800-666-2503.

Marcia Williams: Illustrations by Marcia Williams. Reprinted by permission
of the illustrator.

Library of Congress Cataloging-in-Publication Data

Love, Susan M.
[Hormone book]
Dr. Susan Love's Hormone book: making informed choices about
menopause / Susan M. Love, with Karen Lindsey.
p.   cm.
Includes bibliographical references and index.
ISBN 0-679-44970-1
1. Menopause—Hormone therapy—Popular works.   I. Lindsey, Karen.
II. Title.
RG186.L68   1997
618.1'75061—dc20   96-35120

Random House website address: http://www.randomhouse.com/
Printed in the United States of America on acid-free paper
2 4 6 8 9 7 5 3
First Edition

This book is dedicated to my mother, who never lived long enough to face the hormone dilemma; my life partner, Helen, who faces it with me daily; our daughter, Katie, who I hope will have it solved. It is also for all of the women who crave information to make informed choices about their health.

Acknowledgments

As this book is being completed, I am awed by how many people helped. First I want to thank Jill Kneerim, my agent, who conceived of the book and nurtured it along; and Elizabeth Rapoport, the midwife and editor who helped it be born. Karen Lindsey, my coauthor, has put up with three of these "births" now, and I thank her for her graciousness and enormous talent. Marcia Williams is also part of the team. Her art always captures exactly what I was thinking.

I want to also thank all of the professionals who let me interview them and who read parts of the book for me. Any errors of fact or interpretation happened in spite of their generosity. They include Elizabeth Barrett-Connor, Deborah Grady, Steven Cummings, Gail Greendale, Lynn Rosenberg, Walter Willett, Marie Cargill, and Susun Weed. Special thanks to those readers who sloughed through the penultimate draft: Cindy Pearson, Janine O'Leary Cobb, and Elizabeth De Gracia, and most especially Marcie Richardson, who is still the only gynecologist I truly trust.

I am blessed with a very supportive family. My father, James Love, and his wife, Ruth, are my loyal fans. My sisters, Chris and Betsy, and my brother, Michael, have always been my cheerleaders. I thank them all.

The staff of the Revlon/UCLA Breast Center put up with a lot of extra work because of the book. I want to thank Sherry Goldman, Leslie Laudeman, Shannon Tucker, Lisa Gotori-Koga, and Christi Dearborn. Jean Chou's support kept the research going while I was preoccupied. Special thanks to Kathy Salcedo, who spent countless hours in the library photocopying articles, often long into the night. Her efforts did not go in vain.

Connie Long deserves her own separate thank-you. She was there well into the night slaving over this baby and deserves much of the credit for the fact that it got born at all. I value her loyalty, intelligence, good nature, and goodwill, not to mention her skill.

Finally, I need to thank Brownie, the cocker spaniel, my running partner and shadow whose place is always at my feet. Special thanks and all of my love go to my life partner, Helen Cooksey, and our daughter, Katie Love-Cooksey.

SUSAN LOVE
August 1996

Contents

Introduction

We're the baby boomers. We were born in the 1940s or 1950s, we wanted to change the world in the 1960s, and we didn't trust anyone over thirty. Now *we're* over thirty—well over thirty. And if we haven't changed the world, we've changed a lot of things in it. During the years before we began approaching middle age, a sexual revolution occurred, and we claimed the right to enjoy our bodies. The women's movement made it clear that we had the right to define that enjoyment, and we wanted more knowledge about how our bodies worked. We read books about menstruation and about childbirth. We talked about natural childbirth and about nurse-midwives; we were no longer contented to turn ourselves over to the paternal obstetrician, allowing him to escort us into a hospital room and close the door, from which we would emerge discreetly sanitized, the process of birthing hidden from the world and from ourselves. Now we're approaching menopause, and we want to decide for ourselves how we'll experience this process as well.

But how do we do that? We're faced with all kinds of options, and with them all kinds of questions. If I have terrible hot flashes, do I just have to grit my teeth and bear them—the midlife equivalent of the biblical curse on Eve, "Unto woman he said, I will greatly multiply thy sorrow and thy conception; in sorrow thou shall bring forth children"? Or should I take hormones to stop them? If I take hormones, will I get breast cancer? If I don't, will I get brittle bones, or die of a heart attack? Is there anything besides taking hormones I could be doing? Is there anything I *should* be doing?

I've been hearing variants of these questions over and over in the past few years—from patients, from friends, from my own inner voice as I've hit middle age and begun experiencing the undeniable signs of what was once referred to, in sad whispers, as "the change."

That is why I've written this book. Not to give definitive answers to all these questions—there are no definitive answers, alas—but to explore the context in which the questions arise, to separate the medical from the cultural, the hype from the reality, and the few "definites" from the many "maybes."

The idea that there are no definitive answers can be startling to some people. There has been such a strong tendency in our culture to see menopause as a disease that much of our thinking has been formed by that construct. We expect that diseases will have well-defined causes and treatments. But menopause is not a disease; it's a natural stage in a woman's life. It often carries with it symptoms that range from mildly annoying to debilitating; and coming as it does in midlife, it often coincides with, and interacts with, other aspects of aging. The symptoms may or may not need treatment; the conditions of aging may or may not entail diseases for which a number of methods of prevention or cure exist. We will discuss all of these throughout this book. But keep in mind that one thing you can "do" about menopause is nothing.

Menopause is a change. Not "the" change, but "*a*" change—and your body, in the midst of that change, is in a process of flux for a few years. (Those few years are not actually menopause itself, but perimenopause— a differentiation we'll go into at length.) As this process goes on, you may find that your symptoms or your experience of them changes. The decisions you make about what, if anything, to do for your symptoms may change accordingly. That's fine—you're not marrying your approach to menopause; you're only agreeing to live with it while you're happy together.

Your body isn't the only thing that's constantly changing. Medical scientists are working feverishly to create new drugs for menopause, and to reexamine old drugs. Researchers are studying the effects of lifestyle changes and the role of alternative medicine. Any new finding, positive or negative (or, as is often the case, unclear), may alter your choice. We've seen the startling transformations of medicine at work in our lifetimes. Miracle drugs and vaccines have been discovered, curing and even eliminating once fatal diseases such as polio and smallpox. The meat-and-potatoes diet so beloved of the previous generation turns out to be less healthful than we'd thought. We've learned about the importance of low-fat and "natural" foods. Any decision you make today can be altered by tomorrow's new discovery.

The powers that be in our consumer society have taken full advantage of new discoveries, often interweaving them with our fears of aging and death—and most powerfully with images of desirability created by advertisers. Whether it's the pretty young thing who can't get a date because of her acne or the white-haired woman whose husband can't take her dancing until she takes care of her incontinence, advertising has seized on the vulnerabilities accompanying each stage of life. Aspects of life once considered too shameful to mention are now being talked about openly—as they should be. But too often they're spoken of only in the language of advertising, which, paradoxically, returns them to the arena of shame. Hide your pimples, hide your period, hide your gray hair.

Inevitably, as we begin to talk more openly about menopause, commercialism tries to define the terms of this discussion as well. Turn on your television and you'll see a vigorous sixty-year-old looking wistfully at her grandson, terrified that osteoporosis will keep her from playing with him—and the drug company's 800 number, flashing on the screen, offers her salvation from this dire fate. The drug companies, not surprisingly, want you to take drugs for menopause, and so they need to convince you that it's a disease. Thus they foster the notion that menopause is an illness for which any enlightened woman will seek a cure.

All of this combines into a confusing picture. What are you supposed to do about this new phase in your life? You don't look or feel like a twenty-year-old anymore. (Maybe *you* do, but I certainly don't!) You're approaching menopause, and you've heard frightening things about what's ahead of you. Will you lose your sexuality and your sexual attractiveness? Will you be tormented by constant, debilitating hot flashes? Or maybe you're already having perimenopausal symptoms—hot flashes, irregular or heavy bleeding, mood swings—and you're not enjoying it. You don't like bursting into a sweat during a business meeting. You feel like a friend of mine who muttered angrily, "I've got more tampons and sanitary napkins in my briefcase than medical papers!"

On the other hand, you could be one of the lucky ones whose symptoms aren't so bad. You may not be feeling any discomfort at all. But you're scared. You've read in the newspapers that postmenopausal women are in danger of heart disease or osteoporosis. You see a hunched-over, fragile elderly woman in the supermarket checkout line, and you wonder if that's you in another twenty or thirty years.

Your gynecologist has the answer: hormone replacement therapy. You're told that it will make the hot flashes go away, that it will keep your bones and heart strong. You'll almost certainly be handed a prescription, but not much information about how these hormones work, what they can and can't do, and what their possible dangers are. You walk out of the doctor's office, prescription in hand, and turn toward the nearest drugstore. And then you stop.

Do you really want to take a hormone pill every day for the rest of your life? Hormones are powerful. Are there side effects that you don't know about? Are these things safe? If you take them, will you go on having periods for the rest of your life? Wasn't DES supposed to be a miracle drug? And didn't you read somewhere that estrogen causes uterine and breast cancer?

At the same time, you're nervous about what will happen if you don't take them. Are you condemning yourself to osteoporosis or heart failure? Will you look aged and worn before your time? Didn't that article say hormones keep your skin soft, your hair full? What about your sex life—does menopause kill your libido? If so, will hormone therapy bring it back to life?

You're not a kid anymore; you've been around long enough to know that there's no free lunch. But you don't want to deprive yourself of something that might vastly improve, and even extend, your life.

You're not alone in your confusion. Only 30 percent of women who are given prescriptions for "hormone replacement therapy" ever fill them. They don't throw the prescriptions away; they don't clearly decide against hormone therapy: they just ignore the issue for the time being, or they decide to get more information at some point. They feel they should take the pills, and they feel they shouldn't. The promises of hormone therapy appear to be too good to be true. The questions that nag at you also nag at these women and even at those who do fill their prescriptions: more than half of them stop taking the pills within a year.

If you're one of the women who are confused about whether or not to take hormones, it isn't because age has dimmed your brain cells and you can't put together obvious information anymore. You're confused, at least in part, because the *doctors* are confused. You're getting different, and contradictory, messages. As I'll explain, the prevailing wisdom on hormones has done several flip-flops in the last few decades. Sometimes when I lecture, I hear from a woman who says, "I went through menopause in the 1970s. We were all taking hormones, and then the doctors told us it caused cancer and everyone stopped taking it." There have been so many changes over the last few decades that if you heard one set of "facts" ten years ago, you may be hearing an entirely different set today. The state of our knowledge keeps changing as new studies provide new data—and as the pharmaceutical companies find new ways to interpret the data.

The problem is that there is no easy answer, no clear-cut right or wrong. Hormone therapy is neither a fountain of youth nor an "evil empire." It can solve one problem, but it can create another—sometimes for the same person. I can't tell you in this book whether or not you should take hormones, but I can spell out the pros and cons, examining the various promises that have been made for menopausal hormone therapy, and letting you know what the side effects and dangers can be. Perhaps most important, I can help you judge what weight to give each factor. In other words, I can give you the material with which to make your decision.

One of the things I'll be doing is making a clear distinction between the two concerns for which hormones are prescribed. You may be considering hormones for symptoms you're currently experiencing, such as insomnia or hot flashes. Or you may be considering hormones to help prevent possible future problems, such as heart disease or osteoporosis. These two concerns—short-term relief of symptoms and long-term prevention of disease—have very different implications, and this is one reason for the confusion surrounding menopausal hormone therapy. As you'll see, two or three years on hormones may be perfectly safe, but ten or twenty years can cause health problems at least as serious as those the medications are supposed to prevent.

In the last decade or so, we've redefined health. In the past, you were sick because you had a symptom—you went to the doctor because you had a headache or a broken bone or a fever. With the shift in emphasis to prevention, some of that has changed. Now you can take a test to see whether you have or are "at risk" for a disease, in spite of the fact that you're symptom-free. In some cases, this has been beneficial, even lifesaving. Pap smears have caught cervical cancer in time to prevent it from spreading; mammograms, although less effective, have nonetheless caught breast cancer in some women at earlier stages than would have been possible in the past.

But this shift to early detection and prevention has also created a sense of disease in some situations where no disease exists. Even mammograms have detected harmless conditions that might or might not have grown into cancers, precipitating surgery that might or might not have been needed. And being "at risk" for a given disease does not mean that you'll certainly get it. Whenever medical intervention is used for potential rather than existing problems, it's important to be cautious. You need to ask yourself if the intervention itself could create health problems.

This is a pertinent question when you're thinking about hormone therapy. Even the language is suspect: "hormone replacement therapy" is what it's usually called, suggesting that you've lost something you should get back; you're suffering from a disease, "estrogen deficiency." (If "estrogen deficiency" is a disease, are all men sick?) And a disease, of course, must be cured.

As I've said, I don't buy the idea that menopause is a disease, and I refuse to cooperate with the language that defines it as such. For this reason, I refer to treatment with estrogen or estrogen and progesterone as *menopause hormone therapy* or just *hormone therapy*. You're not replacing "lost" hormones, any more than you're replacing something when you take an aspirin for a headache. You're adding something to relieve a symptom or to prevent a condition from occurring in the future.

At this point, I might have added to your confusion by talking about "symptoms." Doesn't this mean you *are* sick? Actually, it doesn't mean that at all. Over the years, the meaning of "symptom" has become blurred, and people tend to think that a symptom always goes with a disease: your sniffles are a symptom of a cold; your headache is a symptom of flu. But in fact, a symptom is any physical sensation that bothers you: it doesn't have to be a symptom "of." If you have unpleasant sensations in connection with menopause, you have symptoms. You do *not* have a disease.

None of this means that you shouldn't take hormones, either for symptoms or for prevention. For the record, I am not against hormones. I think they are the right choice for many women. What I am against is the knee-jerk tendency of most doctors to hand you a prescription for hormones as soon as you seem to be menopausal, rather than taking a close look at your individual needs, risks, and lifestyle. Given the pressure to prescribe—which I'll describe more in Chapter 2—it's up to you to look into all the ins and outs, and not assume that you've got some nasty condition the doctors can cure with their little pills. It's a complicated business, and not all the answers are in yet.

What I hope to do with this book, then, is to help you understand the factors that should go into helping you make your decision. This book will show you that menopause is a natural stage of a woman's life, not an aberration that needs to be controlled. It will explain how the medical industry has redefined menopause as a disease so that you'll spend money going to doctors and buying drugs to cure it.

At the same time, I know that some of the symptoms you experience during this stage of your life can be uncomfortable, and that your fears of osteoporosis, heart disease, and the other illnesses that come with aging are well grounded. So the book will discuss all these symptoms and diseases, and explain what you can do to address each of them. It will start with the least dangerous approach—lifestyle changes such as exercise and healthy eating habits—and move through to the increasingly more dangerous modes, such as the powerful drugs favored by the pharmaceutical companies and by many doctors.

What this book will not do is provide your answer for you. The "right" answer, or combination of answers, is something only you can come up with for yourself.

And so you stand there, outside the doctor's office, the prescription in your hand, uncertain whether to throw it away or get it filled. In this book, we'll give you information that will help you make that decision.

DR. SUSAN LOVE'S HORMONE BOOK

CHAPTER 1

What Is Menopause?

Before we can discuss how to deal with menopause, we need to have a clear understanding of what it is. If menopause means "the time after your periods stop," why are you having hot flashes while you still have periods? What if you have had a hysterectomy—does that count as menopause? What if you never go through menopause: your doctor just puts you on hormones and you still get your periods?

STAGES OF MENOPAUSE

Some of this confusion exists because there are two different stages of the menopausal process. During *perimenopause,* your hormones are winding down, fluctuating, and often creating the mass of symptoms we think of, incorrectly, as "menopausal." (I'll discuss those symptoms in detail in Chapter 3.) In most cases these are self-limiting and will go away in a few years.

Then there's menopause itself—which is, strictly speaking, your last period (the permanent "pause" of your menses). In the aftermath of menopause, you may also experience some symptoms, but these are typically different from the symptoms of perimenopause. (Menopause itself, by the way, probably lasts for only a few days, and you can never be absolutely certain when it's occurred. Menopause is usually identified retrospectively, when it's been a year since your last period. Everything afterward is, strictly speaking, "postmenopause"—though for some reason this term has never existed as a noun.) To avoid ambiguity, in this book I'll comply with popular custom and continue to speak of menopausal women, menopausal symptoms, etc. Keep in mind that I'm referring to the time after that elusive moment when your last period ends.

The reason I'm making such a fuss about semantics is that terminology can cause a lot of needless fear. One of the reasons many women dread menopause is that they confuse the lesser, often nonexistent symptoms of menopause with the symptoms of perimenopause—and so they think that the most difficult, confusing symptoms will last the rest of their lives. In reality, the vast majority of women experience these two stages very differently.

A study done in 1965[1] found that, with the exception of hot flashes, the symptoms of perimenopausal women were closer to those of adolescents entering puberty than to those of postmenopausal women. When adolescent girls experience weight gain, bloating, and mood changes, doctors assume it's because of high estrogen levels. When women around menopause get the same symptoms, the assumption is that it's caused by low estrogen. Yet it has seemed obvious to me for quite a while that the time right before menopause is the mirror image of puberty. During puberty, this mechanism is starting up. Then, at the other end, when the process is gearing down, the same things happen again. What these two life stages have in common is big hormonal shifts.

Times of hormonal shifts and changes are times of symptoms. Remember the highs and lows of puberty? Your face broke out. You slept half the day. Your brain didn't seem to work the way it used to. You didn't know what was going on with your body. Well, with perimenopause it happens all over again. This too is a time of symptoms in many women—hot flashes, mood swings, fuzzy thinking, insomnia, and, most of all, unpredictability. Fortunately, just as with puberty, these symptoms do end. The hot flashes dry up, just as the acne did. Your sleep patterns return to normal; your brain becomes able to focus again. Nothing lasts forever. Overall it takes about three to six years for each transition, until your body is balanced at a new place. (God help those of you who have teenage daughters going through puberty while you are going through perimenopause!)

Acknowledging the parallels between puberty and perimenopause makes the whole process less strange and scary. You've been through puberty. It may not have been fun, but you survived it. And you did it without any of the wisdom and coping skills you now have. Most of you also experienced the enormous hormonal shifts that accompany pregnancy and childbirth, and you got through those as well. There's no reason to fear perimenopause or menopause. It's just hormones again, and we all know how to deal with them.

Biology of Perimenopause: Puberty in Reverse

What exactly is going on in your body, bringing about all this change? In order to clearly define the phases of the menopausal transition, we need to review a little biology. Okay, I know there are those of you who want to skip the technical stuff. "I don't want a biology class—just tell me what to do!" Feel free to skip the next several paragraphs and pick up again on page 16. For those of you who want to know how it works, read on.

It's amazing to realize how little we actually know about the way a woman's body works. We do know, however, that hormones work together in a wonderful and intricate dance.

At birth your two ovaries contain all the eggs you'll have throughout your lifetime (Figure 1.1). The eggs sit there comfortably for several years; then you hit puberty and the beginning of your years of menstruation. Your hormone levels begin fluctuating wildly before settling down as you reach maturity. The major hormones involved in this process of puberty are follicle-stimulating hormone (FSH) and luteinizing hormone (LH), which come from the pituitary gland (a small gland that lives near the brain, between the eyes); and estrogen and progesterone, which come from the ovaries. In addition, the hypothalamus (part of the brain) produces gonadotrophic-releasing hormones (GnRHs). (Are you still with me? One

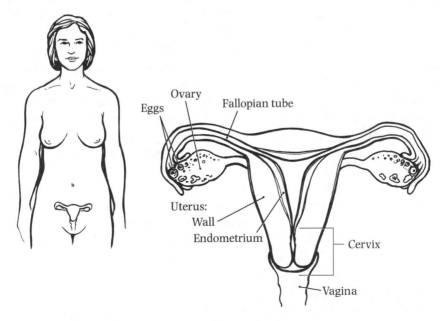

FIGURE 1.1   Female reproductive organs.

friend who read this chapter said it was great until she saw FSH, and then her eyes glazed over. And she was a doctor!)

Now you've left puberty, and you're in your fertile years. Here's basically what goes on for the next three decades. Stimulated by FSH, the follicles (the eggs encased in their little sacs) produce estrogen. When estrogen rises to a certain level, the hypothalamus gets the message and secretes LH-releasing hormone, which tells the pituitary to turn off the FSH and produce a surge of LH. When the LH is at its peak, you ovulate—that is, your body releases an egg from the follicle. The follicle shifts to a new phase (the corpus luteum) and starts to produce progesterone in addition to estrogen. These hormones build up the lining of the uterus. The corpus luteum is short-lived, and its production of hormones soon begins to decline. Once the progesterone in your blood drops to a certain level, you get rid of the uterine lining by getting your period. In addition, these lower levels of estrogen and progesterone tell the hypothalamus to get some FSH going, and the cycle continues. Every month (except for those few months when you're pregnant), your body goes through this familiar dance.

It can take a while for this dance of hormones to get its choreography down (Figure 1.2). One study[2] confirmed that earlier on, girls have longer periods. The follicles don't mature, and there may be a longer time between periods. This seems to be in part because the ovaries aren't yet really producing eggs, and egg production is necessary for a regular "loop" to be completed. Once the whole system gets coordinated, a girl's cycles become regular and her symptoms settle down.

This dance, like most dances, has a few variations. In some months, you don't ovulate. Then there's no progesterone, and your period may actually come early and be lighter or later, or you may skip a period altogether. Your body also requires a certain amount of fat to ovulate; if you're very thin or anorexic, or an athlete who is very muscular with very little fat, you will often lose your period and in essence be in temporary menopause. This time it is literally a "pause," because you'll get your periods back once your fat level increases.

So far so good. But our understanding of the process gets a little fuzzier when you come to the end of your fertile years. The standard line in the textbooks is that when you run out of eggs and you're no longer ovulating, your body stops making estrogen. This causes your FSH to go up as your pituitary tries to kick-start the ovary into producing more eggs. When that doesn't work, everything just shuts down.

Yet often the symptoms of perimenopause (breast tenderness, headaches, increased vaginal lubrication) are symptoms not of low estrogen but rather of *high* estrogen. Some recent studies have looked more deeply into what may explain this phenomenon. A study in 1989[3] fol-

FIGURE 1.2   The hormonal dance.

lowed five perimenopausal women, one of whom had occasional periods every six weeks. Fortunately, the researchers were monitoring her
while this was going on. They discovered that she had low estrogen in
the beginning of her cycle. Her ovaries were just tired. As a result of the
low estrogen, she had symptoms such as hot flashes for a couple of
weeks. Meanwhile, her hypothalamus and pituitary responded to these
low levels by increasing her FSH. Her ovaries woke up in a panic, as
though they had been sleeping on the job, and decided to make up for
their inattention by sending out lots more estrogen—two to three times
the normal amount. And then she ovulated. Now her symptoms were
those of high estrogen—breast tenderness, etc. Her progesterone went
up after ovulation and her period came exactly two weeks late and was
very heavy, because of the extra estrogen. You can see why life at this
stage is so unpredictable. (While working on this book, I experienced
exactly the same cycle as the woman in the study and was relieved to
know exactly what was going on.)

This is often what happens in perimenopause. Sometimes your estrogen
levels are high and your progesterone is low, and you might get symptoms
of PMS. At other times, your estrogen levels shift and you get hot flashes.
Then for several months you're back to normal. So the common explanation—that your symptoms are due to low estrogen—is wrong. Your symptoms are actually caused by *fluctuations* of high and low estrogen.

This also explains why you can't just get a blood test, as some doctors suggest, to tell if you are in perimenopause. Because your FSH goes up with menopause (once your periods have stopped for a year), some doctors will measure your FSH level in perimenopause, hoping to determine whether or not your symptoms are related to menopause. If your FSH is low, they tell you you're not in menopause and they don't know what your symptoms are from. If your FSH is high, they say you're menopausal—even if you're still menstruating.

Are they crazy? No. They simply don't understand perimenopause. A study in 1994[4] confirmed that perimenopausal women show varying patterns. Some women in the study still menstruated, even with increased levels of FSH. Some had increased FSH and normal to low estrogen. Some continued having cycles and had abrupt fluctuations of both FSH and estrogen. Some had typical postmenopausal levels one month and typical premenopausal levels the next month. So testing FSH isn't a really definitive tool for determining your menopausal status.

If you've stopped menstruating for several months, the FSH test might be a little more useful for determining if you've really gone into menopause. But even then it's not 100 percent accurate. Another study[5] found that 20 percent of women who have no period for three months start having their cycles again. I've had patients with breast cancer who were thrown into menopause by their chemotherapy treatments, missed three or four months of periods, and showed high FSH levels—and then got their periods back. There's no foolproof test to determine menopause. The only way we can really do that is the good old-fashioned way. If you haven't menstruated for a year, you're menopausal.

Why hasn't your gynecologist talked to you about the hormonal flux that ushers in both puberty and menopause? Unfortunately, medical texts often don't really explore these two experiences that frame the reproductive years. In one book, for example—a 1,000-page textbook on reproductive endocrinology (endocrinology is the study of hormones)—all I could find on puberty was a single paragraph, which said, in full: "These prolonged menstrual intervals are associated with the frequent occurrence of anovulatory cycles during adolescence and the menopause transition. At these times the aberrant secretions of estradiol and gonadotropin result in an asynchrony of the various elements of the system and manifest as an anovulatory cycle." On perimenopause, in a chapter titled "The Menopause and Perimenopausal Period," this text notes only: "It is surprising that relatively few substantive investigative studies have been performed concerning physiologic and clinical aspects of the perimenopausal period."[6] And that's it—that's all there is.

Biology of Menopause: The Misunderstood Ovary

In a way, you can't blame the doctors for failing to understand what the ovary does in perimenopause. Throughout most of medical history, we have never really understood the ovary itself, and because we haven't grasped the full complexity of this intricate organ, doctors have assumed that after menopause, when the ovary is no longer capable of reproduction, it shrivels up, dries out, and becomes completely useless.

Actually, this misunderstanding can serve as a metaphor for the way our culture sees the postmenopausal woman herself—as nonproductive, dried up, and useless. This is consistent with the common definition of menopause as "ovarian failure." With the assumption that the ovary's sole function is to produce eggs comes an inevitable corollary: When it stops doing that, it's "failed."

In fact, making eggs isn't the ovary's whole function, any more than reproduction is a woman's whole function. The ovary is more than just an egg sac. It's an endocrine organ—an organ that produces hormones. And it produces hormones before, during, and after menopause. With menopause, the ovary goes through a shift. It changes from a follicle-rich producer of estrogen and progesterone into a stromal-rich producer of estrogen and androgen. Stroma is the glue that holds all the eggs together. In youth, you have more eggs and less stroma. As time goes on, you have fewer and fewer eggs but more and more stroma. In its hormonal dance with the hypothalamus and pituitary, the postmenopausal ovary continues to respond to the call of the pituitary. It responds to high levels of FSH and LH with increased production of testosterone as well as continued lower levels of the estrogens estrone and estradiol, and the estrogen precursor androstenedione.[7,8] (I'll discuss this in Chapter 15.) The hormonal dance doesn't end; the band just strikes up a different tune.

Testosterone is, of course, a male hormone. But don't panic: you're not going to grow a beard. Every human being produces both male and female hormones; the proportion differs according to your gender. Much of the testosterone and androstenedione is converted to estrone (a form of estrogen) by an enzyme called aromatase found in fat and muscle. This continued production of hormones varies somewhat from one woman to the next and may well explain some of the individual differences in symptoms after menopause. It also explains why women who have both ovaries removed surgically, thereby losing all of these hormones, have worse symptoms of menopause, and increased vulnerability to osteoporosis[9] and cardiovascular disease.

Jane Cauley, a researcher on menopause, measured hormone levels in the blood of postmenopausal women.[10] She found a lot of variability, but interestingly, neither age nor time since menopause had much to do with it. Hormone production doesn't automatically dwindle with age. Obesity, defined as being at least 20 percent over your ideal weight, was a major determinant of estrogen levels in postmenopausal women. The estrogen levels of obese women were 40 percent higher than those of nonobese women. This is because aromatase is found in fat. However, obesity wasn't the only determinant. Women who were physically active also had higher blood levels of estrone. Although some active women had lower levels of estrogen (because they were thinner), paradoxically, those with more muscle mass had higher estrogen levels. This is probably because muscle also has a large amount of aromatase. In fact, outside of the ovary, the aromatase in muscle accounts for the conversion of 25 to 30 percent of androgens to estrogens, while the aromatase in fat accounts for only 10 to 15 percent.[11] Other organs that can perform this conversion include the brain, skin, hair, and bone marrow. So we're not left without hormones after menopause. Our misunderstood ovaries continue to be productive.

What this all means is that our ovaries serve more than one function. Reproduction is their most dramatic function, but it isn't the only one. These organs have as much to do with the maintenance of a woman's own life as they do with her role in bringing other lives into the world. The menopausal ovary is neither failing nor useless. It's simply beginning to shift from its reproductive to its maintenance function. It's doing in midlife exactly what many people do—it's changing careers.

PREMATURE MENOPAUSE

Some women go through menopause in their thirties—an unusually young age. This is called *premature menopause.* Just as you can start your period early (any time after age nine) and still be normal, you can normally stop menstruating early. Like surgical menopause, which we will discuss below, this leaves you at greater risk for bone loss and higher cholesterol levels. So you might want to take hormones until you reach fifty, the average age of menopause. You can then decide whether to continue on hormones for prevention or gradually taper off, mimicking a natural menopause.

SURGICAL MENOPAUSE

Up to now, we've been talking about natural menopause—that is, what happens to a woman on her own, as she ages without intervention. But there are other ways to go into menopause. The most dramatic is to have both of your ovaries removed. This is called a bilateral oophorectomy, and it may be done independently or together with a hysterectomy—surgical removal of the uterus. Removing the ovaries will result in an immediate menopause. Not only do you experience an onslaught of symptoms because of the sudden change in hormones, but you lose most of your hormones permanently. You don't lose all of them, however. The adrenal gland also produces androstenedione and a little bit of testosterone. This androstenedione is converted to estrogen in fat and muscle. For some women, particularly those who are obese or muscular, this may be enough to counteract symptoms. For others it is not. In addition, there are some data indicating that women who have their ovaries removed have higher rates of osteoporosis and heart disease, even on hormone therapy.[12]

Sometimes only one ovary is removed. If the remaining ovary continues to function, you'll go through menopause at the normal time. But sometimes the remaining ovary stops functioning prematurely (perhaps because of injury to its blood supply during surgery), and you experience premature menopause.

Finally, you may have your uterus out but still retain both ovaries. In that case, as we discuss in Chapter 11, you may go through menopause earlier or right on time. But how will you know? Since you're no longer menstruating, you won't have any missed periods to show that you're approaching menopause. You may get hot flashes, night sweats, or any of the other symptoms we discuss in Chapter 3. But suppose you don't have any symptoms? Generally, you can figure that you'll have gone through menopause somewhere between ages forty-eight and fifty-three. You can consider estrogen therapy if you're suffering from symptoms or if you feel you need it for prevention. You shouldn't wait, however, to adopt a healthy lifestyle. The sooner you start with that, the more it will help prevent all kinds of diseases, whenever you actually go through menopause.

MEDICAL MENOPAUSE

There are other forms of menopause brought on by forces outside your own body. Very often women who have been treated for cancer with chemotherapy go into temporary or permanent menopause. (That condition will be reversed in about 30 percent of cases when chemotherapy ends.) Radiation for colon cancer can also create menopause.

There are drugs that block the gonadotropin-releasing factors that stimulate FSH and LH. They can put you into a reversible menopause. They include Lupron and Synarel, which are usually given for short amounts of time to treat endometriosis or to shrink fibroids before surgery.

These forms of menopause have not been well studied. Nonetheless, it appears that with medical menopause the severity of symptoms is somewhere between that associated with surgical menopause and that associated with natural menopause.

WHY DO WE HAVE MENOPAUSE?

The Theory That "We Weren't Supposed to Live This Long"

The pervasive assumption that the postreproductive ovary is useless probably ties in with our culture's generally negative attitude toward aging. There is a widely held misconception, based on a misreading of statistics, that old age itself is unnatural—that we're not meant to live long enough to go into menopause. According to this argument, in the old days, before human intelligence created artificial, life-prolonging environments, people died of "old age" at thirty or forty. Since we've artificially extended life, we need artificial tools to help make the extra years bearable. Thus we need hormone replacement to address the illnesses entailed by a life that should have been over long ago.

But "average life expectancy" doesn't mean the age at which people usually die. It means something quite different. It's determined by adding together all ages of death and then dividing them by the population. If a lot of people die young, you'll have a low average life expectancy. For example, the average life expectancy in 1640 was thirty-two. This was a time of high infant mortality and widespread poverty that caused malnutrition and the deadly exhaustion of constant work with no time for rest. Among the wealthy, those "who survived to twenty-one could expect to live into the early 60s."[13] It appears that a fairly large percentage of people lived into healthy old age, in fact. During the Renaissance, men in most European countries were considered fit for military service until they were sixty.[14] A late-sixteenth-century English chronicler estimated that in most villages 10 percent of the inhabitants were sixty or older. Antonia Fraser, in *The Weaker Vessel*, cites numerous examples of seventeenth-century Englishwomen who lived into their nineties and beyond: "It would not be not so much the lack of aged persons as the lack of a large middle-aged group which would surprise us about the seventeenth century," Fraser writes.[15]

"Nature," then, has no particular objection to our living past our fertility.

In the article "Overview on Menopause," researcher Wulf Utian offers a look at some of the history of this stage of life. "Menopause," he tells us, "was recognized as a stage in human life at least as far back as the biblical era. Abraham in Genesis acknowledged the fact of reproductive failure when he pondered the prospect that a couple who were 190 years old would be granted offspring."[16] It's unlikely that people really did live for 200 years or more, but this does suggest that they routinely lived past their fertility—that women lived past menopause. Further, Utian notes, Aetius of Amida, writing in the sixth century, observed that women usually menstruated until forty-five, rarely continuing past fifty. He said nothing to suggest that it was strange for a woman to live this long—as he surely would have if most women died before forty. He attributed variations in menstrual activity to age, season of the year, the woman's eating habits and other activities, and the presence of complicating diseases.

The fact that the ovary is an organ with two distinct life phases—first as a source of eggs, then as a maintenance organ—also gives the lie to the idea that nature didn't intend us to live this long. If we were all supposed to be dead by menopause, there would be no natural purpose in the ovary's switching gears like this. It would simply stop working—just as popular mythology believes it does. But it doesn't; it simply starts its new job.

The Grandmother Hypothesis

The anthropologist Margaret Lock, among others, has pondered why menopause exists, from an evolutionary perspective.[17] Why, she asks, is women's fertility limited when men's is not? What advantage is created for survival when women live on after their fertility is over? From studying hunter-gatherer societies, anthropologists[18] have come up with the "grandmother hypothesis." Human children need to be cared for over a long period of time, and so women who were fertile their whole lives would not be able to care as well for their later children. In addition, society needed a group of nonfertile women who could serve as teachers and child care workers and gatherers of food while fertile women were busy having babies. These women, the "grandmothers," were the core of a society and served a necessary function in propagating and maintaining the tribe.

But this theory of evolutionarily predestined grandmothers has little currency in cultures that devalue age. In the United States, we've been particularly prone to this. We deny most of what's good about old age. We deny the elderly their sexuality at the same time that we define sexuality as all-important. We pat the grandmother on the head and send her Hallmark cards, without really acknowledging the deep joys she can have both in her role as grandmother and outside of it. We treat old age as a shameful condition, not as a passage in life. Instead of offering respect for old age, we offer illusions of eternal youth.

I am not trying to deny all the problems that come with aging, or to pretend that aging is all fun. You may lose strength as you grow old. You're susceptible to many more illnesses than when you're young—and you're closer to the inevitability of death. But wisdom, life experience, and the ease of having passed through certain phases of your life and knowing who and where you are—all these have their own value.

MENOPAUSE AS A METAMORPHOSIS

Susun Weed, in her book *The Menopausal Years: The Wise Woman Way*,[19] describes menopause as a metamorphosis, a time when you truly change from one person to another, just as you did at puberty. Such a change is never fun, or even comfortable, but the end result in growth and maturity is usually worthwhile. And indeed we are leading new lives, whether they appear so in clear-cut life changes or not. Often a perimenopausal woman will say, "I don't feel like my old self." To the extent that this means she's feeling unwell, or that she's disoriented by symptoms, the feeling will eventually go away as she moves into and past menopause itself.

But on a deeper level, she feels this way because she *isn't* her old self— any more than the twelve-year-old adolescent is the eight-year-old she was before, or any more than the twenty-year-old is the twelve-year-old or the forty-year-old is the twenty-year-old. Menopause is a transition into a new part of your life: some of your old self will remain—or will return when your symptoms quiet down—and some of it will fade away as it's replaced by new ideas, interests, attitudes, and abilities.

Germaine Greer talks about our truest self emerging from the "chrysalis of conditioning"[20] only after menopause has liberated us from our reproductive bodies. Ursula Le Guin writes that "the woman who is willing to make that change must become pregnant with herself."[21]

I think that's an important consideration when you're thinking hormones—especially if you're considering taking hormones for the rest of your life. If you never experience this change, something gets stunted. Certainly it makes sense to alleviate any overwhelming symptoms. But it seems to me that at some point, you want to experience the transition, to go through it literally to get to that other place. It's a bit like childbirth. Most of us don't want the drug-induced "twilight sleep" our mothers may have had, where they never knew what happened but simply woke up to find a newborn in their arms. Today, some women choose natural childbirth; others want an epidural to help them along; but most women want to experience giving birth if they can. Even puberty is worth experiencing. I think of the young kids doing alcohol, pot, even stronger drugs rather than live through the painful, terrifying, unpredictable experiences of adolescence. You blot out the pain, yes—but at what cost to your spirit? You can create for yourself a state of suspended animation, without pain or confusion, but also without joy, without growth, without discovery.

A NEW PARADIGM

As you can see, how you look at menopause is all in the framing. As long as we refer to menopause as "ovarian failure," "reproductive failure," or "estrogen-deficiency disease," we will have negative feelings and expectations about it. But if we view it as a hormonal shift mirroring puberty, it begins to look much different. As I thought about this concept, I began to see another way to frame women's lives.

Recent studies on young girls have shown that they are full of themselves. (I'm the mother of an eight-year-old girl: I didn't need the studies to figure that out!) They have lots of self-esteem, and they are on top of the world. Then, when puberty hits, they lose it. They become timid. They do less well in school. They become insecure about their bodies. They're not the fearless world-beaters they once were.

Meanwhile, at the other end, what happens to postmenopausal women? Occasionally they get worn down by society's devaluation of them, and they end up mirroring the forlorn figures in the estrogen ads. But when they're able to break through that image, they blossom. They feel themselves capable of changing the world. They no longer feel constrained by the dictates of finding a man for reproduction. They come into their own. Margaret Mead called this stage of life "postmenopausal zest." It has often been postmenopausal women who become leaders—Golda Meir, Indira Gandhi, Margaret Thatcher, Eleanor Roosevelt. It was postmenopausal women who helped get us the right to vote.

What does this say? Maybe the problem isn't estrogen deficiency after menopause—maybe it's too much estrogen before. Dare I say "estrogen poisoning"? Maybe the only way women can become docile enough to couple and reproduce is if they are under the influence of domesticating hormones. Biologically, this would mandate forty years of having cycles. But maybe when our biological responsibility is taken care of, we're allowed to be freed of those domesticating hormones and can reclaim our eight-year-old self again, full of beans and ready to take on the world.

I know you're laughing—or at least smiling. Who knows what's true? But doesn't this view make you feel a whole lot better about menopause?

The time has come for us to reclaim menopause from those who try to define it for us—and to look squarely at those who wish to medicalize it.

CHAPTER 2

The Medicalization
of Menopause

MENOPAUSE AS THE NEWEST DISEASE

We've seen it before. Childbirth was once considered natural. Women gave birth at home, attended by midwives. Then, during our grandmothers' times, childbirth moved from home to hospital and midwives were replaced by doctors. The results weren't uniformly disastrous: for one thing, infant and maternal mortality was greatly reduced. But better pre-natal care would have had an even greater effect while still allowing women to control their own birth processes. And the rate of cesareans went up with hospital births. So did the incomes of obstetricians. Women had once sat up to give birth, assisted by gravity and midwives; now they had to lie helplessly while their doctors did everything. As Western culture has become more and more high-tech, so has birthing. Fetal monitors are used routinely, in spite of studies showing that they have little worth. If you don't get ultrasound, chorionic villus sampling (the newest technique for prenatal diagnosis), or amniocentesis, you are made to feel you are somehow neglecting your baby. The medical profession is slowly recognizing that many women don't like this medicalizing approach, and so there has been a boom in birthing rooms, made to look just like your bedroom at home—but all the high-tech machines are still present, carefully hidden from view.

The medical profession even tried to medicalize puberty. Many of us were put on birth control pills during puberty to "regulate" our cycles—but the cycle is supposed to be irregular at that point of our lives.

And now, right on cue, as the first baby boomers hit fifty, there's a strong push to medicalize menopause. Interestingly, as Sandra Coney points out in *The Menopause Industry,* the medical profession's concept of "treating" menopause was shaped by the advent of tranquilizers and antidepressants in the 1950s. These drugs were first used primarily in mental hospitals, but "there was a bigger market waiting to be tapped and the pharmaceutical companies were not slow to realize it. By the early 1960s, psychotropics were widely promoted to doctors as being ideal for middle-aged women and able to 'cure' the 'symptoms of menopause.' "[1] Though the widespread prescribing of tranquilizers for housewives was soon abandoned, a subtle change had taken place in the public's thought process. Menopause was considered an illness to be treated.

The next step was to shift from the mind to the body. These women weren't crazy, just sickly: they just had "estrogen-deficiency disease." One might think that if estrogen deficiency were really a disease, the doctors would have declared all men chronically ill. But no, this disease was a result of a particularly feminine problem defined in the gynecology textbooks as "reproductive failure" or "ovarian failure." Women in midlife were therefore defined as sick failures—and this notion continues to dominate medical thinking.

It's an ugly and dangerous notion, equating a natural stage in a woman's life with illness. It echoes age-old attitudes about the "uncleanness" of menstruation and childbirth. While men go from youth to adulthood to old age, women progress from uncleanness to disease.

To be fair to the doctors of the mid-twentieth century, they were following a misogynist tradition dating back two hundred years. Earlier descriptions of menopause were fairly matter-of-fact. But by the 1700s, according to Wulf Utian, editor of the journal *Menopause,* doctors began sounding gloomy about menopause.[2] By 1845 a man named Colombat de l'Isère was warning postmenopausal women not to allow themselves to have erotic feelings, since no one could possibly respond to them: "Their features are stamped with the impression of age and their genital organs are sealed with the signet of sterility."[3]

This image has never died out. Over a century later, the gynecologist Robert Wilson wrote a spectacularly popular book called *Feminine Forever.*[4] Its cover boldly described the book as a "fully-documented discussion of one of medicine's most revolutionary breakthroughs—the discovery that menopause is a hormone deficiency disease, curable and totally preventable." (I'll discuss this watershed publication in more detail shortly.)

So it's no surprise that F. P. Rhoades, writing in the *Journal of the American Geriatric Society,* in 1967 called menopause a tragedy: "Many women are leading an active and productive life when this tragedy strikes. They are still attractive and mentally alert; they deeply resent what to them is a cat-astrophic attack upon their ability to earn a living and enjoy life."[5]

In 1985, the International Menopause Society, meeting in France to reach a consensus on how to define menopause, took a less melodramatic approach, describing the climacteric simply as the transitional period from reproductive to nonreproductive status, and menopause as beginning with the final menstrual period, typically occurring around age fifty-one.[6]

Wulf Utian was unhappy with this straightforward medical definition: it lacked the tragic dimension favored by Wilson and company. Menopause, Utian claimed, was an endocrinopathy—an endocrine disease—that had drastic effects on the pelvis and its surrounding tissue. "The longer these effects are allowed to continue without corrective therapy," he warned grimly, "the more likely there is to be an expression of the pathological process."[7]

Today, this controversy continues. Elizabeth Barrett-Connor was one of the first doctors to discover that hormone therapy might protect against heart disease, yet she has consistently warned that "[e]strogen deficiency is not a disease in the same sense as diabetes or hypothyroidism, because every woman who lives long enough will become estrogen deficient."[8] Other doctors, however, still cling to the notion of menopause as a disease. For example, the physician Theresa L. Crenshaw was quoted in 1996, in an article in *The Philadelphia Inquirer*, as saying that menopause "is not a nat-ural condition; it is an endocrine disorder and should be treated medically with the same seriousness we treat other endocrine disorders, such as dia-betes or thyroid disease."[9]

This insistence on viewing menopause as a disease has a number of implications. On a practical level, it implies the need for medication: dis-eases are treated. On a deeper level, it defines older women as aberrant. Pre-menopausal women are normal; postmenopausal women are not.

Indeed, if we insist on defining women as hormonally diseased creatures (as distinct from their wholesomely testosteroned brothers), we might just as well look at our reframing again. "Estrogen deficiency" is, supposedly, a disease from a biological standpoint because, as I'll discuss in depth later, it makes women more susceptible to weaker hearts and thinner bones. But the premenopausal years also have health risks related to estrogen—too much estrogen. Breast and uterine cancer are both caused, in part, by an oversupply of this hormone. So we could argue that, since nature intended us to have ten or twenty children, rather than the two or three most women have, this constant fertility, unchecked by regular pregnancy, keeps all that estrogen circulating and creates its own disease—let's call it "estrogen-surplus disease." Fortunately, however, it's a disease we can cure. We can put all women into menopause at puberty, and give them drugs to reverse it temporarily when they want to have children. In fact, one researcher, Malcolm Pike,[10] suggests that women at high risk for these diseases be put into a reversible premature menopause and then given very low doses of hormones to maintain their hearts and bones. This idea may sound crazy, but is it any more crazy than putting all postmenopausal women on hormones and trying to keep them premenopausal forever?

In fairness, not all the advocates of hormone therapy believe that every woman should be kept premenopausal. Pieter van Keep[11] describes a "milestone" in the history of hormone therapy—the first meeting on the subject held by the Health Foundation in Geneva in 1971. These European scientists and clinicians defined their therapeutic strategy: "We should not aim at making . . . a postmenopausal woman into a premenopausal woman again," they said, refreshingly. But they still wanted us all on hormones. "We should try to make a bad postmenopausal woman into a good postmenopausal woman."[12] So now, not only are menopausal women diseased—some, at least, are also "bad." But we can become both healthy and good by taking the doctors' magic little pills.

This depiction of menopause has crept into the thinking of women as well. A study done in 1986 found that 53 percent of women thought menopause was a medical condition and should be treated medically.[13] That was over ten years ago: the percentage must be far higher now. Studies show that the women most likely to remain on hormones are those who think of menopause as a medical complaint. It makes sense: if you think you have a medical problem, you take pills to cure it. If you think you're going though a normal stage of life, you're far less likely to respond to that by taking medicine.

In the United States, the highest use of hormone therapy is among women who have had their ovaries removed when they had hysterectomies. There are two reasons for this. First, hysterectomies are often done on women who are comparatively young—in their mid-thirties or early forties. In this case, the women tend to want to take hormones at least until the time they would have probably gone naturally into menopause. Second, women who have hysterectomies later, at around the time of menopause, generally have a stronger sense of menopause itself as a medical condition, since it's been instigated by a medical procedure. Their symptoms have been brought on by a medical process, not a natural one, and it seems reasonable to treat them medically. (Few postmenopausal women have hysterectomies, and those who do generally have them because of cancer, which usually rules out hormone therapy; see Chapter 8.)

Many other women believe that menopause is a disease because their doctors treat it as a disease, insisting that a woman patient should take hormones simply because she is approaching menopause. I would often discover, in the course of getting a new patient's medical history, that she was taking hormones; she'd be surprised when I asked why. "Well, because you're supposed to be on it," she'd say. When I probed further, some women would indeed tell me they had awful hot flashes, extreme swings of mood, or some other very troublesome symptom. But some would turn out to have had no symptoms at all. Their doctors simply told them they should be on hormone therapy, and they complied. Many of these women have told me they expressed uneasiness to their doctors about continuing the hormones and wanted to stop, only to be told emphatically that they should remain on the medication for the rest of their lives.

The American College of Obstetrics and Gynecology's "Premenopausal Office Visit Form" has a list of the benefits of hormone replacement therapy, and the concerns and risks involved. It has boxes to check off, attesting that counseling was done. To be fair, it even mentions counseling about symptomatic relief for hot flashes (if estrogen is contraindicated). It allots a space for the regimen planned and chosen and the date started. There is *no* space for "patient's opinion" and *no* box is provided to be checked if the doctor and patient decide against it.

Even people you'd expect to be skeptical about Western medicine often buy into the idea that menopause must be "treated." A forty-five-year-old friend of mine (who eats health food, takes herbal remedies, and avoids doctors like the plague) told me she'd been lucky so far because she hadn't needed any estrogen. But she knew it was in her future and said that when the time came she'd try to take natural estrogen. When I asked why she was so sure she'd need it, she said, "I'll need it to manage my menopause, of course!" It apparently hadn't occurred to her that she might not need to "manage" anything. I've come across this frequently—people in the alternative medical movement who accept without question the basic premise that all women need estrogen, and quibble only about which kind.

CROSS-CULTURAL STUDIES AND THE "DISEASE MODEL"

Looking at other cultures highlights something very important. If menopause is a disease, its worst symptoms seem to be limited to white women in Western cultures. I think this is a crucial point. Until menopause became big business, American women were always told their symptoms were in their heads. With the new business of hormone therapy, there's been a complete flip-flop. Not only have the symptoms become "real," but all women are expected to experience all symptoms, and with the same degree of severity.

Yet individual and cross-cultural differences in women's experience of menopause suggest something far more complex. Diet and reproductive history probably influence what symptoms a woman has, and social factors influence how she interprets her menopause. So we need to look at the whole experience.

Menopause in Japan: Differences in Lifestyle

Margaret Lock did a survey of menopausal symptoms in Japan.[14] She was astonished to find that the Japanese had no word for a hot flash. Instead, they used words that encompassed a range of changes in body temperature, including suddenly flushing after drinking alcohol, a sensation experienced by a large proportion of East Asians of both genders. The most common symptom, experienced by 52 percent of the women in Lock's study, was stiff shoulders: it's almost as if these women literally felt the weight of the world on their shoulders. Twenty-eight percent had headaches. Less than 20 percent had other symptoms. Only 9.5 percent had hot flashes, and only 3.2 percent had night sweats.[15]

Interviews with doctors confirmed these findings. Thirty doctors were questioned for this study, and all said that the symptoms their menopausal patients complained of most were shoulder stiffness, headaches, and dizziness. The equivalent words for hot flashes were near the bottom of their list of symptoms; some didn't even include them at all. "Every Japanese doctor interviewed during the survey and since that time confirms that hot flashes are not symptoms about which Japanese women consult a doctor," writes Lock.[16] Women hadn't been going to their doctors with menopausal symptoms: when they did go, they consulted primary care physicians, not gynecologists or psychologists. Yet Japan is an extremely health-conscious nation with a high doctor-patient ratio and universal health insurance, with easy access to health facilities.

But changes are brewing. For the past two years, the subject of menopause has suddenly been taken up repeatedly in Japanese women's magazines. The supposed long-term benefits of hormone therapy have been emphasized, including its alleged effectiveness against dementia, stroke, heart disease, and osteoporosis. Many articles have indicated that hormone therapy can help women recover their youth. The medicalization of menopause is creeping into Japan.

Japanese women have a life expectancy of nearly eighty-two years—higher than ours. It's true that, like American women, Japanese women have osteoporosis at twice the rate of men—in part, at least, because they live longer. Yet osteoporosis—a bone-thinning disease that typically affects people in their late seventies and eighties—is only half as common among Japanese women as among American women. What makes this really fascinating is that most Japanese women have lower bone mass than Caucasian women. If osteoporosis were only about bone mass, they'd have more, not less, of it—as you'll see in Chapter 5. As for coronary heart disease, the mortality rate of Japanese women is a quarter that of American women. The mortality rate from breast cancer is a fourth to a third that of North American women. Japanese women drink little alcohol, exercise continuously throughout their lives, and rarely smoke. Apart from a high consumption of pickled foods, they eat a well-balanced diet with a lot of soy products and no milk. (See Chapter 12 for a discussion of the amazing qualities of soy.) It's beyond me why they'd want to interfere with what seems like a winning system by introducing hormone therapy.

Biological Differences

Not all the differences are based on diet, however. Other studies of different cultures demonstrate that at least some cross-cultural differences are biological. Jews from North Africa living in Israel experience few symptoms, while Jews of European ancestry have symptoms similar to those of Americans. In 1990, one study[17] looked at two groups of Indonesian women who experienced few hot flashes. The researchers had hypothesized that the women who migrated and became acculturated into urban life would get more hot flashes, but in fact they turned out to have no increase in symptoms.

The Mayan Indians have no symptoms with menopause, even though they have the same hormonal changes as white women.[18] Since they live in a tropical climate, one might expect them to have hot flashes, but they don't. Even when researchers asked very specific questions, the Mayan women didn't express any familiarity with the symptoms they were being asked about. In fact, like the Japanese, the Mayans have no word for "hot flash."

Cultural Influences

In addition to biological differences, the cultural milieu has a powerful effect on the experience of menopause. One study[19] looked at the Rajput women of Northern India. These women, who are kept in strict purdah during their fertile years, are restricted far less once they reach menopause; they are then permitted to move freely about the village. They experience no unpleasant menopausal symptoms. The study concluded that the two facts were related: if menopause improves the quality of your life, either you experience no symptoms or those you do experience are so minor compared with the rewards that you don't mind them.

The studies of Mayan women confirmed this view. Like the Rajput women, they also look forward to menopause, which frees them from constant pregnancy and childbirth. Is that why they have no hot flashes? Several studies[20] conclude that menopause is actually a biocultural event: lifestyle differences like diet and reproductive histories as well as cultural views of older women play a large role in how women experience menopause.

This biocultural effect was demonstrated in 1994, in a study of women and their physicians in a village in Thailand.[21] The interviewer was a native, which was important because the researchers wanted to be certain they understood the nuances of the language. In this village, the women all saw both menopause and menstruation as a natural part of life. Their word for menopause translates roughly as "no more babies." They tend to welcome it, since it relieves them of the burdens of menstruation, pregnancy, and childbirth. Since it signals the beginning of old age, they feel they are now able to free themselves from the menstrual taboos that accompany fertile years in their culture. They have greater independence, and most of the premenopausal women interviewed were looking forward to menopause.

Perimenopausal women in this study did report symptoms, but for the most part they didn't find them very troublesome. About a quarter of these women experienced hot flashes—a condition for which they, like the Mayans and Japanese, don't have a specific word. They described it as a burning sensation inside the body or on the skin. It made them uncomfortable, and they became irritable. Dizziness and headaches were the most common symptoms, and the headaches sometimes kept them from concentrating, which affected their work—this was the symptom that most bothered them.

Most believed their symptoms were temporary and didn't seek medical help, feeling comfortable with letting nature take its course. On the infrequent occasions when a woman's symptoms were so severe that she wanted help, she went to a healer, an herbalist, or a village elder.

Their doctors, however, had a different attitude. A middle-aged gynecologist in the village, Dr. Chaaj, told the interviewers that menopause should not be treated as a natural event but as a state of estrogen deficiency that causes heart disease, osteoporosis, and other illnesses. He wanted to persuade these women, who did not even "treat" menstruation with sanitary napkins, to treat their "deficiency" with estrogen pills. "Hormone replacement therapy is used to promote quality of life in the industrialized countries," Dr. Chaaj explained, "and its use in Thailand will ensure that women have a happy postmenopausal life."[22] He attributed this belief to the medical literature he'd read, mostly from the West. The fact that the women in his village were already having perfectly happy postmenopausal lives without hormone intervention didn't seem to faze him.

He was not alone in his attitude. Altogether fifteen Thai gynecologists were interviewed, and all saw menopause as an estrogen-deficiency disease that should be treated with hormone therapy. They felt that Western technology was superior to traditional village values.

The Experience in England

Lest I leave you with a biased view—that all women in other countries are going through menopause happily but are being badgered by doctors to take drugs—we should look at the other side of the coin. In 1983, a book about hormone therapy called *No Change*, by Wendy Cooper, was published in England.[23] It set off an explosion among Englishwomen who had long been complaining about menopausal symptoms. After Cooper's book came out, more and more Englishwomen began to seek out hormone therapy. Unlike women in the United States, who were having hormones thrust on them by their doctors, the British women asked for hormone treatment but were often denied it.

The experiences and views of 3,117 women receiving hormones at 21 menopause clinics in the United Kingdom were cited in an epidemiological study in 1988.[24] The article quoted one woman who was grateful for "the chance to talk to an understanding doctor about the symptoms that were physically and mentally draining but didn't seem important enough to take to an ordinary doctor. My own doctor gave me the impression that I had to live with it. . . . The very fact that some interest is being shown in the distressing symptoms I was suffering and someone was trying to do something about it was very comforting." Until then, she had been convinced that "the medical profession thinks that middle-aged women are neurotic idiots with hypochondria."[25] This suggests an interesting possibility. It may be that some women need support during perimenopause and menopause and that the medical profession interprets this as a need for drugs. Hormone therapy is still used less in the United Kingdom than in the United States: only 7 to 10 percent of women in the United Kingdom take it, as compared with 32 percent in the United States.[26]

BIG BUSINESS

If so many cultures experience menopause as a natural stage of life, why is it being turned into a disease? As I've said, this is at least in part because diseases need treatment and treatment costs money. Unfortunately, the medical world is no freer from the manipulation of big business than the rest of us are—and the pharmaceutical industry is very big business indeed.

Although we might like to think of the medical profession as pure and the drug industry as altruistic, we live in the real world. Drug companies want first and foremost to make money. They are expert at marketing to us as well as to doctors. If corporations can make us believe that smoking will make us sexy and that waxing the kitchen floor will save our marriages, they can make us believe anything. Doctors are as susceptible to marketing as the rest of us. Drugs and diseases go in and out of fashion, just as lipstick shades and car models do.

We also cling to the idea that because medicine is "scientific," doctors are always right. But science itself is never pure: it changes with new discoveries and with new social values. Tonsillectomies, which were so popular when we were kids, are rarely done today. Ulcers, once thought to be caused by stomach acid, are now treated with antibiotics, because we've learned that they're caused by a bacterial infection.

One of the most powerful marketing techniques used to influence both doctors and patients is the manipulation of fears of aging and death. In our youth-oriented culture, we tend to act as if we can stay young forever as long as we do everything right. We think that death is optional. Time challenges that illusion. In spite of all the hair coloring, wrinkle creams, and miracle vitamins, we do age. Menopause, that undeniable harbinger of middle age, eventually comes to any woman who's lucky enough not to die young. You start to get hot flashes, or rushes of heavy bleeding—often disruptively severe, always a reminder that youth is gone. And then you're offered a lovely little pill that can make it all go away.

That little pill has been around since the 1940s, and for many women, it *has* been lovely. For years it was given to patients who suffered from hot flashes and vaginal dryness, offering real relief for extreme symptoms. But during the past several decades, pharmaceutical companies have seen an opportunity here and have tried to capitalize on it: why confine their pills to the relatively few women with severe symptoms, when they could offer them to all women in menopause?

Marketing Eternal Femininity—and More

The drug companies began by creating a fancy name: "hormone replacement therapy." This was a nice touch, suggesting that something should be there but has been taken away, and that they can give this something back to you. The idea of "hormone replacement therapy" is consistent with the language that marketing has created everywhere: you can smell "naturally fresh" by using an artificial deodorant; you can have "home-baked goodness" by buying a packaged food; you can prolong youth by "replacing the hormones nature has taken away."

Getting all women in menopause to take hormones required identifying a purpose for the medication beyond simply alleviating severe symptoms. It meant mythologizing those symptoms, and, more, it meant creating new claims for hormone therapy. The pharmaceutical industry began to encourage the idea that estrogen could do more than relieve present symptoms—that it could also prevent a large range of problems, from wrinkles to heart disease.

Paula B. Doress-Worters, in the preface to *The Menopause Industry*, called hormone therapy "a product in search of a market."[27] Part of the strategy, she says, was to promote hormone therapy "not simply as a palliative for the discomforts of menopause but also as a panacea for 'psychological problems' supposedly related to the change of life. Such claims were unproven but were treated as common knowledge." The postmenopausal older woman was depicted as "asexual, neurotic, and unattractive."

The pharmaceutical companies were incredibly lucky to discover a spokesman for this view, a gynecologist in Brooklyn named Robert Wilson. His book *Feminine Forever* (1966),[28] written for laywomen, was heralded for years as the book that was changing women from dried-up relics of their lost youth to vibrant, joyful, perennial twenty-year-olds. Wilson told the story of his mother's menopause: "I was appalled at the transformation of that vital, wonderful woman who had been the dynamic focal point of our family into a pain-racked petulant invalid. I could feel the deep wounds her senseless rages inflicted on my father, myself, and the younger children. It was this frightful experience that later directed my interest as a physician to the problem of menopause." He went on to describe a second crucial event. A local woman had drowned herself in the reservoir because, the "town gossips" told him, she had "gone mad" with the change of life. Wilson apparently accepted the diagnosis of the town gossips; it did not occur to him that there might have been reasons other than menopause for a middle-aged woman's suicide.

In his book, Wilson also told how he had confirmed that estrogen could keep women looking eternally young. He examined a fifty-two-year-old patient and was struck by how youthful she seemed. He asked her her secret, only to find that she was still using birth control pills because she was still menstruating. Wilson was amazed and immediately became a zealot about the wonders of estrogen. "I therefore believe that menopause prevention far transcends the purely clinical aspects of the subject. It even transcends any narrow view of sex as such. What is really at stake is a subtle and almost metaphysical factor—a woman's total femininity."

Wilson's book became a best-seller, first in the United States and later in Europe, selling over 100,000 copies in a few months. In 1969 a survey conducted by the International Health Foundation[29] of four hundred women in five European countries found that the popularity of *Feminine Forever* directly influenced the extent to which hormone therapy was used in each country. "The more publicity there had been in a country, the higher the percentage of perimenopausal women who had heard that medical treatment existed to lessen the problems of the climacteric." Although estrogen was being prescribed for short-term, self-limited symptoms, the implication was that if you stopped taking it, the symptoms would all come back. To remain feminine forever, you had to stay on estrogen forever.

Sales of Premarin, the most popular formulation of estrogen, soared as women sought this fountain of youth. Dr. John Lee, a gynecologist in San Francisco, tells of being given a free copy of Wilson's book by a pharmaceuticals representative.[30] In fact, the makers of estrogen soon started funding Wilson's lectures to women's groups. Barbara and Gideon Seaman, who are experts on estrogen, have written about Wilson's private trust, the Wilson Foundation, established to promote the use of estrogen.[31] Wilson's foundation received $1.3 million in funding from pharmaceutical companies. In 1964—two years before Wilson's book was published—the foundation had received $17,000 from Searle, $8,700 from Wyeth-Ayerst Laboratories, and $5,600 from the Upjohn Company, all of which made hormones that Wilson promoted for the treatment of menopause.

While Wilson proselytized to menopausal woman, the pharmaceutical companies continued their barrage on the doctors. Medical journals ran ads showing dour old women who perked up immediately on estrogen. Combinations of estrogen and the tranquilizer Librium were formulated and advertised "for the problems that bother *him* the most." Presumably the job of the doctors was as much to keep husbands happy as to make women patients feel better.

Wilson shared this focus. He saw "estrogen-deficient" postmenopausal women as the source of most of society's woes: "The transformation, within a few years, of a formerly pleasant, energetic woman into a dull-minded but sharp-tongued caricature of her former self is one of the saddest of human spectacles. The suffering is not hers alone—it involves her entire family, her business associates, her neighborhood storekeepers, and all others with whom she comes into contact. Multiplied by millions, she is a focus of bitterness and discontent in the whole fabric of our civilization."[32] Reading his book, one wonders why he stopped short of blaming the sinking of the *Titanic*, World War II, and the fall of the Roman Empire on postmenopausal women.

The Worm Turns—For a While

But even with all this hype, sales of Premarin have still been subject to the vicissitudes of medical knowledge. The ups and downs of prescriptions for estrogen reflect the flip-flopping advice in medical books. A study done in 1993[33] examined changing information in gynecological textbooks, internal medicine textbooks, a pharmaceutical text (written by Goodman and Gilman), and the *Physicians' Desk Reference* (*PDR*) over the last sixty years.

Until the mid-1970s, as we've seen, estrogen was used mostly to treat existing menopausal symptoms—hot flashes, mood swings, etc. In 1975, 28 million prescriptions for Premarin were written in the United States. Then, in 1975, suggestions appeared that women were at risk for heart disease and that hormone therapy could help lower the risk. (Studies in the 1950s had suggested that estrogen could prevent atherosclerosis in animals fed a high-fat diet.)

As a result, a study was launched—of men. Don't ask me why the first effort to determine the effects of estrogen on the heart was done with men; the logic eludes me. But the fact remains that the first and (to date) only completed randomized controlled study (see page 68) of estrogen and heart disease was done on men who had had heart attacks or angina, the crushing pain that indicates heart disease.[34] (Two studies on women are ongoing now.) The men were given high doses (2.5 milligrams and 1.25 milligrams) of Premarin in the hope that it would lower their risk of repeat attacks. It didn't—in fact, it was correlated with more heart attacks. The doctors became concerned that the same effect would occur with women, so they decided that women who were at risk of heart disease should not receive Premarin. (The subtle notion that biological differences between women and men might cause them to respond differently to the same drugs apparently hadn't occurred to these doctors.)

Other studies[35] were starting to show that use of estrogen could lead to endometrial cancer. Doctors immediately stopped prescribing estrogen for women, except for those who had had hysterectomies and therefore did not have uteruses that could be harmed. (This fact, as you'll see in Chapter 4, becomes important when we look at the pool of women who have been studied to see the effects of long-term use of Premarin.) By 1980, sales had fallen to 14 million.

The decline in prescriptions for Premarin was only a temporary lull. The drug companies once again had an answer: Add another drug. In the early 1980s, gynecologists began to prescribe estrogen combined with an oral progestin called Provera, which was shown to protect the uterus. (They had no idea whether the progestin had any effect on heart disease, because there were no studies on this, but naively assumed that its only effect was on the uterus.)

With the successful addition of Provera to the mix, estrogen sales began to rise again, hitting 16.6 million by 1983—an improvement, but still a plummet from the levels of 1975. The makers of Premarin needed a new approach to counteract the bad publicity from the association of estrogens with cancer—and to add even more women to their lists. The baby boomers might not all embrace the promise of eternal youth, but they were increasingly health-conscious and concerned with preventing disease. So the drug companies picked up on another aspect of Wilson's theory: without estrogen, all women were doomed to osteoporosis.

There had been some preliminary studies suggesting that estrogen therapy could decrease the risk of osteoporosis if taken over the long term. Marketing on this basis might be just what was needed to rehabilitate the drug before the baby boomers reached menopause. The pharmaceuticals industry was savvy enough to recognize that marketing a disease is the best way to market a drug. Osteoporosis suited their needs: it has no symptoms until you have fractures, which means you can have it for years and not know until it's too late. If the baby boomers could be convinced that without drugs their bones would slowly and silently deteriorate, they'd be more likely to take drugs at the first hint that menopause was approaching. The pharmaceutical companies started placing ads in the medical journals, showing wheelchairs, X rays of crooked spines, and pathetic-looking women with dowager's humps. They funded medical meetings and lectures about osteoporosis.

These scare tactics were extremely successful. In less than ten years, women and doctors were viewing osteoporosis as a "female disease" (although it occurs in men and women), the inevitable fate of women who did not take estrogen after menopause.

This approach continues into the present. Merck, the company that makes Fosamax (a new nonhormonal treatment for osteoporosis), stated in its annual report of 1995: "Consumer research shows a growing level of awareness and knowledge about osteoporosis. We have been aggressively working to educate consumers about the disease and the importance of early diagnosis and appropriate treatment with organizations such as the National Osteoporosis Foundation, the Older Women's League, and members of the European parliament. We have established the Bone Measurement Institute, a non-profit organization, to increase the accessibility and affordability of bone measurement technologies. Merck has also provided funding for the first world summit of osteoporosis societies."

And Merck funded more studies. It even ran commercials on television, aimed at the public rather than just doctors. One showed a healthy-looking grandma who's just been diagnosed with osteoporosis looking wistfully at her grandson and wondering how long she'll be able to play with him. Another commercial showed wishbones being pulled, just on the verge of breaking.

These public education efforts have been very successful. On June 15, 1995, *The Wall Street Journal* reported that "Charles H. Chestnut, a researcher [on osteoporosis] and Professor of Medicine at the University of Washington, says that when he gave presentations of his work at scientific meetings two decades ago, 'there would be three or four people in the audience, and most of them were the next speakers.' " Now the disease is hot.[36] Chestnut said that research funding had increased dramatically and that his presentations now drew hundreds of scientists. Researchers credited media coverage of the disease in the early and mid-1980s for generating public awareness, along with efforts of the NIH and other scientific groups.

In spite of all this media blitz, messages to doctors about who can benefit from estrogen, and who is at risk, have kept changing. These mixed messages are demonstrated in one gynecology textbook.[37] In 1961, the authors cautiously advised that estrogen therapy might protect against cardiovascular disease, adding in the editions of 1965 and 1971 that it should be given to women who have a family history of heart disease. In the 1975 edition, however, as a result of the studies on men, they said that it should not be given to women with a history of heart disease. In the editions of 1981 and 1988, they went back to their earlier position: "Women with a family history of heart disease should be treated with hormone therapy."

Yet in 1996 the package insert that came with Premarin said that "estrogens should not be used . . . [i]f you have had any heart or circulatory problems."

Because of all the changes of attitude—often based on bias rather than on hard evidence, as I'll explain in Chapter 4—doctors are getting, and giving, mixed messages. Further, when they want to update their information, they don't always turn to the latest scientific studies. Instead, they often turn to sales representatives for drug companies or to medical meetings that may be funded by drug companies. In 1995, meetings sponsored by pharmaceutical companies rose 31 percent. Pfizer, which doesn't make any HRT products, led the industry in promotional expenditures in 1995, spending $364 million on sales representatives and $93.7 million for events. Pfizer made 2.7 million sales calls to doctors in 1995; American Home Products, the parent company of Wyeth-Ayerst (the makers of Premarin), was second in the total number of sales calls (mostly to doctors): 2.4 million.[38]

At the time of this writing, in 1996, Wyeth-Ayerst was funding the reception at the annual American Medical Women's Association meeting. (This promised to be a real gold mine: women and doctors at the same time.) It funds a postdoctoral fellowship in clinical epidemiology and women's health at the University of Maryland.

Such practices are not limited to the United States. In the United Kingdom, the National Osteoporosis Society, with the kind support of the Lilly Women's Health Initiative (Lilly has a new drug for osteoporosis coming out soon) is "inviting applications for research funding to encourage young researchers to develop their interest in osteoporosis and menopause issues."

Medical journals are replete with ads selling doctors on the wonders of particular drugs. *Menopause*, the official journal of the North American Menopause Society, has ads for hormone therapy scattered among its articles, proclaiming the benefits of various hormone therapy drugs. Doctors are as susceptible to advertising as the next person, especially if they think that a treatment will make their patients younger, happier, and healthier. I'm not saying that doctors are lazy. At a time when doctors must struggle to keep current with a vast and proliferating body of research, it's easy for them to let their attention be drawn to information that's neatly packaged for ready absorption. At any medical meeting, one of the most popular spots is the exhibits area, where drug companies put up elaborate booths and give away anything from cappuccino to tote bags stuffed with information about their latest products. In fact, many of the speakers at these meetings are also provided, or at least paid for, by the drug companies' representatives. A drug company doesn't tell a speaker what to say, but a recent study[39] showed that a medical audience is influenced by a sponsoring company; one month after a talk, most members of the audience prescribed more of a drug produced by the drug company paying for lunch than other drugs for the same purpose. In most teaching hospitals, the main teaching rounds provide lunch courtesy of local drug representatives. A hospital in San Francisco called me while I was writing this book and asked if I'd give a talk; my secretary told them my fee and they responded, "Is she on the drug list?" (a list of speakers whose fees the drug companies have agreed to pay), intimating that if I were (I'm not, to my knowledge), they could get me my fee.

THE RISE OF THE GYNECOLOGIST

Along with changes in the profile of estrogen have come changes in the profile of the doctors prescribing it. In 1971, 27 percent of the doctors prescribing estrogen were gynecologists. In the 1980s, that percentage started to increase, and by 1991, 60 percent of these prescriptions were given by gynecologists. Two decades ago, general practitioners wrote 37 percent of prescriptions for hormones; today they write only 20 percent. Internists have gone from 17 percent to 12 to 15 percent. Thus most of the prescriptions for menopausal hormone therapy today are given by gynecologists, and comparatively few by internists and GPs.

At first glance, this seems logical: menopause is a slowdown of the reproductive process, and that's the domain of gynecology. But think again. Estrogen therapy is being given to prevent heart disease and osteoporosis—hardly gynecological problems. And while some menopausal and perimenopausal symptoms are gynecological—vaginal dryness, for example—others aren't. Hot flashes and night sweats are really vasomotor conditions and thus may be more in the realm of the internist or primary care doctor.

Why, then, aren't more internists and GPs prescribing hormones? It may be that they simply aren't bothering to prescribe because the gynecologists, who are often women's chief health care providers, are doing it anyway. But there may be something else going on. Advertisers are marketing hormones most heavily to gynecologists, possibly because they know that's where women turn most often. And gynecologists derive some benefit from putting you on hormones, so they're more likely to buy into the advertising. Once you stop having babies, you don't often need to see a gynecologist—unless you're on hormone therapy. Not only do you have to see the gynecologist every six months for a refill, but, as you'll see later, women on hormones are more likely to need many more revenue-generating gynecological procedures such as endometrial biopsies, D and Cs, and of course hysterectomies. (I thought I might be unduly cynical about this until a gynecologist friend of mine wrote me that she'd come up with the same theory; she ruefully added, "And to think I prescribe this pill daily.")

In addition, gynecologists are trying to reframe themselves as primary care doctors. Until the last ten or fifteen years, women went to gynecologists only for pregnancy and for gynecological surgery. Otherwise, internists and GPs did everything, including Pap smears and even some surgery. But as we've turned more and more toward managed care, relying less on specialists than we used to, gynecologists have been trying, with some success, to position themselves as women's primary care doctors.

On the face of it, their success seems like a triumph for feminism. But in fact, in many areas of women's medical concerns, gynecologists don't have the best training. They're not experts in breast disease, in high blood pressure, or in osteoporosis. Internists do have some specialized training in these areas. As gynecologists try to increase their training and internists add gynecology to their repertoire, we'll see an increasing turf battle emerging over who owns women's bodies. And menopause clinics will proliferate. I suspect they'll all find themselves enthusiastically supported by the pharmaceutical companies.

In fact, some of the pharmaceutical companies are planning to step up their involvement in medical practice by delivering services themselves. In July 1995, Wyeth-Ayerst (the maker of Premarin) and Merck (the maker of Fosamax, a drug for osteoporosis) announced the formation of a joint venture company to develop disease management programs for women's health in areas such as prenatal care, menopause, osteoporosis, and family planning. "Disease management" is the fancy name for specialty centers focused on one disease. This new company plans to market its disease management programs to employers and managed care organizations such as HMOs. You can imagine the possibilities. Is this conflict of interest, or just good business? I'm not sure.

THE MEDIA

The drug companies and the medical profession are not the only sources of mythology and misinformation. The popular media have certainly contributed their share. On the nightly news, tentative new findings in small studies become transformed into miracle cures. The media often confuse news stories and advertising, touting a new product's claims as if they had been proven. As recently as December 1995, the cover of *Reader's Digest* boldly touted Premarin as "the pill that keeps women young." Meanwhile, the package insert for Premarin says, "You may have heard that taking estrogens for long periods (years) after menopause will keep your skin soft and supple and keep you feeling young. There is no evidence that this is so and such long-term treatment may carry serious risks."

The media have been aided and abetted by the corporations who produce the drugs and devices used in medical interventions. When a new study comes out that might call the safety of hormone therapy into question, the pharmaceutical companies send out a news release to the media offering expert spokespeople who will discuss the flaws in the study. For example, in 1995, when a study from Harvard validated earlier studies showing that postmenopausal estrogen might increase the risk of breast cancer, American Home Products lined up a prestigious crew of scientists to attack the Harvard results. One of them, Leon Speroff, a professor at Oregon Health Sciences University in Portland, immediately sent out a letter to the media urging caution in interpreting the study. "As a physician/researcher who treats and studies menopausal women, I've witnessed firsthand the hysteria that can be generated as a result of unbalanced study data—particularly related to breast cancer." Speroff wasn't paid to write this by American Home Products, but he has done clinical work for the company.

American Home Products also distributed its own meta-analysis rebutting the Harvard study.[40]

On the other hand, when a study showing a beneficial effect of hormone therapy comes out, the drug companies make sure it gets a lot of press: they'll hand out copies of the study to doctors and the media and offer to pay the authors of the study to speak at national medical meetings and press conferences. They rarely pass out the less favorable studies. This means that doctors and the media get an unbalanced impression. Before you know it, interesting preliminary data become accepted as dogma.

The claims that the pharmaceutical company experts make are often belied by the products' own package insert (which is required to use language approved by the FDA). Take a look at the small print in the ads in women's magazines for Premarin, Prempro (a combination of estrogen and progestins by the maker of Premarin), or any other estrogen—or, if you're already taking one of the drugs, at the insert that comes with your own pills. The Prempro insert reads in part: "Some research has shown that estrogens taken without progestins may protect women against developing heart disease. However, this is not certain. The protection shown may have been caused by the characteristics of the estrogen-treated women and not by the estrogen treatment itself. In general, treated women were slimmer, more physically active, and were less likely to have diabetes than the untreated women. These characteristics are known to protect against heart disease."

Do you see any drug companies stepping forward to set straight the public misconception that a connection between hormones and preventing heart disease has been proven? They're not actually lying, but they're not actually being truthful either.

As I've pointed out earlier, there are many competing interests in this business. Researchers want to get more research money and more fame, and so they have a tendency to make their own studies sound better and more important than those of their colleagues. The university where a study is done wants more donations from its wealthy patrons, so it too wants to make all of its discoveries sound bigger and better. The media—and the medical journals, for that matter—would rather publish studies that show positive results than negative results, and they would rather publish studies on drugs than on changes in lifestyle. Take, for example, the journal *Maturitas:* from 1978 to 1985, this international journal for the study of the climacteric had ninety-six articles related directly to hormone therapy, but only seven on nonhormonal medication.[41]

In evaluating research in this area, you need to question what hasn't been studied as well as what has been. If most research on treating menopausal symptoms is based on evaluating the role of hormones rather than of, say, lifestyle, it isn't surprising that doctors and consumers develop a bias toward hormone therapy.

Further, experts who don't follow the party line are often not published. Jerilynn Prior, an endocrinologist, tells of having a colleague call and ask her to do a chapter in a book on menopause.[42] When she told him that she didn't believe all women needed to be on hormones, she was told that they'd find another author. Barbara Seaman, an expert on estrogen who is often cautionary, found that "in the 60s, 70s and 80s most discussions of menopause permitted several points of view. As a result of the vested interest pharmaceutical advertising supports, the conservative view on hormone therapy is no longer admitted on talk shows and is rarely seen in magazines that seek advertising. . . . In the 90s I have given interviews to scores of magazine writers, only to have my comments removed from the final copy. In the 90s I have been called by and booked on all three network morning programs, only to be canceled out with some lame excuse."[43]

Women's magazines are encouraged to run stories on osteoporosis and heart disease, and they run plenty of ads for hormone replacement therapy. It's probably not a coincidence. Within the past year, *Prevention* magazine, a popular health monthly, has run at least two major articles in favor of hormone therapy. They've also run ads for Premarin in the same issue. When they ran an article discussing the use of soy protein as an alternative to estrogen for decreasing hot flashes, there were no Premarin or Prempro ads in the issue.

The women in the ads for hormones keep getting younger and younger. The drug companies aren't actually saying that you'll look thirty-five forever if you take estrogen, but having a woman who looks thirty-five in the ad says it without words. Cigarette companies don't say that smoking will make you sexy, either—they just show very sexy women smoking.

Is it any wonder that you can't figure out what's really going on? Obviously a lot of people are invested in this "disease" and its treatment, and it's important to be aware of all of them. It's unfortunate that corporate profits and media fads should determine anyone's medical treatment—or lack of treatment. But they do, and just as consumers need to distrust the glittering promises of car companies and perfume manufacturers, they need to question the promises of the pharmaceutical industry, filtered through the agency of well-meaning doctors and superficial media coverage.

WHY PREMARIN?

From the earliest days of estrogen "replacement" therapy, one product—Premarin—has dominated the market in the United States. You'll hear more about Premarin in this book than about any other kind of estrogen. The fact that so many doctors have been persuaded that their patients need estrogen doesn't explain why, in the United States, one brand of estrogen dominates all others. The credit for that goes to drug companies' "positioning." The story of Premarin is perhaps the best example of the power and influence of pharmaceutical companies.

Remember that in 1975, 28 million prescriptions were given for Premarin in the United States. After the dip following bad publicity linking estrogen with endometrial cancer, sales of Premarin slowly climbed again. By 1992, there were 31.7 million prescriptions; in 1995, prescriptions had gone up to 44.3 million. Between one sixth and one fourth of all postmenopausal women take Premarin. It's become the most frequently dispensed brand-name pharmaceutical in the country.

Premarin was studied initially because it was more readily available than other preparations and because the manufacturer, Wyeth-Ayerst, provided it free to researchers. Wyeth-Ayerst also sponsored research using its product. Premarin is the subject of nearly 90 percent of the estrogen studies (over 3,000 studies to date). Now doctors argue that they prefer to prescribe Premarin because it's been studied more than the others. This is true, but the situation has become highly self-perpetuating. When new studies are planned, such as the Women's Health Initiative (see page 67), they tend to study Premarin because they want to concentrate on drugs in common use, and, again, because the pharmaceutical companies will provide the drugs free. Wyeth-Ayerst has agreed to donate over 100 million tablets of Premarin and medroxyprogesterone (a progestin) or placebo to the National Institutes of Health, which funds the Women's Health Initiative. Wyeth-Ayerst has also funded the $40 million study called the Heart and Estrogen-Progestin Replacement Study (HERS), which is investigating Premarin for women with preexisting coronary artery disease. It is also funding a $16 million study to investigate whether Premarin can prevent or delay Alzheimer's disease. It's hard to break out of this mode and start testing new things. Doctors say, "We'll put you on Premarin because we know more about it." And something new, which may actually be better for you, never gets a chance.

The maker of Premarin has done other things to maintain its dominance. Premarin sales hit $850 million in 1995. Premarin (or conjugated equine estrogen, as it's formally called) comes from the urine of pregnant horses, a fact its manufacturers have used for twenty years to block FDA approval of any generic equivalents that have been developed. (A generic CEE was approved in Canada in 1996.) They argue that Premarin contains six dominant estrogenic compounds (horse estrogens), including one that is missing from the proposed generic equivalent. They contend this is a key factor in the drug's effectiveness. The manufacturers of the generic versions claim that their product is just as effective, but they've been unable to include this particular horse estrogen. Regardless of the truth of the matter, the difficulties in mimicking horses' urinary estrogen has kept Premarin on top.[44]

I don't mean to make either the drug companies or the media sound like the Evil Empire. They're all doing their jobs, and in many ways we benefit from that. The fact that 90 percent of new medicines are discovered by drug companies doesn't mean that these medicines aren't valuable, and the media do provide the public with important information about diseases and treatments. But the limitations built into what both institutions are doing mean that you, too, have a job—to be as fully informed as possible, to be aware of biases in research and reporting, and to make up your own mind.

CHAPTER 3

"What Does It Feel Like?"

IDENTIFYING SYMPTOMS

Problem 1: Variations—We Are Not All the Same

Perimenopause, the three to six years before the last period, is extremely individual: each woman experiences this transition in her own way. This is not surprising. Each of us had her own experience of puberty. Some of us have had PMS while others have sailed through their years of menstruating. Some of us had morning sickness with pregnancy and others didn't. I know some women who claim they knew they were pregnant from the moment of conception, and there are stories of women who never knew they were pregnant until they went into labor. Hormones and hormonal shifts affect each one of us in her own unique way, so it's only natural that perimenopause and menopause will be experienced highly individually. There's a wide range of possible symptoms, limited only by your imagination.

Women are usually able to recognize which of these symptoms are actually related to their hormones and which aren't. Doctors are not always so perceptive. One of my patients, a lawyer, was in the midst of a fairly humdrum meeting with a client one day and suddenly got palpitations and shortness of breath. She covered as best she could, and as soon as the client left she called her husband, a doctor. Could this be the start of menopause? she asked. He asked if she'd felt hot or had turned red, and when she said no, he said it couldn't be menopause; it was just nerves. When it happened again later in the day she started to get scared and went to an emergency room. She ended up seeing a team of specialists and having a battery of tests, none of which turned up anything. She asked the doctors several times whether this episode could be related to menopause. And to a man, all the doctors were adamant. These were not menopausal symptoms. Absolutely not. When she finally got home that night, she told her Latina housekeeper about her symptoms. "Oh, señora, that's just your change," the woman laughed. "It happened just like that to my sister." And, of course, the housekeeper turned out to be right. What my patient had experienced was, as she herself had suspected, a variant of a hot flash. Though it was an unusual variant, it wasn't so unusual that an astute doctor shouldn't have at least considered the possibility. But remember that gynecology book we talked about in Chapter 1, with only one sentence on perimenopause? You don't learn what you're never taught.

So the doctors aren't the experts about hormonal symptoms: you are. Your intuition about symptoms at this time of life is probably right. You've been living in your body for almost fifty years and you know it pretty well. Though some symptoms are more common than others, the range is enormous. I have listed in Table 3.1 some of the symptoms that have been reported by various women at various times to Janine O'Leary Cobb,[1] who has been writing a newsletter on menopause for twelve years. This should show you that whatever you're feeling is probably normal. But don't be alarmed if your symptoms don't appear here. It doesn't mean that you're crazy or that you've really got some deadly, exotic disease. You'll want to check with your doctor to rule out anything serious, but it probably just means you've got a particularly unusual symptom.

On the other hand, you may not have any unusual symptoms—or even any of the usual ones. Ten percent of women don't experience perimenopause at all. They just stop menstruating. And this can seem the weirdest "symptom" of all, because we're so conditioned to think of menopause in terms of hot flashes, vaginal dryness, and wild mood swings. When one of my friends, an intelligent woman in her mid-forties, was told by her gynecologist that she seemed to be in menopause, she denied it. It was true she hadn't had a period in months, but she wasn't having flashes, her mood was fine, and nothing else in her body had changed. The poor doctor had an awful time convincing her that she wasn't premenopausal; she was just lucky.

The duration of perimenopausal symptoms also varies, although they rarely go on for more than a few years. Sonja and John Mckinlay, Boston researchers, were critical of most of the studies of women's experience of menopause because the studies looked only at women in medical settings. Women who go to doctors are usually having symptoms—that's why they're there. So the Mckinlays did their own five-year study in Massachu-

TABLE 3.1   Perimenopausal and Menopausal Symptoms

Menstrual irregularity
Hot flashes and/or flushes; night sweats
Dry vagina
Insomnia and/or weird dreams
Sensory disturbances (vision, smell, alterations to taste)
Funny sensations in the head
Lower back pain (crushing of vertebrae)
Waking in the early hours of the morning
Onset of new allergies or sensitivities
Fluctuations in sexual desire and sexual response
Annoying itching of the vulva (area around vagina)
Sudden bouts of bloat (waistline expands by two to three inches for an hour
    or two)
Chills or periods of extreme warmth
Indigestion, flatulence, gas pains
Rogue chin whiskers
Overnight appearance of long, fine facial hairs
Bouts of rapid heartbeat
Crying for no reason
Aching ankles, knees, wrists, or shoulders
Waking up with sore heels
Thinning scalp and underarm hair
Graying scalp and pubic hair
Mysterious appearance of bruises
Sudden inability to breathe ("air hunger")
Frequent urination
Urinary leakage (when coughing or sneezing, or during orgasm)
Prickly or tingly hands with swollen veins
Lightheadedness, dizzy spells, or vertigo
Weight gain, and in unusual places (on the back, breasts, abdomen)
Sudden and inappropriate bursts of anger
Sensitivity to being touched by others ("touch impairment")
Inexplicable panic attacks
Tendency to cystitis (inflammation of the bladder)
Vaginal or urethral infections
Anxiety and loss of self-confidence
Depression that cannot be shaken off
Painful intercourse
Migraine headaches
Easily wounded feelings
Crawly skin ("formication")
Disturbing memory lapses

Table adapted from J. O. Cobb, *Understanding Menopause* (New York: Plume, 1993), p. 20, with permission of author.

setts, following 2,570 perimenopausal women. They found that the average length of the perimenopausal or transition period for these women was about three and a half years. About 10 percent of the women went from pre- to postmenopausal in a very short time—less than six months. They had fewer symptoms, particularly hot flashes, than the average woman in the study, and about 20 percent of naturally menopausal or surgically menopausal women reported that they never had hot flashes at all.[2]

According to most studies, about 5 percent of women continue to have hot flashes well into menopause or even for the rest of their lives; the rest have them off and on over about two to five years. Other symptoms of perimenopause are also usually short-lived. Even vaginal dryness can be transient. Generally, the body gradually rebalances at a lower level of estrogen.

Menopausal symptoms, on the other hand, are usually persistent. These include symptoms that really come from living at a new level of hormones rather than just adjusting to the shift. They include vaginal dryness that persists or occurs several years after the last period, urinary difficulties, and persistent decrease in libido.

It's interesting to note the degrees to which women are troubled by symptoms. In the Mckinlays' study, only 16 percent felt that their hot flashes were really bothersome, 12 percent were upset by night sweats, 7 percent by problems with menstrual flow, and 3 percent by vaginal dryness. More women rated their symptoms as somewhat bothersome: 33 percent for hot flashes, 25 percent for night sweats, 5 percent for problems with menstrual flow, and 10 percent for vaginal dryness.

Some situations affect the severity of symptoms. You'll recall from Chapter 1 that surgical and medical menopause are more likely to give you abrupt and more disturbing symptoms. But of course none of this is carved in stone. You may have your ovaries removed and sail through your postmenopausal years symptom-free; you may have a natural menopause and flash till you're ninety.

Problem 2: Are You Perimenopausal or Just Getting Older?

Another problem with delineating perimenopausal and menopausal symptoms is that so many other things are happening at this stage in your life. Thus it's not always easy to sort out what causes what. You go through major life changes at middle age: your children leave home, your parents become ill and die, and your body begins to sag, wrinkle, and otherwise remind you of your lost youth and your own mortality. Stress can cause depression, and it can also throw your hormones out of whack.

Further, your body goes through other physical changes at middle age. Many symptoms attributed to menopause are actually just symptoms of aging. A doctor named Bungay in England sent a questionnaire to 1,120 women and 500 men.[3] Never mentioning menopause, he listed a number of symptoms and asked each respondent to note how many of them she or he had ever experienced. Much to his amazement, he found that the only symptoms that affected women more than men were hot flashes and vaginal dryness. All of the other symptoms, including many that we think of as perimenopausal, affected men as much as, or more than, women. Many of these symptoms turned out simply to be signs of aging. For example, loss of appetite, crawling or tingling sensations in the skin, headaches, and difficulties with intercourse affected men and women about equally.

Other experiences did appear to be related to menopause, however. While both men and women had crises around midlife that involved loss of confidence and difficulties in making decisions, perimenopausal women seemed to have more trouble with these than did men or postmenopausal women.

PERIMENOPAUSAL SYMPTOMS

Perimenopausal symptoms are usually transient, but they are often more troubling than menopausal symptoms. You can have any of these symptoms in varying degrees of severity or mildness, and you may experience the same symptoms differently at different times.

Let's look in depth at some of the more common perimenopausal symptoms. Later, in Chapter 11, I'll discuss how you can cope with them.

Hot Flashes

Hot flashes aren't confined to perimenopause, or even to women. Men with prostate cancer who are treated with estrogen sometimes get hot flashes when the treatment stops. And men who have had their testicles removed will also experience hot flashes, as will men put on tamoxifen to treat breast cancer. Niacin, too, can cause hot flashes in both men and women. However, since hot flashes are so frequent in perimenopausal and menopausal women, they are inevitably associated with menopause in people's minds.

The usual description of a hot flash goes something like this: You're sitting there minding your own business when all of a sudden you get a strange feeling and then your whole face and neck are hot, and maybe sweat breaks out on your upper lip or the nape of your neck, or even all over, and your heart starts racing. You pick up something to fan yourself with, or you think about tearing your clothes off—but before you know it, it's gone and you're drying out. Not a terrible experience when you're alone at your computer, but an extremely disorienting one in the middle of a presentation to the board of directors or a class of sixth-graders.

Hot flashes are the most common symptom of perimenopause in the Western world. We know they're related to estrogen, because estrogen medication gets rid of them—though the relationship is probably more complicated than simply a question of low estrogen.

Studying them hasn't been easy for researchers. They can't schedule you for a 2:30 lab appointment, then sit you down and say, "Okay, will you have a hot flash now, please?" They have to draw blood while you're there, hoping you'll have a hot flash or two while they're doing it.

In spite of this obstacle, some good studies have been done. One important study found that the flash is initiated not in the ovary but in the hypothalamus—the part of the brain involved with the pituitary and menstrual cycling.[4] That makes sense. The hypothalamus is located next to the thermoregulatory center, the thermometer in the brain that regulates your body's core temperature.

This gave researchers a clue about how exactly a flash works. Apparently what happens when you get a hot flash is that the normal mechanism overshoots. Normally, if you get hot, how do you cool down? Your face gets red, because blood rushes to the vessels nearest the surface so that they can release heat more easily, and you sweat. A hot flash is misnamed: it's really an attempt by your body to cool down. Researchers think that hot flashes happen when the set point of the thermoregulator gets abruptly shifted. It's as though somebody has walked by and pushed the thermostat in your head down to 55 degrees. Your brain says, "Uh-oh, you're 98.6 degrees now—that's too hot!" and immediately tries to cool you down by increasing your heart rate and the blood supply to your skin so that you blush and sweat. You may not have actually been too hot, but you will cool down.

One study[5] documented that 30 percent of women have hot flashes within three years before menopause. By one year before menopause, almost 50 percent of women have had at least one hot flash. By four years from their last period, however, only 20 percent of women were still having hot flashes. And 50 percent of women never experience hot flashes at all.

Howard Judd, an endocrinologist at UCLA, recorded the hot flashes of twenty perimenopausal women for two weeks.[6] Of a total of 1,041 hot flashes, the average flash lasted about three and a half minutes, but they ranged from five seconds to sixty minutes. On average, each woman flashed three or four times a day.

The menopause researcher Ann Voda questioned women about their flashes.[7] Most women in Voda's study described an aura or premonition before a flash started. Either a woman's heart rate went up or she felt a sensation in one spot—for example, behind one ear—just before it happened. The average age at which the flashes began was forty-five in women who had had surgical menopause and forty-eight in those whose menopause had occurred naturally. (This reflects the fact that a surgical menopause usually occurs earlier than a natural one.) There was no particular predilection for day or night flashing. The number of flashes varied greatly. One woman had 241 hot flashes in a two-week period; another had 2. One woman who had had 59 flashes in two weeks had 51 of them between 10 A.M. and 10 P.M.; another had all of hers between 4 P.M. and 2 A.M. There were two women who just had long flashes. The flashes lasted between thirty seconds and four minutes; the women who had the most flashes had the briefest ones.

The researchers were surprised at where women felt their hot flashes. Over half of the flashes started in the neck, head, scalp, and ears; 68 began in the neck or breasts; 59 below the breasts; 114 all over; 19 in the neck and above the breasts. Not all these women experienced flashes consistently in the same areas, though some did. One always had her flashes in her earlobe and cheek.

With regard to intensity, 455 flashes were rated as mild, 358 as moderate, and 116 as severe. *Mild* meant that a flash was barely noticeable, was quick, and didn't interfere with anything. *Moderate* meant that it was warmer, noticeable (with obvious perspiration in certain areas), and longer-lasting; often the woman tried to end it by taking some clothes off. *Severe* meant that a flash was intensely hot and caused the woman to stop what she was doing immediately, remove as much clothing as she possibly could, and seek a way of cooling down. It caused profuse perspiration, often over the entire body.

When women in this study were asked what they did to relieve the flashes, they said that they fanned themselves or drank cold liquids, but nothing really helped much. There was no single common trigger event. Many of these women got flashes when they were asleep; some got flashes chiefly when they were very emotional. One woman's flashes responded to the temperature of the air around her: when it got hotter, they lasted longer.

Many had considered themselves "cold-blooded" before the onset of hot flashes. They had usually been colder than the people around them. They'd always had to dress warmly, especially before going to sleep; they wore socks to bed. When the hot flashes began, their overall body temperature changed. They now slept in light nightwear or in nothing. They disliked skin-to-skin contact with other people because they felt uncomfortably warm. They cut back outdoor activity during the hot summer months and used more air-conditioning than they had in the past.

This study and others confirm that there seem to be as many variants of hot flashes as there are women who have them. Some women experience waves of heat and drenching sweats followed by chills, but sometimes the chills come first. For some it's nothing more than a transient sensation of warmth; for others it's a perpetual heat wave. Sometimes flashes are accompanied by feelings such as tension, anxiety, heart palpitations, and nausea. Sometimes they aren't exactly flashes, but rather an overreaction to a normal stimulus. You're doing an exercise that usually makes you sweat a bit, and suddenly you're pouring sweat. Or you're in a room that's slightly stuffy and you suddenly feel as if you're in the Amazon forest.

Hot flashes aren't always awful. Many women don't mind them at all. Since I started writing this book, I've been getting frequent hot flashes myself, and I'm rarely bothered by them. Sometimes there will be a band of sweat across my upper lip. Most of the time I just feel as though I'm blushing, although I don't necessarily look that much redder. On rare occasions, I have to rip off as many layers of clothes as I can without getting arrested for indecent exposure. Once I was heading toward downtown Los Angeles on the freeway and found myself pulling clothes off as I drove. Of course it was L.A., so no one noticed.

When I do something that would normally make me a little warm, like running across campus because I'm late for a lecture, I become very hot and sweaty. I often end up lecturing with my jacket off.

I don't find my hot flashes particularly distressing. In a way, I like having them: they're a badge of honor, a sign that I'm a perimenopausal woman. (Of course, if they were more severe, I might feel differently!) I never hide the fact that I'm having them. If someone asks why I've just removed my jacket in this cool room, I say, "It's okay—I'm just flashing." I now wear a button stating boldly "These are not hot flashes I am having, they are power surges."

In *The Menopausal Years: The Wise Woman Way,*[8] Susun Weed describes hot flashes as useful—a way to get extra heat out of your body now that you're no longer menstruating. Some women said they were actually happy about having hot flashes. To them, flashing signaled a quick, easy transition into menopause—almost as though they were flushing themselves out, allowing themselves to get on quickly with their lives. Without hot flashes, they believed, menopause was a longer, less comfortable process.

There are even cases of women enjoying the actual sensations of hot flashes. Sadja Greenwood, author of *Menopause Naturally,*[9] interviewed a large group of women about hot flashes and found that between 2 and 3 percent liked "feeling the heat as energy traveling through their bodies." My coauthor's aunt had hot flashes during a cold winter and appreciated the extra warmth.

Night Sweats and Insomnia

Night sweats are hot flashes that occur in the middle of the night. Typically, you wake up in a pool of sweat, having soaked your nightclothes and bed linen. Sometimes your heart is racing and it is very difficult to get back to sleep. At other times you can change your nightclothes and go right back to sleep. Or you may not even wake up at all. I find that I just wake up a little damp in the morning, having slept through the whole thing. Needless to say, if your night sweats keep you awake, you will grow increasingly tired. This can lead to mood swings and anxiety.

Some clinicians have attributed all of the insomnia of perimenopause to night sweats. But there probably is something else going on as well. While most night flashes cause waking, 40 percent of wakening is not associated with hot flashes. Most people awaken once or twice in the night, but they usually go right back to sleep. The perimenopausal woman often can't. It's this lack of sleep rather than the hot flashes or night sweats that drives many women to seek relief, medical or other. Hot flashes can usually be dealt with (see Chapter 11), but it's hard for a sleep-deprived woman to go to work or take care of her family.

Heavy Bleeding and Fibroids

Perimenopause brings changes in your menstrual cycles. For one thing, your periods often become irregular. The most frequent sign of the coming change is shorter periods. During your fertile years you usually have a cycle of about twenty-eight days. But in perimenopause, as in puberty, it's very normal to have wildly irregular cycles—twenty-one to twenty-five days between cycles and then sixty days before the next cycle. This can be confusing and alarming. Your period is late, and you wonder if you're pregnant. Or you're sitting in your office, and you suddenly feel that telltale dampness . . . but it's been only a couple of weeks since your last period. Once you've gotten used to the irregularity, and remember to take tampons or pads with you everywhere, irregular periods are usually not too much of a problem, though they can still be annoying.

Heavy bleeding, however, is a different story. It's the most distressing symptom most women report, the symptom that usually has them running to the doctor—and rightly so. Often, it's transitory. You may have a couple of heavy months and then stop, or have a heavy flow one month and a light flow the next and then a heavy flow again the next.

Other women are bothered by bleeding between periods. This can range from slight spotting to flooding, and it can last for a few days or continue without stopping.

Heavy bleeding can interfere with your life: it can make you anemic; it can make it nearly impossible to leave the house. Most alarming is the fact that though it's usually associated with hormonal shifts, you can't be certain that that's the case. It could be a symptom of something more serious. You should always check with your doctor and make sure. One of my old friends, a college professor, had heavy bleeding that she ignored because she assumed it was menopausal, and she ended up dying of endometrial cancer—cancer of the lining of the uterus.

You should consult a gynecologist if your periods come more than every twenty to twenty-one days, if they last more than seven to eight days, if you bleed between periods, or if your periods become much heavier than they used to be. To pinpoint the cause of abnormal bleeding, you'll need an endometrial biopsy. This is an office procedure in which a catheter the size of a pencil is passed into the uterus and a small bite is taken from its lining. This is usually uncomfortable but not too painful. Some women will have uterine cramps or bleeding as a result. This is the easiest and most cost-effective way to make sure your bleeding isn't caused by endometrial cancer or hyperplasia (see Chapter 8). The biopsy can also indicate if you're ovulating. If it doesn't confirm that the bleeding is caused by hormonal shifts, then you'll need further evaluation. Your gynecologist may then do a vaginal ultrasound (putting a specially shaped ultrasound probe into your vagina to get a picture of the uterus) or hysteroscopy (putting a pencil-thin instrument into the uterus that allows the gynecologist to see the endometrium, the lining of the uterus). The traditional D and C (dilation and curettage) is hardly ever used for diagnosis anymore, because it isn't necessary.

Cancer, fortunately, is the least common cause of abnormal nonhormonal bleeding. Other, more likely, suspects are polyps and fibroids, which are anatomical problems.

Polyps are small outgrowths of the lining of the uterus. The surface of a polyp can erode and lead to bleeding. Polyps can be seen on ultrasound and snipped out easily through a hysteroscope.

Fibroids are also outgrowths of the uterus. They're very common: over 30 percent of women have them by the time they reach fifty. Nothing needs to be done about fibroids unless you're having symptoms. They are self-contained balls of uterine tissue that can grow quite large. They can be found under the surface of the uterine lining (submucosal), in the middle of the uterine wall (intramural), or on its outer edge (extramural) (see Figure 3.1). Where they're found determines the symptoms they cause. The surface of submucosal fibroids will sometimes erode and cause bleeding. This bleeding may be hormonally related, in which case it will get worse with your period. Taking hormones won't usually help the bleeding, however,

FIGURE 3.1   Anatomic uterine problems.

because it is basically caused by an anatomical problem. Submucosal fibroids can be identified by vaginal ultrasound or hysteroscopy and can usually be removed at the time of hysteroscopy with an instrument called a resectoscope. Unless a fibroid is unusually large, there is no need to have a hysterectomy (see page 173).

Even if fibroids don't bleed, they can create other problems. Sometimes they can become enormous—even as large as a basketball. If that happens, you get symptoms because they take up so much room. They lean on your bladder, so you have to urinate constantly. They can cause indigestion. They're not cancer, and they're not going to spread—it's purely a question of discomfort.

Fibroids tend to get bigger as you get closer to menopause, and then they usually shrink after you go through menopause. So if your symptoms start at around forty-eight, you might want to try to hold off two or three years till your body gets rid of them for you. I know many women who are playing a waiting game, hoping they'll reach menopause before their fibroids become so bothersome that they're driven to drugs or surgery (see page 170).

The most common cause of heavy bleeding or abnormal periods in perimenopausal women is hormonal fluctuations that result from an imbalance of estrogen and progesterone. When you have an anovulatory cycle (one in which no egg was released), you don't produce any progesterone. The estrogen causes a buildup in the lining of the uterus, which then sheds irregularly as your estrogen levels go down. It's too much estrogen that leads to heavy bleeding in this situation. This problem can sometimes be diagnosed by vaginal ultrasound but is more commonly diagnosed by endometrial biopsy. It's actually a process of elimination. If it's not polyps, fibroids, or cancer, it's probably hormonal. And if it responds to hormonal treatments, it's probably hormonal.

Mood Swings

You know the image: the middle-aged woman is suddenly sullen and bitchy; her friends are aghast and her long-suffering husband explains sadly, "She's going through the change." It was this notion of the distressed, anxious menopausal woman, so prevalent in the 1950s, that inspired a popular drug called Menrium, a combination of the tranquilizer Librium and estrogen (variants are still available today; see page 255).

Menopausal mood swings do occur, but not everyone gets them, and they're not always overwhelming. Many women describe perimenopause as similar to PMS. If you have mood swings—or just moods—right before your period, then you'll probably experience them during perimenopause.

Serious psychological problems such as depression and deep emotional distress are another matter. Several different studies suggest that these are not a common symptom. Major studies of a total of 13,000 women in Norway,[10] Canada,[11] and Massachusetts[12] found that perimenopausal women did not experience an increase in psychological symptoms. In the Mckinlays' study, women who had a long and symptomatic perimenopause were more likely to feel somewhat depressed—which is hardly surprising. Other studies also suggest that mood changes are minimal.

But women's experience of menopause varies widely, and what studies call "minor symptoms" may not be so minor to the women who have them. I think that there probably are some women whose brains are very sensitive to hormonal fluctuations. They're the ones who get postpartum depression and terrible psychological PMS, and they might also react to menopausal hormone changes, particularly if their menopausal situation comes on suddenly rather than gradually; for example, if they have had their ovaries removed. Studies show that women who have had hysterectomies are more likely to experience menopausal-related depression. That may be caused by a reaction to losing a body part, or by the sudden loss of hormones. It also occurs in women who have received chemotherapy for breast cancer. Women who have been on estrogen therapy and quit abruptly—rather than tapering off slowly—are also more likely to experience mood swings. Sometimes drugs like Lupron, which throws you into artificial menopause, can have that effect. The brain reacts to many chemical neurotransmitters that are related to the hypothalamus and thus to the menstrual cycle. We all know that there is a correlation between your hormones and your moods (ask any woman or anyone who has lived with one), but we really don't understand it.

What tends to happen in these cases is an interaction through which outside emotional stress becomes exacerbated by internal chemical events. The hormonal changes don't actually cause the depression, but they change your body's equilibrium, so that a situation that would normally upset you a little upsets you a lot, and a situation that would normally upset you a lot devastates you. (This is similar to the change in temperature set point we saw with hot flashes.) For example, my coauthor, before her hysterectomy, was taking Lupron to stop her heavy bleeding. She was going through a family crisis and was already anxious and depressed. On the Lupron, she suddenly found her depression deepening and found herself becoming furious over small irritations. After the hysterectomy, she stopped taking Lupron and went on estrogen. Her mood went back to the level it had been at before, though the family situation remained the same.

Since we have so few studies on it, I can't prove this, but I'd be willing to bet that this is also what happens with puberty: the erratic hormonal activity intersects with outside issues in a girl's life and intensifies her moods. (I should note here that, while the infamous "swings" are usually discussed in terms of negative moods, they can also happen with positive moods: the mildly funny television show is suddenly hilarious, or the pleasant evening of bowling is wonderfully exciting.) I doubt that these subtle variations in mood are easily detected in large cross-sectional studies that are usually able to pick up only diagnosable psychological problems, such as clinical depression. Nonetheless, many women do experience this sense of imbalance in their moods.

My coauthor's situation illustrates the difficulty in identifying emotional states connected to menopause. Even at the level of clinical depression, this isn't easy to ferret out. As I've said, menopause occurs at a time when stressful changes are often taking place in people's lives. Children are growing up and leaving home—or staying at home as adults because of problems with marriages, finding jobs, or other troubles. Parents are elderly, growing more feeble, facing lingering illnesses, and dying. Spouses or lovers may leave or become ill. The loss of youth can be devastating to middle-aged people in a culture that idolizes youth. The fact of oncoming menopause, quite apart from any of its physical effects, can be distressing, signaling the end of your fertile years and the end of an era in your life. Whatever combination of these things a woman is going through can cause periods of depression, just as it does with men.

The British researchers J. Greene and J. Cooke carried out an investigation of how a range of stresses affect postmenopausal women.[13] They found that stressful events in a woman's life accounted for more psychological and physical problems than did her menopausal status.

Of course, life stress may have a direct biochemical effect on estrogen levels. There is some evidence that women who are depressed have lower estrogen levels, which go up when the depression lifts. In fact, a recent study showed a lower bone density in women who were depressed, another sign of decreased estrogen levels. It may be that feeling distressed triggers hot flashes in some women. Certainly we've all experienced hormonal changes with anxiety: you worry that you might be pregnant, and then your period is late.

Different women have different coping abilities before menopause, and those differences remain during and after this stage. If you're good at coping with stress, you won't suddenly lose that capacity with menopause. And often the anticipation of menopause is far worse than its reality. One study showed that premenopausal women had more negative attitudes about menopause than did women who had already been through menopause.[14] Seventy to 80 percent of the women in the study said they were relieved to reach menopause.

There is also a danger in underestimating the degree of psychological distress you're experiencing. Mood swings and fluctuations can be uncomfortable and unnerving, but actual psychological problems are disruptive and can take over your life. These can be triggered by menopause or can become intolerable with the additional stress of menopause. If you're in doubt, consult a therapist. Just as you don't want to take drugs unnecessarily for a normal life transition, you don't want to suffer needlessly from a treatable disorder—and emotional distress is treatable.

Fluid Retention

Fluid retention is another common symptom of menopause, and it can be very frustrating. You diet and exercise rigorously, step on the scale, and find you've gained five pounds! This happens premenstrually to many women of all ages, but often it begins in perimenopause in women who have never experienced it before. We don't know why this happens: I wonder if the body is trying to make sure it has enough fluid on board to take care of extra bleeding and sweating.

Like bleeding, fluid retention can happen one month and not again for the next several months, or it can happen for several months until you're convinced it will go on forever, and then suddenly it will stop.

Memory Problems and Fuzzy Thinking

You go upstairs to get something, and by the time you get there you can't remember what it is. You run into an acquaintance in the supermarket and can't for the life of you remember her name. Your brain just doesn't seem to be working right. Often your doctor will attribute this to lack of estrogen, but the evidence that menopause causes memory loss and fuzzy thinking is hard to quantify.

Some of the memory loss experienced around the time of menopause is caused by age, not hormones. When women over forty experience it, doctors tend to attribute it to menopause. In one study,[15] a range of men and women were shown a list of things and then asked to repeat them. Younger people did better than older ones, but nobody looked to see how much this differed between genders, if at all. Men have memory loss as well, and there are no studies indicating that their loss is less than women's. We do know that as people age, long-term memory remains better than short-term memory. You'll forget the name of someone who works in your office today; you'll remember the name of someone who worked in your office thirty years ago.

Again, it's hard to separate any effects of hormones on your ability to think clearly from the effects of the stresses of midlife. We do know that some aspects of perimenopause contribute indirectly to memory problems. Loss of sleep, stress over heavy bleeding, or constant severe hot flashes can bring on or exacerbate forgetfulness.

Fuzzy thinking is not uncommon in times of hormonal flux in general. Remember when you were pregnant? With big hormone shifts, there are certainly changes in your ability to concentrate and remember things. We all expect it. Postpartum fuzzy thinking can even be worse, although we chalk a lot of it up to lack of sleep. But rest assured that it all evens out again, and your brain does go back to normal.

The menopause researcher Barbara Sherwin found that even at different points in the menstrual cycle women have different levels of memory.[16] When your hormones are low, you do better at spatial, "male" things; when they're high, you're better at verbal, "female" things. But we're talking about really subtle changes. You may not notice them at all, or if you do, you'll think it's part of PMS. There's no reason to believe, for example, that your verbal memory is actually impaired in the phases of the menstrual cycle marked by low levels of estrogen.

Estrogen activates and progesterone apparently depresses the central nervous system. But although few studies have really looked at the effect of estrogen in normal women, those that have show no association between lower hormone levels in general and cognitive functioning.

We've all seen the headlines: "Estrogen helps memory!" "Estrogen helps you think!" These are mostly from a number of small studies (usually looking at only twenty women at a time) on memory loss in menopausal women. There have been two kinds of studies. In one type, the researchers take women who are on hormones and women who aren't, give them a battery of tests, and then compare the results. They find that women on hormones do a little better on some of the tests. It's hard to know what this means. The women on hormones are usually healthier, better educated, and of a higher socioeconomic status than the women who aren't. So it may not be the hormones causing the difference.

The other approach to studying this problem is to look at women who are about to have hysterectomies in which their ovaries are to be removed. Barbara Sherwin did one such study.[17] First she tested the women a month before the surgery. After surgery, she divided them into two groups. Half got estrogen and androgen; half got estrogen alone, androgen alone, or a placebo. Three months later she tested them again. The ones who got hormones did better on the memory tests than did those who got a placebo. Though these findings are interesting, it was a very short study. We don't know if the effect of hormones on someone thrown abruptly into menopause is the same as on someone who has a natural, more gradual, menopause.

Also, each of these studies used a combination of different tests. For instance, Elizabeth Barrett-Connor studied a group of women in the community of Rancho Bernardo.[18] The women who had used estrogen for at least twenty years had higher scores on one test but lower scores on the other tests. This suggests that estrogen might help maintain some aspects of short-term and long-term verbal memory, but it does not improve, and might even be bad for, visual spatial memory. It's certainly not a cure-all for memory problems.

In any case, the studies don't seem to be turning up differences in women's own awareness or experience. For example, a study by Jerome Yesavage at Stanford[19] looked at seventy-two women who were on estrogen and seventy-two who weren't. The women were given a list of sixteen names and asked to memorize them. On average, the women on estrogen could remember four names and the others could remember three. Yesavage called that a "significant difference." In terms of statistics, he's right. But it's probably not too significant in terms of the women's lives. None of the women could remember ten names, as they probably could have done when they were twenty.

Such memory problems as exist are probably fairly short-term, even among women whose ovaries are gone. Animal studies appear to confirm this. In one study, researchers removed monkeys' ovaries, then put half of them on estrogen. They found no difference in the monkeys' memory, but the monkeys on estrogen had slightly better attention spans when tested.[20] However, the differences lasted only for a short time: within three months, the monkeys who were not given estrogen had caught up to the others. So either the monkeys got better at the test with practice, or some attention deficit comes from abrupt change of hormones, and then evens out.

My conversations with postmenopausal women lead me to think that most of the fuzzy thinking and memory changes are short-term. We may not be able to avoid the toll the years take, but we're certainly as good as the monkeys at compensating. As we did with puberty and pregnancy, we do get back on an even keel.

Headaches

Migraines are definitely related to hormones, but exactly how and why they strike is unclear. Some migraines—particularly the kind that are related to the menstrual cycle—tend to go away after menopause. Some women have their first migraine during perimenopause; in some others, migraines become worse after menopause. Generally, a migraine has to do with blood-vessel constriction in the brain. Most commonly you notice an aura: this may cause a change in your vision, a blind spot, or even difficulty talking. This will be followed within about twenty minutes by a headache.

We know that migraines are more common in women than in men and that they start at puberty, so there's obviously a hormonal element. But it doesn't seem to be consistent. Nor do we know whether estrogen or progesterone is the culprit. Both affect blood-vessel constriction in the brain. Estrogen tends to dilate vessels; progesterone has the opposite effect. Hormone therapy sometimes alleviates the problem, but at other times it makes migraines worse. Obviously, we don't really understand migraines.

Many other kinds of headaches are related to hormones; these may well increase during perimenopause.

MENOPAUSAL SYMPTOMS

Though the majority of symptoms that have been called "menopausal" occur right before menopause, during the perimenopausal years, some do occur afterward. They may be short-term, but in some cases they last for the rest of a woman's life.

Vaginal Dryness

The image of the postmenopausal woman as "drying up" and becoming asexual refers to the common notion that with menopause you will lose all sexual lubrication and therefore all interest in sex. Although this is thought to be a universal symptom of menopause, it actually isn't. One study of 1,109 women showed that only 20 percent of postmenopausal women reported vaginal dryness, and only 15 percent of those were bothered by it.[21] Another study[22] reported that 45 percent of postmenopausal women and 25 percent of pre- and perimenopausal women complained of vaginal dryness. Some of the differences may have to do with how many surgically menopausal women were in each study. But in either case, this problem occurred in less than half of the women.

Vaginal dryness is not unique to menopause. Furthermore, it's not always a big problem when it does occur: one study showed that 80 percent of women with vaginal dryness felt satisfied with their sexual relationships.[23] (Since the study didn't include questions about whether or not the women were sexually active, it may be that at least in some cases this answer reflected the fact that the women didn't have or want a sexual relationship.) What I find most interesting is the fact that vaginal dryness also seems to be transient in many women. As with many of the other symptoms we have been discussing, it often improves when your hormones come into balance again. Unfortunately, though, this isn't always the case. For some women dryness continues after menopause, and it tends to worsen with age.

Vaginal dryness probably results from changes that occur in the genital area at lower levels of estrogen. The vagina and surrounding connective tissue can lose elasticity. The vagina can get smaller, thinner, and more fragile. It bleeds more easily if it's scratched, and it can get very sore and raw.

In addition, the acidity of the vagina can change, increasing the possibility of infection. The cervix gets a little smaller, and you can experience less lubrication with sexual arousal. This tends to be particularly true of women who are not very sexually active—the old principle that "if you don't use it, you lose it." Regular intercourse stretches the vagina out and increases blood supply and lubrication. Even regular masturbation will decrease symptoms of dryness and irritation.

I think vaginal dryness (sometimes called vaginal atrophy) is often overdiagnosed. It can be extremely alarming to a woman who has no symptoms to be told by her gynecologist in the middle of a pelvic exam that she is "drying up down there." One woman I know had a vague sense of something being different in her vagina and went to her gynecologist. He examined her and found nothing wrong, but decided she was a candidate for vaginal dryness and gave her estrogen cream to prevent it. While it's true, as we'll discuss in Chapter 15, that the dosage of estrogen in vaginal cream is low, it's still medication, and I think it's foolish to use it when you don't need it.

Studies show that women who have had a surgical menopause and women who undergo menopause as a result of chemotherapy have more problems with vaginal dryness than women who undergo a natural menopause. This again is probably caused by the lack of the testosterone and estrone that the ovary provides.

Skin Changes and Wrinkles: Is It Menopause or Age?

As part of their effort to sell youth, the drug companies often imply that estrogen keeps your skin young. They use young-looking models to sell the product, intimating that these are menopausal women made youthful by estrogen, and that if you use estrogen, you'll look like these near-nubile women. As with many other ads, the actual language doesn't lie—they never say that estrogen will prevent wrinkles. As I mentioned in Chapter 2, the package insert for Premarin clearly states that it does *not* help your skin, and even lists as one of the side effects "a spotty darkening of the skin, particularly on the face." But the picture does the lying for them: that smooth-skinned, youthful beauty isn't saying, "My mom uses estrogen."

Loss of estrogen doesn't cause wrinkles and sagging. Age does that, in both women and men. Too much exposure to the sun, and smoking, will hasten the process. The most important factor for youthful skin is your genes, however. If you are born with the right genes and stay out of the sun and don't smoke, you'll have the best chance at staying youthful-looking for a fairly long time.

There are only a handful of scientific studies on estrogen and skin changes, and they show little or no relationship between the two. One study from Spain[24] showed that estrogen didn't prevent the expected loss of collagen with age. Another study looked at collagen content in the skin of women who were taking estradiol and testosterone.[25] The ones who were on hormones had slightly more collagen in their skin than the ones who weren't. There was one other, larger study looking at collagen in both bone and skin. These researchers found differences in bone, but not in skin.[26] Although these studies are interesting, they don't tell us anything immediately useful, since we don't know exactly how collagen is related to wrinkles, sagging, and aging skin. One theory is that estrogen doesn't actually prevent wrinkles and sagging but rather causes the skin of your face to retain fluid, making it a bit more puffy and thus filling out some of the lines you've earned over the years.

Weight Gain

One of women's greatest fears is that menopause will cause them to gain weight. In a society that's neurotic about being thin, women panic at the thought of weight gain. In fact, women usually do put on some weight with menopause, but it's hard to determine the exact cause. As we discuss in Chapter 12, you need fewer calories to maintain your weight as you grow older. If you also decrease your activity, as people often do in middle age, then you're bound to gain weight. But more important, you're likely to see your weight shift. It's as if all those years of gravity finally take their toll and you find that your hips, lower abdomen, and bottom are bigger than you remember. Although you can't stop gravity, you can keep your weight stable with exercise and a reasonable diet.

Urinary Problems

Since there is a larger elderly population today than in the past, we're hearing more about incontinence (leakage of urine). As you can see from all the television commercials for Depends, this is a problem that comes with aging, and it can happen to both women and men. It's more common in women, however, and in many cases is probably related to menopause.

There are many kinds of urinary problems. You may have pain when you urinate (dysuria). Sometimes you'll have a sense of urgency—you feel as though your bladder is desperately full—but when you try to urinate, only a little comes out. Or you suddenly have to urinate so badly that you can't hold it. You might also experience frequency, a constant need to urinate. All of these symptoms have been linked with menopause in the public's mind. Is this association accurate? One study did show that the vast majority of urinary problems after menopause were in women who had had hysterectomies.[27] Whether the urinary problems came from the surgery itself or from these women's lower hormone levels is not clear, however.

There are two kinds of incontinence. One is *urinary incontinence*, which affects 10 percent of postmenopausal women. The urethra, the tube that carries urine from the bladder out of the body, has estrogen receptors. After menopause, the urethra gets thinner, and some of its tissue shrinks. This causes it to lose strength. When you need to urinate and feel a lot of pressure in your bladder, you tighten up the muscles that hold it in till you can get to the nearest toilet; but a weakened urethra can't help hold it in as well, and you'll get leakage.

Stress incontinence is probably the most common urinary problem in women between ages sixty and seventy-five. It occurs when you lose a little bladder control if you laugh, cough, jump, sneeze, or bear down. This tends to be related to muscles and to having had children, rather than to low estrogen levels. In rare cases, there's a loss of sensation: you don't know you have to urinate and aren't tightening the muscles, so the urine comes out. There are of course factors other than the urinary tract related to stress incontinence. You may be bedridden and unable to get to a bathroom. Or you may have arthritis in your hands that's so severe you can't get your underpants down in time.

Not all incontinence is permanent. As with vaginal dryness, some women have a temporary problem while their hormones are readjusting and then are fine again.

Studies have tried to determine if women on hormones have fewer urinary tract infections, but so far they haven't found any connections.

Libido

Does menopause quash or quicken your love life? We all know that the most important sex organ is the brain. It's a little difficult to judge what the effect of menopause is on sexual interest and sexual behavior because they appear to be relatively independent of natural estrogen levels. No correlation has yet been found between estrogen levels and sexual interest.

What is the origin of the idea that after menopause you lose interest in sex? It comes from small, widely reported studies. Most of the sexual problems studied have come from clinical samples—women who had gone to the doctor because of some health concern and so had problems of one sort or another already. There have been very few well-designed studies of sexual interest in healthy people. The famous sexologist Alfred Kinsey and his colleagues interviewed women throughout their life cycles, and they found that there was a decline with age in incidence and frequency of marital intercourse, and of intercourse to the point of orgasm. But there wasn't a decline in women's solitary sexual activity until well after sixty.

A study done in 1972 showed also a gradual decrease in sexual activity with age, particularly between forty-five and fifty-five, in both men and women.[28] A British study in 1985 showed that men reported a greater sexual loss of interest in their late forties and fifties than women did.[29] This would suggest that loss of sexual interest and reduced sexual activity are signs of age or of a partner's lack of interest, not signs of menopause. And maybe this is why some of those women engaged in solitary sexual activity.

One study[30] of sexual behavior in sixteen women over the course of their menopause found small but significant decreases in sexual activity, sexual thoughts, and vaginal lubrication, but not in frequency of orgasms or in sexual enjoyment. In another study, 70 percent of women between forty-five and fifty-six reported being sexually active, with no differences between the pre-, peri-, and postmenopausal women. Women between fifty-five and sixty-five were less sexually active than younger ones. And the major physical problem they discussed was vaginal dryness, which can cause discomfort with intercourse and thus affect sexual behavior.

In Chapter 2, I mentioned a study of women in a village in Thailand.[31] This research looked at sexual behavior in a different cultural context. Some women in the study experienced a decline in libido, but they didn't see that as a disadvantage: they felt released from having to worry about sex.

So while it seems that menopause either contributes to or coincides with some lessening of sexual desire, not everyone experiences that, and not everyone who does experience it considers it a problem.

Sometimes menopausal symptoms, rather than menopause itself, contribute to sexual problems: vaginal dryness, night sweats, hot flashes, etc.

Again, surgical menopause may affect sexual desire and attractiveness. After hysterectomy, whether or not her ovaries have been removed, a woman can lose interest in sex. She may also lose a degree of sexual desirability. There seems to be some biological basis for this. Studies of monkeys show that the male is no longer attracted to a female who has been hysterectomized.[32] But when the vaginal secretions of nonhysterectomized female monkeys are rubbed on the one who had the hysterectomy, the male regains interest. These secretions contain pheromones—aromas that are sexually stimulating. After hysterectomy they are no longer produced in the female. We do need to be careful about drawing conclusions about human sexuality from animal studies, since so much of our sexuality is psychological and sociological. But we can't rule out the possibility that the loss of pheromones affects male sexual responsiveness—or, for that matter, female responsiveness—to a woman.

In addition, hysterectomy alters the relationship of the vagina to the surrounding tissues. (Once something is taken out, the other organs shift to fill in the space.) This may affect how intercourse feels to both partners.

Another consequence of hysterectomy and removal of the ovaries has been postulated by the researcher Barbara Sherwin, who thought that a lack of testosterone may be what causes problems with libido.[33] In 1985, Sherwin and her colleagues found that giving testosterone to women who'd had their uteruses and ovaries removed enhanced the intensity of their sexual desire and arousal and the frequency of sexual fantasies. However, there was no evidence that testosterone affected the women's physiologic response or interpersonal aspects of their sexual behavior. The effect appeared to be more on motivation than on activity. Most of the articles about the effect of testosterone on libido are not scientific studies, just theories. This hasn't stopped one writer, Susan Rako, from writing a popular book—*The Hormone of Desire*—about the wonders of testosterone.[34] She writes about herself and many women she has consulted with (see Chapter 15), but she lacks the scientific data that might prove her case.

As I've pointed out before, menopause is a major change. You're unlikely to "feel like your old self" and more likely to feel like a new self. This may include new ways of being sexual and intimate. Some women feel more able to have sex with abandon, since they no longer have to worry about birth control; others feel less driven by their hormones to have sex. Everyone is different, and everyone's response is different. The most important point is that you feel comfortable with yourself and your libido. If you don't, then give yourself permission to explore ways of changing the situation. I'll discuss a few of these ways in Chapter 11.

CHAPTER 4

Prevention and Risk:
Understanding Research

Once upon a time, you went to the doctor because you were sick. If you felt okay, you didn't worry; you assumed that nothing was wrong and you went about your business. But in the past twenty years, there's been a strong focus on stopping disease before it starts. With this emphasis on preventive medicine, the concept of health has been redefined. As one cynic has said, "If you think you're healthy, you just haven't had enough tests done yet." Prevention has saved lives and forestalled needless suffering. But it has also fostered a boom in medical technology that has made health care decisions more complex and confusing. We have far more options about health care than our mothers and grandmothers ever had.

This hasn't been an unqualified boon. We started to realize this when daughters of women who had taken DES to prevent miscarriage in the 1940s showed an increased rate of vaginal cancer, while the mothers themselves had a disproportionate incidence of breast cancer. The original high-dose birth control pill caused strokes. The radiation therapy given to cure acne of the chest in the 1950s caused breast cancers that began to emerge in the 1990s. Understandably, though, the medical industry has preferred to focus on the more positive aspects of scientific progress.

Nowhere has the concept of preventive medicine caused more confusion than in the area of menopausal hormone therapy. In Chapter 3 we talked about the short-term symptoms of perimenopause and menopause. When treatment of such symptoms is called for, it is, for the most part, used for only a few years. Taking hormones for three to five years for the symptoms that you're having now, and then tapering off over six to nine months, may well make sense. For symptoms such as vaginal dryness that can sometimes be lifelong, very small doses of hormones, applied locally, may be the right choice (as you'll see in Chapter 11). But when we move into prevention, the issue gets trickier. Do you want to take hormones for the rest of your life to prevent diseases that you may or may not get? This question hinges on several others. Can hormones really prevent osteoporosis and heart disease? Is it safe to take these drugs for twenty or thirty years? Do we really know whether they cause breast cancer?

Let me make one thing very clear at the outset: there are no large prospective randomized controlled studies of postmenopausal women and hormones. That kind of "gold standard" research, which I'll explain shortly, hasn't yet been done. And therefore there are no real answers. In spite of the cheery reports on television, we really don't have much direct information on the effect of postmenopausal hormones. The first such study, the Women's Health Initiative, is going on now but won't give results until the year 2008. Since you and I want to know what to do now, we'll look at the data that are available. This is circumstantial evidence, if you will, and like all circumstantial evidence, it's flawed and subject to interpretation. That's why this issue is so confusing.

In this chapter I'm going to try and explain to you the circumstantial evidence: how the studies are done and what their limitations are. My goal is not only to help you understand what weight you should give the studies that have been done, but to help you evaluate the ones that you'll hear about after this book comes out. In other words, I'm going to help you become a more discerning consumer of health news. I want to warn you now, however, that many of you will find this boring. If you want to, you can skip to Chapter 5. My feelings won't be hurt. And you'll be in good company— most doctors don't understand these nuances either. Those of you who want to be one up on your doctor and want to really understand how to analyze one of these studies, read on. And those of you who aren't sure, come on in. Read what you want and skip what you don't.

There are many ways to conduct studies. But doing a completely accurate, comprehensive study is next to impossible. There are too many variables in studying even the simplest disease or life stage. To understand how accurate a study is, you need to be able to look at all its elements. It may be weak in one area, stronger in another, and excellent in a third. It's sort of like comparing the different grades for a school composition. One composition may get A for spelling, B for handwriting, and C for content. Another might get B for spelling, C for handwriting, and A for content. Although the average grade is B in both cases, the composition graded C for content may not be half as good as the one graded A for content. There are different aspects of a study that make it more or less credible.

Unfortunately, most doctors don't really understand study design. (Statistics and epidemiology are the courses most students sleep through in medical school.) And doctors are as prone to self-deception as the rest of us: they tend to believe the studies that feed their biases and discount the ones that don't. Further, as we discussed in Chapter 2, their source of information is often a drug company—which means that their bias is usually in favor of hormone therapy. Thus their overall tendency has been to overestimate the benefits and underestimate the risks of long-term use of hormone therapy.

This same tendency is reflected by the media—whose relationship to corporate interests is strong ("Tonight's weather is brought to you by . . .")— and they are even less able than doctors to critically analyze the strengths and weaknesses of studies. We've all had the experience of reading in a newspaper that some study shows that drug X causes disease Y, only to read in the same paper a few days later that a new study proves it doesn't. The reporters often don't understand the nuances of the study, and the researchers have their own bias in presenting the results. Rarely do news reports point out flaws in the design of a study. And even when they do, we often hear what we want to hear. Recently I read an article in *The New York Times* about a study that had been started, looking at the effect of estrogen on Alzheimer's disease. The article clearly stated that the current data were preliminary and thus this big, well-designed study was necessary. That day at lunch a friend of mine overheard a woman in a restaurant saying to her companion, "Did you hear that estrogen can cure Alzheimer's disease?" All of these factors create widespread confusion about hormones and their effect on the prevention and risk of disease.

KINDS OF STUDIES: WHICH ARE MOST RELIABLE?

There are two main categories of studies, each with its own strengths and weaknesses. One is the *observational study.* In an observational study the researcher observes people doing what they might normally do, but doesn't intervene. The second is a *clinical trial,* or *interventional study,* whose purpose is to test a certain drug or treatment, so the researcher has the subjects change their behavior (by taking a pill, perhaps) and records the results. There are a few varieties of each of these studies.

Observational Studies

Observational studies can be cross-sectional studies, cohort (follow-up) studies, or case control studies.

In a *cross-sectional study*, a large number of people are asked about their symptoms at a given moment in time. One study might survey a number of fifty-year-old women who have had bone-density tests and find that 50 percent of them have low bone density. That will provide a sense of the usual bone density of a fifty-year-old. It won't, however, provide any idea about why they have a given bone density—and, as you'll see in Chapter 5, there are significantly different possible reasons.

In a *cohort,* or *follow-up, study,* a particular group of people are observed over time. For example, a study could look at 100 forty-five-year-old women and measure their bone density for the next ten years. This is sometimes also called a longitudinal study, since the women are followed over time. This would provide a better idea of whether all the women lost bone density at menopause or whether only some did. On the other hand, the data would be limited to those 100 women, who might or might not be representative of the population as a whole. If a cohort is large enough, the researchers can compare people with a given condition and people without it. The Nurses' Health Study in Boston, Massachusetts, is a cohort study that has carefully followed a group of 121,700 nurses since 1976.[1] The nurses fill out questionnaires about their health every two years. The researchers periodically analyze different diseases or risk factors in this group. Because the number of subjects in this study is so large, the data obtained are very powerful, but the study still has limitations. The researchers have no control over the behavior of the women in the study. They can't, for example, decide who gets hormones, or who gets mammograms; they can just ask questions. So the study might include some women at risk for breast cancer who aren't getting hormones or who are getting more frequent mammograms, and this will skew the results.

Cohort studies can be either retrospective or prospective. *Retrospective* studies look at the medical histories of a certain number of people, some of whom have a particular condition and some of whom don't. The researchers then try to determine how many of them had a certain risk factor. For example, they might look at women diagnosed with Alzheimer's and find out how many of them took estrogen at menopause.

Prospective studies start on the other end. They take a group of subjects and follow them forward over a period of years. For example, a prospective study might take a group of women who have been on estrogen at some time in their lives and compare them with a group who haven't, to see how many develop breast cancer in the next ten years. Prospective studies are generally thought to be more accurate than retrospective studies, which depend on the participants' memories; depending on memory is chancy at best, and the difficulty is compounded when the subject being studied has a disease like Alzheimer's. But prospective studies are more difficult to conduct, and more time-consuming.

A *case control* study looks at a group of people with a certain condition, comparing them with another group of people who don't have the condition but who are similar to them in other ways. For example, you might take a group of people recently diagnosed with lung cancer and match them up with people of the same age and sex chosen randomly out of the phone book to see how many people in each group carried cigarette lighters when they were in their thirties. And you might learn that, indeed, more people who carried cigarette lighters got lung cancer. But there's always the chance that factors you don't know about or don't understand will enter into the equation. For instance, you might conclude that the plastic in cigarette lighters causes lung cancer, completely missing the fact that people who carry cigarette lighters use them to light cigarettes, and it's the cigarettes that cause the cancer.

This, of course, is a fanciful example, invented to illustrate my point. But there are many actual cases of such mistaken leaps of logic. And something like this may be happening now in some of the studies looking at estrogen replacement, heart disease, and osteoporosis. We've noted that women who have hysterectomies are more likely to be on long-term estrogen therapy and also that most women with hysterectomies have also had their ovaries removed. This was particularly true in the 1970s and 1980s, when the fact that estrogen increases the risk of uterine cancer had just been proved. It was for this reason that 60 to 80 percent of the women in the large studies of estrogen therapy were those who had undergone surgical menopause: they no longer had uteruses at risk from estrogen. But women who have had surgical menopause tend to be fairly young—in their early thirties or forties—so the women in these studies are often younger than women who experience menopause naturally. Thus the subjects in the studies are at higher risk for osteoporosis and heart disease, and therefore the benefits of hormones in preventing these diseases in these women may not be the same as for women who go through a natural menopause and are at lower risk in the first place.

A particular group may be chosen for an observational study because of convenience—e.g., researchers might question all the women who live in the same retirement village to study the relationship between estrogen and breast cancer. But this creates some limitations. It may not be clear why some women were put on estrogens and others weren't. Asking them would be of limited use, because they themselves may not know—many patients simply do what the doctor tells them to without asking questions. This can introduce enormous bias, as you'll see when we look at one such study in more detail later on.

Clinical Trials or Interventional Studies

Clinical trials, or interventional studies, are actually studies of treatment. (By definition, clinical trials are prospective.) Everyone in such a study is given a certain treatment to see what happens. The problem is that in order to tell if something works, you need a *control group*—people who haven't been given the treatment—for purposes of comparison. Sometimes researchers will use "historical controls," meaning that they'll look at what the results of a previous treatment were and see if a new treatment makes a difference. The problem with this type of study is that you don't really know what made your patients different from those in the past. For example, the survival rate of women with breast cancer has improved, even with conventional treatment. So if you tried a new treatment and saw a small improvement, you wouldn't know if that was from the treatment or whether it was just another instance of the fact that women do better now.

Our hypothetical study of a retirement village would be even better if researchers gave the "experimental" group estrogen and the "control" group a placebo (inert pill). This would be a *controlled study.* You could compare the results in one group with the results in the other, but you wouldn't know if the two groups themselves were really comparable. For example, if by chance all the women with a family history of breast cancer were in the experimental group, the results could be inaccurate.

It would be a much stronger study if researchers could take the women in the retirement village and randomly pick a number of them to take estrogen, and then follow them for ten years to see who got breast cancer. That way we could be sure that the women given estrogen weren't by coincidence those at low risk for breast cancer, thus biasing the results. The study would then become a *randomized controlled clinical trial.*

Randomization is a concept that most people don't understand. *Randomized* doesn't mean "accidental" or "capricious"; it means that each person in a given group, large or small, had an equal chance to be chosen for a study, or that each person had an equal chance to be chosen to receive one treatment or another. In a randomized study, each subject's treatment is picked randomly, usually by a computer, to eliminate the possibility that subjects will be chosen on the basis of situations they're already in, skewing the results. If all of the women who exercise were put on one treatment and all the couch potatoes on another, the first treatment would end up looking a lot better than it really was.

If neither the researchers nor the subjects know who's taking which pill, there will be no temptation to treat one group differently, perhaps by performing more mammograms on the group taking estrogen. That type of study is called *double-blind* because both the researchers and the subjects are in the dark as to who's getting what treatment.

A *prospective randomized double-blind controlled* study is the "gold standard" of studies. It has the fewest flaws and is thus the most reliable. There's still the problem that women who choose to participate in such a study may not be like the rest of us—most people, after all, prefer to know what treatment they're getting and don't want to risk being given nothing or a placebo. But it's the closest we can get to good data.

As I've said, the Women's Health Initiative is a randomized controlled double-blind study started several years ago to investigate the effect of Premarin and the progestin Provera, calcium, vitamin D, and a low-fat diet on heart disease, breast cancer, and osteoporosis. When it's completed in the year 2008, we'll have the type of data about the risks and benefits of these treatments that we've all been longing for. Until then, we're forced to rely on more limited studies.

WHO'S IN WHAT STUDY?

Aside from knowing what kind of study you're looking at, you need to be aware of who's in the study. In this case, you need to know how a study defines "hormone use." Some studies take into account how long a woman has used hormones; others don't. Some simply compare women who have taken hormones with women who have never taken them, without considering how long the hormones were taken. Such a study ends up lumping together someone who took hormones for three months and someone who took them for thirty years. Other studies lump together women who have taken different doses and preparations of hormones. Some studies compare women who are currently taking hormones with women who took them in the past.

All of these studies may have different results, depending on how estrogen relates to the particular disease being studied. If estrogen prevents heart disease by lowering levels of the cholesterol that gradually clogs arteries, you'd expect that taking it for ten years would put off your risk for heart disease for ten years. On the other hand, if its effect is mostly on dilating clogged coronary blood vessels at the time of a heart attack, you'd expect that only a women who was taking it at the time of her heart attack would get any benefit.

We also need to be aware of what is called *selection bias.* A study is biased if the people in it are not typical of the general public. As you'll recall from Chapter 2, the approach to giving estrogen therapy to women with a risk of heart disease has been contradictory over the years. Originally, there were two things that worried researchers about using estrogen to prevent heart disease. One was the study we discussed in Chapter 2, in which estrogen was given to men who had heart attacks.[2] Not only did the estrogen fail to reduce their likelihood of further heart attacks, it actually seemed to make their risk of future heart attacks a bit worse, and doctors feared that it would have the same effect on women with heart disease. Doctors were also concerned when it became clear that the early high-dose birth control pills, especially when used by women who smoked, caused an increase in heart disease and strokes. They feared that estrogen treatment for menopause would have the same effect.

These two concerns made doctors reluctant to give estrogen to women who had high blood pressure or were otherwise at risk of heart disease. So until fairly recently, they didn't. Nor did they give estrogen to women who were at risk of breast cancer, because of a suspicion that the hormones would promote the cancer. This is why the women getting hormones have been at low risk for heart disease and breast cancer to start with. This selection bias—studying women at low risk to start with—means that all observational studies are likely to end up *overestimating* any benefits in terms of controlling heart disease and *underestimating* dangers in terms of contributing to breast cancer.

Perhaps most important, we need to understand the *healthy woman effect*. Studies have shown that the kind of women who take hormones are the kind who also do other things to take care of their health.[3] They go to the doctor frequently. If they have high blood pressure, they take care of it. They exercise; they eat a good diet; they don't smoke. They tend to be better educated and to have a higher socioeconomic status. It's these motivated women, with a healthier lifestyle, who get put on hormones and studied. They read the magazines; they go to the doctor and say, "I read about high blood pressure in this article. How do I prevent it?" In fact, women who take estrogen therapy have a decrease in *all* causes of death, even those that have nothing to do with estrogen, like injuries.[4] Women who aren't on hormones, on the other hand, tend not to go to the doctor till they're sick, not to exercise, not to reduce fat in their diets, etc. They therefore tend to be less healthy. Because of the healthy woman effect, if we do an observational study and note that the women on hormones have less disease, it's hard to tell whether it's because estrogen makes women healthy, or because healthy women take estrogen. It will only be through a randomized controlled study with the same number of couch potatoes in each group that we will know the answer.

In addition, there is the *compliant woman effect*. Women taking estrogen replacement therapy are by and large compliant people—they do what the doctor tells them to do. A study of men and women who had heart attacks showed that participants who were compliant about taking their prescribed placebo had the same reduction in the risk of heart attack as those who took drugs—and both groups did better than those who didn't take their placebos regularly.[5] We don't really know what this means. It isn't just the well-known "placebo effect," which shows that to some extent what you believe is happening to you influences what actually does happen. The compliance effect is more like the "healthy woman" effect. If you're someone who follows the doctor's orders, you not only take your pill religiously every day, but also exercise religiously, avoid high-fat foods, and generally do the other things your doctor tells you to do. Also, because most women don't stay on hormones (only about 25 percent of the women who start on estrogen are still taking it five years later),[6] those who stick with them over the course of many years in a given study are a select group for that very reason.

WHAT IS THE STUDY STUDYING?

Since women who are on hormones are more likely to go to the doctor, they're also more likely to get mammograms and other screening for cancer. It's possible, therefore, that when these women get breast cancer they're more likely to be diagnosed earlier, which means that they'll get treated earlier and have a higher survival rate. Thus a study might turn up an increased incidence of breast cancer, but not an increased death rate. These are two different things. One study might look at how many women on hormones get breast cancer, while another might look at how many women on hormones get breast cancer and die from it. It's very important to know what a study has been set up to determine. This is known as its *endpoint*. When you're looking at the results of a study, you need to ask yourself what its endpoint is. That endpoint may or may not be relevant to your life.

There's a well-known example of this. A study examined the benefits of hip replacement surgery versus simply nailing a patient's broken hip back together. The endpoint was to determine how many days patients from each group had to spend in the hospital. The researchers found that patients who had hip replacements had longer hospital stays—which, given the study's endpoint, meant this procedure was not as good as the other. If they'd looked at which procedure gave the patient a better chance of walking, however, they'd have come to the opposite conclusion. No one asked the patient with a broken hip—who probably would be perfectly happy with an extra day or two in the hospital if that meant being able to walk out of it. This is why it's so important to look at exactly what the endpoints of a study are, and to make sure that they're as relevant to you as they are to the researchers.

HOW SERIOUS IS "INCREASED RISK"?

When you hear the results of a study on preventing a disease, you need to know how common the disease is, at what age it's likely to occur, and what your personal risk is.

For example, ovarian cancer can be very deadly, but it's not very common: about one in eighty women over forty will get it. If you are at double that risk, your chance is one in forty. Breast cancer, by contrast, has a lifetime risk of one in eight. Doubling that risk gives a chance of one in four—a much higher probability of developing the disease. A greatly increased risk of a rare disease may have less overall effect on a woman's health than a modestly increased risk of a more common disease. It's easy to get overly alarmed when a headline blasts that a certain treatment doubles your risk of a deadly disease if you don't take into account how common or uncommon the disease is.

It's also critical to look at the average age of people who get a disease. You may not want to take a drug like estrogen for thirty years to prevent a disease like osteoporosis that you're not likely to get till you're eighty, especially if you're at risk of other life-threatening medical conditions.

WHEN SHOULD PREVENTION START?

There are two ways to approach prevention, and they have very different implications. *Primary prevention* means treating people to prevent a disease that they may or may not get. The idea is to try to keep the disease from happening at all. This is the rationale for giving all women over fifty hormones to try to prevent them from developing heart disease.

Secondary prevention means treating someone who already has a disease, in order to prevent the problem from recurring or worsening. For example, a woman who has had a heart attack at sixty-five may be put on estrogen to try to prevent a second heart attack.

Primary prevention has its advantages: obviously, you're better off not getting the disease in the first place. But it involves subjecting people to new risks in order to prevent something that may not happen at all. Thus many women who would never have had heart attacks at all will take estrogen for twenty or thirty years, and they may suffer from side effects of the treatment—side effects that include breast cancer. With secondary prevention we're treating only those we know will benefit. But there's the risk that people will suffer more severely because they developed the condition in the first place: some women will die from the original heart attack, or be seriously weakened by it.

Since each approach has its risks, doctors often try to reserve primary prevention for those who are at higher risk for the disease—those for whom there is likely to be more benefit than risk. Therefore, one of the major questions about hormone therapy is whether to take it now or wait until later, and that brings us to our next question.

CAN WE PREDICT WHO IS AT RISK?

Risk factors are conditions that increase your likelihood of getting a particular disease—for example, smoking increases your likelihood of getting lung cancer. Having a risk factor doesn't necessarily mean that you'll get a disease, nor does not having any risk factors mean that you're home free. In fact, few risk factors are as dramatic or as clear-cut as the connection between smoking and lung cancer. Knowing your risk factors is just a tool for making an educated guess.

It's also important to realize that having a risk factor for a disease doesn't necessarily mean that you're going to get it sooner than anyone else. If most people have a one-in-ten chance of getting a disease at age fifty and you have a factor that doubles the risk, this means that you have a one-in-five chance of getting the disease at fifty—not that you'll get it at twenty-five. Certain risk factors do, however, mean you're more likely to get a disease prematurely—for example, hereditary breast cancer often strikes younger women than the more common, nonhereditary kind.

This is something you need to be very clear about when making a decision. You may feel very different about an increased risk of a life-threatening illness that will hit you when you're fifty, when you could reasonably hope for another twenty-five or thirty years, as opposed to one that will strike when you're eighty, when you're more likely to die of other causes anyway.

It's sometimes hard to apply these numbers to yourself, since your issues are rarely just about one factor. You might have a history of breast cancer and also have high blood pressure, or you might have a lot of both breast cancer and heart disease in your family. We will talk more about how to weigh your individual risks in Chapter 16.

DISEASE OR RISK FACTOR?

Sometimes, instead of studying a disease itself, researchers study a risk factor for that disease. For example, instead of trying to learn how many children who see the Joe Camel billboards will end up dying of lung cancer (a study that could take decades to complete), we could look at how many of the kids who see the billboards start smoking. We know that not all of those children will die of lung cancer, but we also know that a lot more smokers than nonsmokers get lung cancer, and that most people who get lung cancer die of it. A risk factor used as the endpoint of a study is called an *intermediate marker*—we're looking at an early stop along the road to the disease.

But we need to be careful not to confuse these two kinds of endpoints. It's important to know what affects risk factors, but it's equally important not to confuse risk factors with diseases. Even with something as clear-cut as cigarettes and lung cancer, the equation isn't exact: not all smokers get lung cancer, and not all people who get lung cancer smoke. With less clear-cut risk factors, this is even trickier. Are we measuring how many women get fractures of the hip, or what happens with their bone-density tests? Are we measuring heart attacks or cholesterol levels? Not everyone with high cholesterol will get a heart attack. In addition, if a drug improves heart disease because it dilates clogged blood vessels rather than lowering the cholesterol that causes the clog, the studies looking at cholesterol alone might misinterpret the drug's effect on heart disease. Even with a good study like the PEPI study, which I'll discuss in depth in Chapter 6, this is a problem.

HOW BIG IS THE STUDY?

Finally, we need to know the size of the study. If there's a big difference in the effect of a treatment, it will show up in a relatively small study. If, for example, a treatment decreases the death rate from stroke by a third, that will become obvious after studying 100 women, 50 getting the treatment and 50 a placebo: three times as many women in the treatment group will be alive after, say, ten years. But if the effect is smaller, it will take a larger study—a study of more women—to demonstrate that. For example, the Nurses' Health Study, looking at 121,700 women, reported in the summer of 1995 that estrogen and progesterone therapy increased the incidence of breast cancer by 70 percent in women between sixty-five and sixty-nine.[7] (This doesn't mean that 70 percent of women on hormone therapy got breast cancer; it means that 70 percent *more* women on hormone therapy got breast cancer than women not on hormones.) Within a week, a second study came out from Seattle, stating that there was no increased risk of breast cancer in women taking estrogen and progesterone.[8] The media took these parallel studies as showing that scientists can't make up their minds. In fact, the second study was too small to show a 70 percent effect—it included only 1,029 women. It could only have shown a 250 percent difference (2.5 times as many) between the two groups.[9] It didn't contradict the Nurses' Health Study at all.

All of this isn't meant to confuse you, but to demonstrate why data can be confusing. Needless to say, those who believe in estrogen for everyone will be inclined to quote the studies that feed their bias and ignore the weaknesses in those studies. The same is true of those who feel that estrogen is dangerous. Doctors often haven't the time to analyze studies closely, and so they may accept uncritically the results they want to believe.

In the next chapters, we'll discuss the diseases that have been related to menopause in women, how common they are, what their risk factors are, the age at which they occur, what it's like to have them, and what the studies show about preventing them. We'll address the strengths and weaknesses in all the studies, to help you decide the issues for yourself with the best information available.

CHAPTER 5

Osteoporosis: Are We All
Going to Crumble?

Osteoporosis (defined as brittle bones—a definition I'll get into later) is one of the new "in" diseases. Doctors and drug companies love it for two reasons—there is a test that can diagnose people at high risk (more about that later), and there are drugs to treat it. As we pointed out in Chapter 2, the pharmaceutical companies find it easier to market a disease than a drug. Thus they've bombarded gynecologists—and the public—with images of humped-over old women unable to cross a street without help.

Certainly such women exist—but they're far more common in Premarin ads than in everyday life. Look around you at an airport or in a supermarket—you'll see very few elderly women with pronounced dowager's humps. Osteoporosis is no fun, and I'm not making light of it. But our fear of it is out of proportion to its reality. Only about 25 percent of women will ever develop osteoporosis.[1]

Why has osteoporosis gotten a reputation as a women's disease—even a symptom of menopause? Men too can get osteoporosis, if they live long enough. In fact, I recently came across an article in a medical journal bemoaning the fact that we weren't paying enough attention to osteoporosis in men. All the studies were being done on women—even the animal studies used female monkeys.[2] The article was right: the studies do focus on females. This isn't a result of some feminist plot to get even for the years of male-only studies. The studies have focused on women because that's the kind of research the drug companies have funded.

But osteoporosis is an equal-opportunity disease. Weaker bones are a fact of aging. Some people are more likely to develop osteoporosis than others: more women have it because more women live into advanced old age, and because women start out with smaller bones.

THE BONE HOUSE

To understand osteoporosis, it helps to know a little about bone itself. Bone isn't static. It's continually being added to and remodeled. How this process works is fairly complicated, but I'll try to explain it using a metaphor (itself rather complicated) borrowed from the Old English epic *Beowulf*, in which the body is called the "bone house." (In medicine, we speak of the bones' "microarchitecture," implicitly accepting this powerful image.)

In the beginning, your skeleton is like the first small house a couple move into when they're just starting out. It's perfect for two people, but soon the kids start coming and it begins to get cramped. So our young couple, being fairly prosperous, decide to remodel. First they have to do some demolition. Then a cleanup crew comes. Next, a construction crew builds a playroom for the kids. This whole process takes at least six months (see Figure 5.1).

Your skeleton remodels itself much the same way. There are bone-remodeling units, called *osteons,* which function like the construction crew. These osteons consist of *osteoclasts* (the demolition crew), *reversal cells*—also called *mononuclear cells* (the cleanup crew)—and *osteoblasts* (the rebuilders). Once an area of bone is activated (a process we as yet don't understand, in which the bone is tagged for remodeling), the osteoclasts arrive and spend the next couple of weeks resorbing a predetermined amount of bone in that spot (see Figure 5.2). When the osteoclasts have finished, the mononuclear cells come and clean up the surface to prepare it for new bone formation. Then come the osteoblasts. They begin to fill the newly cleared-out area with new organic matrix, called *osteoid* (a jellylike substance that frames the new bone). After a delay of twenty-five to thirty-

FIGURE 5.1   The "bone house."

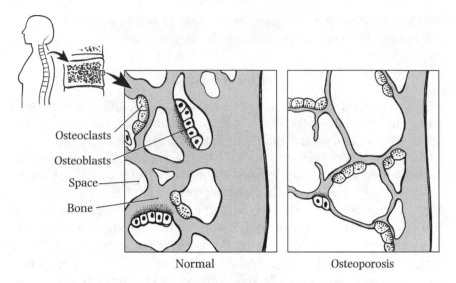

Osteoclasts

Osteoblasts

Space

Bone

Normal   Osteoporosis

FIGURE 5.2   Osteoclasts and osteoblasts in (*left*) normal bone
and (*right*) osteoporosis.

five days, this osteoid becomes mineralized—it turns to bone. A complete
remodeling cycle takes several months.

This bone remodeling continues throughout your life. During the first
twenty to thirty years of life, there's more building than demolition (as in
the first twenty years of our couple's marriage—they might tear down the
garage to build a kid's room and a playroom). There may be a crisis now
and then that calls for more remodeling, such as a fracture or broken bone
(just as a house might get damaged in a hurricane). By about age thirty-
five, you have all the bone you're ever likely to have.

BONE DENSITY

Peak Bone Mass

The amount of bone that you have by thirty-five is called your *peak bone
mass.* Although you'll continue to remodel when it's necessary, from here
on you'll be losing more bone than you build.

Your own peak bone mass will depend on a variety of factors. One factor
is your genes; identical twins raised in different circumstances tend to have
very similar peak bone masses.[3] We might compare this genetic component
of peak bone mass to the amount of money the couple had in the bank to
buy the house in the beginning.

Your diet is another factor. If you take in enough calcium and vitamin D
in your early years, you'll build more bone than if you don't. This dietary

factor could be compared to investments made by our couple to increase the money available for the house.

Exercise also plays a role. The more you exercise, the more bone you'll build—just as our couple might put in overtime hours in order to earn more money for the house.

Turnover and Bone Loss

Bone turnover never stops completely. In fact, after about age fifty, it increases, though it's not quite coordinated. The building team (the osteoblasts) becomes less and less capable of completely refilling the holes left by the demolition crew. Some women (though not all) experience more rapid loss of bone around menopause; this is thought to be due to increased activity from the osteoclasts, which become hyperactive and penetrate too deep into the bone, perforating it and making it brittle. This results in a less stable structure, disrupting the microarchitecture, which can lead to fractures. Basically, it's like having termites eating away at the framework of your house and weakening it.

The peak amount of bone you started with and the rate of this loss will determine the density of your bones. Density will be very different in different individuals, cultures, races, and sexes.

The correct term for *low bone density* is *osteopenia*. Osteopenia is only one factor in osteoporosis and the fractures that result from it. Another factor is the microarchitecture of the bone. As the osteoclasts demolish or resorb more bone than is rebuilt, the architecture becomes more fragile. Just as a flimsy house is more drastically damaged by a hurricane than a sturdier house, a fall or some other injury will do worse damage to a fragile bone than to a sound one.

Some kinds of bone are more susceptible than others to turnover and loss. As they weaken, the wrist and the hip become more vulnerable to fractures. Vertebral bone—the bone in your back—doesn't really fracture or crack but rather collapses on itself. This makes you lose height and, if enough vertebrae are crushed, gives you a dowager's hump. It usually takes four to five crushed vertebrae before you notice a difference (see Figure 5.3 later in this chapter).

Hormones and Bone Density

What do hormones have to do with bone? All of these stages of bone maintenance we've been speaking about need fine-tuning. Hormones help do this job. What's interesting about the hormones that affect bone is that they appear to regulate calcium metabolism rather than bone remodeling itself. Calcium is important throughout the body, and the body has a precise mechanism for making sure that there's enough calcium for the heart and other cells. The major hormones involved in the process are parathormone (from the parathyroid glands), calcitonin (from the thyroid gland), and vitamin D (from the skin). (You usually don't think of vitamins as hormones, and most aren't, but vitamin D actually is, in that it's secreted by one organ and travels through the bloodstream to affect another organ—which is the definition of a hormone.)

There are other hormones that influence calcium less directly: thyroid hormone, adrenal hormones, estrogen, progesterone, and testosterone and other androgens (male hormones). These are set in motion by the parathyroid glands—tiny structures in your neck, behind the thyroid. These glands monitor the amount of calcium in the blood. If it goes below a certain level, they go into action and secrete parathormone. This tells the kidney to hold on to calcium and not let it flush out in the urine. They convert inactive vitamin D to active vitamin D (see below), which helps you absorb more calcium from your food. And they tell the osteoclasts to resorb more bone and release the calcium into the bloodstream. Since calcium in the blood is used by every cell in the body to maintain its integrity, they decide to sacrifice calcium in the bone in order to maintain calcium in the blood—somewhat like burning the furniture to keep a cabin warm when you run out of firewood. This becomes important to older women (and men) who may not be getting enough calcium or vitamin D in their diets. The resulting lower blood level of calcium sends the parathyroid glands into action and starts increasing bone loss. Getting enough calcium and vitamin D in your diet can prevent this type of bone loss.

The thyroid gland produces calcitonin and the imaginatively named thyroid hormone. Calcitonin inhibits osteoclasts and slows down remodeling, maintaining adequate bone mass. Unfortunately, this helpful hormone decreases with age and with menopause. (One of the new treatments for osteoporosis involves a synthetic form of this hormone—see Chapter 15.) Thyroid hormone can cause increased breakdown of bone if it's too high. This can result from having an overactive thyroid or from taking thyroid medication for many years at too high a dose. (If you've been on a thyroid hormone such as Synthroid, you should have periodic blood tests to monitor your thyroid function and make sure the dose isn't too high.)

Vitamin D is always present in our skin, in an inactive form. Sunlight will activate it. It can also be obtained through certain foods. Vitamin D helps the intestine absorb calcium from food; it also helps the kidneys reabsorb calcium from urine. Thus it's an important regulator of blood calcium levels. If you don't get enough sunlight, you'll get rickets, a disease in which the bones soften. This sometimes happens in nursing homes in the Northeast, where sunlight is limited in winter and residents have little need to go outside. However, if you get too much vitamin D (more than 1,000 milligrams a day), it will leach calcium from your bones and so increase bone loss.

Adrenal hormones called *glucocorticoids,* or *steroids,* help your body deal with stressful physical events. They're also sometimes taken as drugs. *Steroids* make bone overly responsive to parathyroid hormone and vitamin D so that calcium can be mobilized in an emergency. This, of course, increases bone loss.

As far as we've been able to determine, estrogen has a less direct effect on bone. It blocks the bone-resorbing effect of parathormone and stimulates the release of calcitonin and vitamin D. Progesterone also seems to have some effect on bone—possibly by blocking the effect of the adrenal hormones. Finally, androgens like testosterone, produced in women by the postmenopausal ovary, stimulate osteoblasts and can build bone. (This is in part why men have a higher peak bone mass to begin with—they have much more androgen, produced by their testicles.)

There's still a great deal about bones that we don't understand. What tells the remodeling to go on in one place and not another? Why do black women have denser bones than white women? What determines the microarchitecture that is so critical to fracture prevention? As we discover more about the active maintenance of strong bones, we'll be much better able to prevent the problems that occur when they go awry.

So, What Is Osteoporosis?

The definition of *osteoporosis* has gone through many permutations over the years. In the old days, osteoporosis meant fractures caused by thin bones. The current definition—agreed on by an international consensus panel of medical experts in the field—has changed the focus. (These panels are generally funded by government agencies, sometimes with the help of drug companies.) Osteoporosis is now "a disease characterized by low bone mass and microarchitectural deterioration of bone tissue, which lead to increased bone fragility and a consequent increase in fracture risk."[4] In other words, you've got brittle bones that are more likely to fracture. The problem with this definition is that the "disease" is not an actual fracture but only an increased risk of fracture. This is like defining heart disease as having high cholesterol rather than having a heart attack. Needless to say, this new definition has increased the number of women—and men, for that matter—who have "osteoporosis."

Although this new disease has two components—bone mass and microarchitecture—one of them is virtually ignored: the bone's microarchitecture. There's a reason for this. Microarchitecture is ignored because we can't measure it; we can measure only bone density. And if the microarchitecture is strong, you'll be less likely to get fractures. So the definition is beginning to shift again: we're hearing low bone density itself, without microarchitectural deterioration, referred to as osteoporosis. It's true that people with very high bone density don't tend to get fractures unless they receive a serious blow to the bone. But not everyone with low bone density gets fractures. By these new standards, you could live a perfectly comfortable life for thirty years after menopause with a "disease" you never knew you had.

This might be funny, except it can cause patients needless fear. I got a frantic call once from a patient who'd just learned she had "severe osteoporosis." I asked if she had any broken bones, or was hunched over, or had any other symptoms. No, she said, she was fine. But she'd just had a bone-density test that showed low density, and the doctor had told her she had this terrifying disease and needed to stop playing sports. The poor woman was devastated.

I have serious problems with this whole business. Why not define low bone density as a risk factor for osteoporosis, rather than as osteoporosis itself? That puts it in perspective: it's a warning sign that might be useful so you can begin to consider ways to keep the disease itself from occurring.

This is an important issue, for a number of reasons. For one thing, as we begin to learn more about genes, we're finding genes that cause a person to metabolize calcium in a certain way or to have lower bone density.[5] Again, this can be useful as a warning signal. But it raises a disturbing question. Will the presence of this gene itself soon be called a disease? If so, how will all this play out on both the practical and the psychological level? Will insurance companies refuse to insure someone with this "disease"? Does a woman who feels fine and has no problems or discomfort, and may never have any, really have a disease? By these standards, most of us are probably "diseased" one way or another.

To me, a "disease" is a clear-cut condition that lessens comfort or well-being. Maybe there's some use in broadening the definition, but if we do that, we should at least be clear about exactly what we're saying.

Once you're told you have a disease, you're going to start looking for a treatment. The drug companies and the doctors know this, and I think it is part of the driving force behind some new "diseases." For example, women who learn from a test that they have low bone density are more likely to be on hormone replacement therapy than those who haven't;[6] they think that without the hormones they're bound to end up with a broken hip or a rounded back. They're rarely given adequate information about what bone density really means.

Measuring Bone Density?

As you can see, the ability to measure bone density has changed the way we look at osteoporosis. In the past, the only tool available was the X ray, which couldn't identify low bone density until it was at least 30 to 50 percent below normal. But now we have techniques that can measure density with far more accuracy.

There are a couple of tests used for screening women for low bone density. Both are painless. *Single-proton absorptiometry* was developed first and is still used by many doctors. Now there's *dual-energy X-ray absorptiometry* (DEXA). This is a better tool for gauging bone density (though not necessarily twice as good, as its name might suggest). DEXA can measure the bone density of the hip and spine, the areas usually involved in fractures. It can detect a loss of as little as 1 percent of bone mass from year to year. But it has several limitations. It measures only the lumbar spine—the lower back. It can't measure the thoracic, or upper back, which is the part involved in vertebral crush fractures. It sometimes overreads bone density when there are benign calcium deposits in the area (such as those that result from arthritis). And it can't detect fractures. This is a serious limitation, since spontaneous fractures in the vertebrae are the basis for a lot of real osteoporosis—dowager's hump and loss of height.

To detect crush fractures, doctors take a standard X ray of the upper back. Crush fractures are irreversible, and with two or more of them you fit the original definition of osteoporosis. Even then, however, you might not actually feel anything—as we said earlier, it takes four to five of these fractures for you to notice any difference in your posture.

A new type of ultrasound that examines the heel, still in the experimental stage at the time of this writing, may allow us to measure bone density.[7] It would be less expensive than DEXA and would use no radiation. But we don't yet know how accurate it will be.

Far more useful than any of these would be a test that could measure microarchitecture as well as bone density; with such a test, we could more accurately diagnose the risk of fracture. To date, though, we don't have it. It would also be helpful if we could measure the *rate* of bone loss or turnover.

The key to determining the risk of osteoporosis will be a combination of all these factors—how much bone you have, how strong it is (microarchitecture), and how fast you're losing it. At the moment doctors can learn this only by repeating a bone-density test after three or four years to estimate the rate of loss. Obviously, you'd have a much better way to gauge your danger of fracture if they could predict the loss in advance.

There are now two urine tests that can monitor bone resorption (the demolition crew). During resorption, bone breaks down into small collagen fibers, some of which are released in the urine. When you're breaking down bone rapidly (regardless of whether you're also building it up at the same time), the level of portions of these collagen fibers in the urine increases. One urine test, Osteomark, measures one such type of fiber in the urine; Crosslaps measures another. Other blood and urine tests of resorption are being developed. These tests can't detect osteoporosis per se. (You could have very low bone density and not be actively losing bone and thus have a normal test; or you could have temporarily high bone turnover as a result of a healing fracture and thus have a high test.) Nonetheless, they can give you more information about your current rate of loss if your bone density is low. They're mostly being used to monitor the effects of drug treatment. If a drug is actually decreasing bone loss, the urine levels of the breakdown products should also go down.

These new tests are just the beginning. Expect to see many more sensitive ways to monitor bone formation and bone loss in the near future.

"Normal" Bone Density

We don't in reality know what "normal" bone density should be. For women, "peak bone density" has been defined as the typical bone density of a thirty-five-year-old. Anything else is defined as abnormal. But that may not be a reasonable definition. Smooth skin is "normal" for a thirty-five-year-old. Does this mean that wrinkles are "abnormal" for a sixty-year-old? Is gray hair abnormal? The rest of your body changes, so why should bone be the same in your sixties as it was in your thirties?

The way experts came up with the definitions of osteopenia (low bone mass) and osteoporosis was by going backward. They measured the bone densities of women who had developed fractures due to osteoporosis. Then they looked at the data and saw that 90 percent of the fractures occurred in women whose bone density was below a certain number.

This number is called the *fracture threshold.*[8] Researchers determined that between ages forty and forty-nine, 5 percent of women are below the threshold; between ages fifty and fifty-nine, 20 percent are below it; between sixty and sixty-nine, 45 percent are below it. The goal of the osteoporosis researchers is that everyone should maintain bone density above the fracture threshold. To do this, 50 percent of seventy-year-old women and 75 percent of eighty-year-olds would need treatment.

The *T score,* which is reported on a bone-density test, is the number of standard deviations (level changes) between a given bone density and the density of a normal thirty-five-year-old. According to the current definition, set by the National Osteoporosis Foundation and others, *osteopenia* is 1 standard deviation (that is, one step away) from the bone density of a normal thirty-five-year-old woman. *Osteoporosis* is defined as more than 2.5 standard deviations from the density of a normal thirty-five-year-old. *Severe* or *established osteoporosis* is bone density more than 2.5 standard deviations from that of a normal thirty-five-year-old plus one "fragility fracture."[9]

So when you hear that *x* women have osteoporosis, what you're often finding out is that *x* women have a bone mass that's 2.5 standard deviations below that of a thirty-five-year-old. Likewise, when you hear that there are now many more women with osteoporosis than there were in the past, part of that increase is nothing but a change in definition. Needless to say, the broader the criteria used to define osteoporosis, the more women will fall into that category. It's as if you were deciding on a definition of *tall*. If you define *tall* as "over six feet," you'll have far fewer tall people than if you define it as "over five feet." This will be very useful to you if you have an investment in the existence of a lot of tall people. The level of bone density that defines osteoporosis has been set rather high, with the result that most older women will fall into the "disease" category—which is very nice for the people in the business of treating disease.

If you define osteoporosis as more than 2 standard deviations below the bone density of a normal young woman (a slightly looser definition than the figure I mentioned above, 2.5 standard deviations), then fully 45 percent of white women over age fifty have the condition at one or more sites.[10] (As I noted earlier, black and Asian women have different degrees of bone density from white women—and most studies, predictably, are done on white women.[11] Interestingly, because Asian women have low bone density, being Asian is often listed as a risk factor for osteoporosis—in spite of the fact that they actually have far fewer hip fractures than white women.)

MENOPAUSE AND OSTEOPOROSIS

It used to be thought that all women have a considerable decrease in bone at menopause, when their estrogen levels shift—and so "estrogen deficiency" was said to be the cause of osteoporosis. This was based on cross-sectional studies of bone density in women of all ages. It's now becoming clear that the process isn't this simple. Longitudinal studies following individual women's bone density over time have shown that although some women lose a lot of bone with menopause, others lose comparatively little; also, some bone loss starts earlier.[12] One Danish researcher[13] did a study using urine tests to measure calcium loss and concluded that some people are naturally "fast losers" and others are naturally "normal losers." About 35 percent of women are fast losers and will indeed lose a lot of bone with menopause, while others will lose bone more gradually. A longitudinal British study did repeated bone-density tests on a group of women at four-year intervals and found that there was a great variety in the rate of loss from woman to woman.[14] In addition, there was a wide variation in which bones the loss occurred. The researchers also noted that they had been unable to predict from their initial study who would be fast or slow losers.

Some studies have shown that people tend to start losing bone more quickly when they get to their seventies.[15] If these studies are correct, it may make more sense to focus on bone density when a woman is seventy, rather than when she's fifty. Undoubtedly there's a range of loss from woman to woman, as well as from age to age. Anyone who presents osteoporosis as a single, inevitable disease that occurs in all women at menopause is oversimplifying enormously.

There's another problem with the studies on osteoporosis that have been done on women—the same problem that exists in virtually all studies of menopause. Studies of both animals and humans have used subjects whose ovaries have been removed. This castration creates an environment far different from that of the body of a woman who has had a natural menopause. We can't simply assume that what is true for one group applies to the other.

Women and animals who have had surgical menopause have twice as much bone loss as those who have had natural menopause. As we noted in Chapter 1, the ovary produces much more than just estrogen, and it continues to produce hormones after menopause. And at least one study has shown that even women who retain their ovaries after hysterectomy have lower bone mass than women who haven't had hysterectomies.[16] This may be because the uterus produces vitamin D as well as prostaglandin,[17] which seems to be important for bone health. (Prostaglandin is a fatty acid that acts like a hormone.)

All of this tells us that estrogen is only one of several factors connected with bone density. Women with the same hormone levels have different degrees of bone loss. Some get osteoporosis and others don't. Even some women on estrogen get fractures. It doesn't add up to a neat little scenario in which women who don't take estrogen get osteoporosis and women who do take estrogen keep their strong bones.

There are other studies that bear this out. The Mayan women discussed in Chapter 2 live for thirty years after menopause, but they don't get osteoporosis—they don't lose height, they don't develop a dowager's hump, and they don't get fractures.[18] At first the researchers thought this must mean that these women had higher levels of estrogen or androgen, or possibly that they had higher peak bone density, than white American women. So they studied fifty-four postmenopausal Mayan women, analyzing their hormone levels and bone density. They found that these women's estrogen levels were no higher than those of American white women—in some cases, they were even lower. The bone-density tests showed that bone loss occurred in these women at the same rate as in white American women. The only significant difference the researchers could find was that the male hormones produced by the ovaries were less affected by menopause in these women: pre- and postmenopausal women had the same levels of testosterone. This suggests that testosterone may also have a role in bone loss.

If loss of androgen is indeed a factor, that would also explain why women whose ovaries have been removed have more osteoporosis, since the ovaries produce some testosterone, and why having your ovaries removed before age thirty-five strongly affects bone loss, even if you're taking estrogen.[19] In one experiment mentioned in Chapter 2, Malcolm Pike, a researcher at the University of Southern California, placed a group of premenopausal women who were at high risk for breast cancer on a contraceptive regimen that included chemical (and reversible) menopause, with replacement of estrogen and periodic progesterone. After six months, they all showed bone loss. When he added a small amount of testosterone to their regimen, the bone loss was reversed.[20]

According to yet another school of thought, progesterone may be an important component in bone strength.[21] All this underscores the fact that the story of osteoporosis isn't about estrogen alone.

RISK FACTORS FOR OSTEOPOROSIS

What's Your Risk of Low Bone Density?

How does this all apply to you? How can you figure out how likely you are to get osteoporosis? To some extent, this depends on your own life history.

In your early years, your risk factors for low bone density are those that would lead to low peak bone mass (see Table 5.1). If you start with less bone, you're likely to drop to a dangerously low level sooner when you start to lose bone. Peak bone mass, as we mentioned, is probably largely genetically determined. A recent study showed that daughters of women with osteoporosis had lower bone density than is normal for their age.[22] Large-boned people have more bone mass than small-boned people and are less affected by bone loss, since they have more to spare.

Whether you reach your genetically determined peak, however, can depend on other factors. Chief among them are a diet with adequate cal-

TABLE 5.1   Risk Factors for Low Bone Density

Thinness
Small frame
Advanced age
Family history of osteoporosis
Early menopause
Abnormal absence of menstrual periods (amenorrhea)
Anorexia nervosa or bulimia
Diet low in calcium
Use of certain medications, such as corticosteroids and anticonvulsants
Inactive lifestyle
Cigarette smoking
Excessive use of alcohol
Caucasian ancestry

cium and vitamin D, and adequate exercise. If you're sedentary, you lose bone. Even if you're sick in bed for as short a time as a week, you'll lose bone—though it will grow back when you get back to normal, especially if "normal," for you, involves standing and walking a lot. Bones need gravity to grow. (That's one of the things scientists are worried about with astronauts: weightlessness in space may look like fun, but it isn't doing their bones any good.)

Other lifestyle issues that will affect both your peak bone mass and your subsequent bone loss are use of tobacco, alcohol (more than three drinks a day), and caffeine, all of which decrease bone density. Being overweight, as we have mentioned, actually enhances bone strength, perhaps because it puts more stress on the bones. In addition, fat converts androgens to estrogen, thus contributing to higher bone density. Weight-bearing exercise (for example, jogging and walking) and strength training (lifting weights to increase your muscle mass) will help to increase bone. It might be that the Mayan women, who have worked in the fields their whole lives, have developed strong muscles, and that may be more crucial than their thinning bones.

There are certain medications that can affect your peak bone mass and subsequent bone loss. Taking steroids such as prednisone or cortisone for a long time is likely to decrease bone mass. Steroids are commonly used to treat diseases such as asthma, rheumatoid arthritis, lupus, Crohn's disease, and ulcerative colitis. (These last two diseases can create additional problems of their own, because they're intestinal diseases that affect the absorption of calcium and vitamin D.) Insulin-dependent diabetics generally have lower bone mass. People with heart disease who take Lasix (furosemide), a diuretic that causes more calcium to be excreted in urine, also have lower bone mass. (Not all diuretics have this effect, however; in fact, Thiazide actually helps the body hold on to calcium.) Aluminum-based antacids also decrease calcium absorption. (Calcium-based antacids, on the other hand, are themselves excellent calcium supplements—we'll discuss this in Chapter 12.) So read the label on any antacid very carefully.

As we mentioned earlier, thyroid replacement medication, if given in too high a dose, decreases bone strength.

What You Really Want to Know: What's Your Risk of Fracture?

The factors we've discussed so far are all risk factors for low bone density. But remember that low bone density is itself only an intermediate endpoint, and it doesn't automatically mean you'll end up with broken bones. Risks factors for *fractures* are a different matter (see Table 5.2).

An ongoing longitudinal cohort study, by the Study of Osteoporotic Fractures Research Group (SOF),[23] has shown the complex interaction of various risk factors that lead to fractures. This study is looking at 9,703 nonblack women, age sixty-five and older, who have had measurements of bone density in the heel and wrist. The study is planned to go on for several years, but there are some early data. After one and a half years, fifty-three of the women had fractures. As might be expected, the number of hip fractures was inversely related to the bone density: the women with lower bone density had more hip fractures. But bone density turned out to be only part of the problem. Even after it was adjusted for, the researchers found that the risk of hip fractures doubled for each ten years of a woman's age.

TABLE 5.2   Risk Factors for Fracture

Maternal history of hip fracture before age eighty
Previous fracture after age fifty
Tall at age twenty-five
Health fair or poor by your own rating
Previous hyperthyroidism
Current use of long-acting benzodiazepines (tranquilizers)
Current use of anticonvulsants
Ingesting high doses of caffeine
Spending less than four hours a day on your feet
Inability to rise from a chair without using your arms
Poor depth perception
Poor contrast sensitivity
Rapid heart rate at rest (greater than 80 beats per minute)
Current weight less than at age twenty-five

The study showed that some of that risk had as much to do with frailty, weakness, and falls as with low bone density. If you don't spend time on your feet, you're not getting the weight-bearing pressure your bones need. If you can't get out of a chair without using your arms, your leg muscles are weak. Poor depth perception and other vision problems are independent risk factors—probably because they mean that you trip more easily. If you have low bone density but you never fall down, you probably won't break your hip. To repeat, then, some of the risk factors have to do with the likelihood of falling rather than with bone density.

How likely you are to have fractures depends on how many risk factors for fractures you have as well as what your bone density is. Compared with a woman with no risk factors, women who had only two of the above risk factors had a risk of about 1.1, or essentially normal. Women with no more than two risk factors but normal bone density for their age had hardly any risk of fractures. But women with five or more risk factors and low bone density had twenty-seven times the risk of getting a fracture.

Since there are other, equally important risk factors for osteoporosis and fractures, why is there such an intense focus on bone density? Why aren't we hearing about the other problems?

First, since bone density is (unfortunately) the only risk factor we can easily measure, it's the one we try to control. And it does make sense to try to control bone density; the problem is that you end up with an inflated view of the value of bone-density tests, and of medications that can affect bone density. A medication that slows down bone loss may stabilize your bone density but may not keep you from getting life-threatening fractures in your old age. Second, we're not hearing about other factors because there's not much money to be made on them. For instance, I recommend that women with low bone density monitor their use of alcohol and tranquilizers, consult a doctor and start a weight-bearing exercise program and improve their diet, make their houses fall-proof, correct failing vision, and possibly put pads on their hips to cushion a fall—but none of these approaches offers much chance for profits.

WHAT IS IT LIKE TO HAVE OSTEOPOROSIS?

Most women today who are considered to have osteoporosis have no symptoms at all. Brittle bones per se don't usually cause pain or disability. The problems come when a woman with osteoporosis has a fracture. But even then, not all fractures are the same. Different types of fractures vary in terms of how common they are, the age at which they appear, and the disability they cause.

A white woman at age fifty has a 17 percent chance of having a hip fracture at some point in her life. (With white men, it's 6 percent.) The chance of a vertebral fracture is 15 percent in women (5 percent in men). The chance of a wrist fracture is 16 percent in women (2 percent in men). If you add these figures up and factor out the women who get more than one fracture, the chance of getting one of those three fractures is 39 percent for women. That figure is often used as the risk of fracture from osteoporosis.[24]

But there's a big difference between these fractures—both in the age at which you're likely to get them and in the amount of disability they cause. If you fracture your wrist, it's painful and inconvenient, but it isn't the same as breaking your hip.

Wrist Fractures

Wrist fractures typically occur when you fall on an outstretched hand. The average age for a wrist fracture is sixty-seven. Of the women who sustain a wrist fracture, only 1.9 percent are estimated to become dependent as a result.[25] One of the main studies on wrist fractures was done on women from Olmsted County in Minnesota,[26] which has a cold winter climate; but since most wrist fractures occur when people fall outdoors, often when it's snowy and icy, this study may well overestimate the chance of getting a wrist fracture in, say, Los Angeles.

A wrist fracture isn't very painful. Your wrist is put in a cast for several weeks, and you usually recover full mobility. The major importance of a wrist fracture is that it may be an early indicator of decreased bone density, giving you time to do something before a more disabling fracture might occur.

Vertebral Fractures

When you have a vertebral fracture—a disruption of one of the bones in your spine—you typically don't even know it's there at first. Such fractures are usually diagnosed when a woman in her seventies has a chest X ray for some other reason, and the film shows a wedging or crushing of the vertebral body (see Figure 5.3). In Denmark, about 55 percent of seventy-year-old women are found to have a crush fracture of at least one vertebra on a routine chest X ray.[27] In Rochester, Minnesota, about 40 percent of white women have at least one wedge fracture by the time they're eighty.[28]

An acute vertebral fracture may cause severe back pain, but that pain seldom lasts more than three months and can usually be managed with an over-the-counter pain reliever such as aspirin or Tylenol. Many vertebral

Normal vertebrae   Vertebrae with   Hip fracture
                      wedge fractures

FIGURE 5.3   Osteoporotic fractures.

fractures cause no pain at all. In a random sample of seventy-year-old Danish women,[29] those with wedge fractures had no more pain than those without them. The fracture rarely requires hospitalization. This kind of fracture can cause problems, however. Because fractured vertebrae never regain their normal shape, multiple vertebral fractures may lead to a humped-over posture, loss of height, and some functional limitations such as difficulty in reaching a top shelf, cleaning house, and finding clothes that fit.

Depending on what study you read, the lifetime risk that a fifty-year-old woman will get a vertebral fracture ranges from 5 to 15 percent; and 7 to 15 percent of vertebral fractures will cause significant pain. About 1.5 percent of women who get these fractures will become dependent as a result.[30] This variation may be in part a result of the different lifestyles, diets, and genes of the women involved in the different studies.

Loss of height may occur from vertebral fractures, but these fractures aren't the only cause of the loss of height that comes with age. Muscular atrophy, vertebral remodeling, disk deterioration, and poor posture all contribute to loss of height. In fact, we're all shorter by about an inch at the end of the day. (I guess everything settles.)

Hip Fractures

Hip fractures are the ones that cause most problems. The average fifty-year-old white woman has an 18.4 percent lifetime chance of having at least one hip fracture; the average age for a hip fracture is eighty. In 13.7 percent of cases, a woman will have another fracture, either in the other hip or in the same hip. This explains why you sometimes see the figure 33 percent reported as the risk of hip fracture. Of women with hip fractures, 19.3 percent will require a long stay in a nursing home, and 10.2 percent will become functionally dependent, needing help with the activities of daily living. On average, this 10.2 percent will remain dependent or will need to stay in a nursing home for seven to eight years.[31]

Again, all these statistics are for white women. Black women have a lower risk. That may be because of their genes, their body-fat composition, the more stable angle of their hips, their degree of physical activity throughout their lives, or any combination of these factors.

Among Asian women there is a different, and intriguing, pattern. Though they show low bone density on tests, they have fewer hip fractures than white women. This may be because they're short and their hip and leg bones come together at a different, more stable angle.

The difference in the extent of impairment that fractures, even hip fractures, entail is amazing. I have two very good examples from within my own family of how variable the problems can be. My stepmother was seventy-seven years old in 1993 when she went traveling in Cambodia with my father. During the trip she fell and broke her hip and elbow when she was pushed down by a thief trying to steal her handbag. She flew back to Los Angeles, where we arranged for her to have her hip fracture nailed. She recovered promptly and a year later went back to Cambodia to finish the trip that had been cut short. She suffered some short-term disability from the fracture, but it hasn't really affected her life.

On the other hand, when my mother-in-law was eighty-four, she broke her hip when she suddenly fell one day while washing the dishes. She had a hip replacement and a short rehabilitation in a nursing home. She returned home but was never able to be totally independent. A year later she broke the other hip, and after a second hip replacement returned to the nursing home, which she has never left. In her case, however, she was becoming more and more frail, and the hip fracture was the last straw. (She has since developed Alzheimer's disease and is still in the nursing home as of this writing.)

Fractures and Aging

Hip fractures don't occur in a vacuum. They're related not only to bone density but also to whether you fall. Your likelihood of falling is influenced by how good your balance is, whether you get dizzy, and whether you're particularly frail. Also, it's inaccurate to blame all of the subsequent disability and dependency on the hip fracture alone.

More than 90 percent of hip fractures occur in people over seventy, and the average age is eighty. You'll often hear that by ninety, one of out three women has a hip fracture. Although this is true, most of us won't live long enough for that to happen—the average life span of white American women is 78.9 (that of white American men is 72).

I'm not trying to dismiss the danger of osteoporosis, or to suggest that we shouldn't try to prevent it. But I question the assumption that you should try to prevent it by taking a drug for twenty to thirty years that may significantly increase your danger of dying earlier of another disease.

PREVENTION

Should You Have a Bone-Density Screening?

If you want to find out whether you're at high risk for fractures later in life, you might consider a bone-density test.

There's a lot of talk now about screening women routinely for bone density—like getting regular mammograms to detect early breast cancer. But such screening is of limited usefulness unless it leads to appropriate therapy. If you discover at fifty or so that you have low peak bone mass, it may encourage to you to take calcium and start a good program of weight-bearing exercise—things you should be doing anyway, but sometimes you need a little push. And, of course, it could push you in the direction of long-term hormone or drug therapy.

But it's important to understand the limits of the information such a test can give you. First of all, you should be careful about how you interpret the results of a single bone-density test. There have been some good longitudinal studies showing that these tests are far from conclusive. One five-year study[32] of women's wrist and vertebral density showed no relationship between original bone density at age forty-five or fifty and rate of bone loss, so we can't assume that the people with low bone density are "high losers": low bone density and high loss of density are two separate problems. If you start out with $100 in your piggybank and never spend it, you'll still have $100 in ten years. On the other hand, if you start out with $1,000 and spend a $100 a year, you'll have none of it left ten years later.

If you're someone who turns out to be a high loser, you could have normal, or even high, bone density at age fifty, before the accelerated loss of bone has begun. If that's the case, you might well end up with fractures in your seventies. On the other hand, if you show low density in your original test, you still may not be a high loser, and you might never have a fracture. So all a screening test can do when you're forty or fifty is give you a hint that you might be at greater risk for fracture.[33] (Your bone density may have some relationship to your risk for breast cancer; see page 299.)

However, this screening is the best we have at the moment. You should look at your personal risk factors for osteoporosis and fractures and decide whether, considering the limitations, it's worth it to you to have a bone density test. And you can decide with your doctor what lifestyle changes you should undertake and whether you would be willing to take drugs. If you are not going to act on the test, it may not be worth taking. Most women aren't at risk, and the test is expensive.

If all this isn't confusing enough, here's another complication. Although the tests can predict bone density, no long-term randomized controlled studies have really examined the effect of treatment—hormone or other—on fifty-year-old women with low bone density. There's been no study in which fifty-year-olds with low bone density who haven't had any fractures have been put on a treatment and monitored for subsequent fractures. Yet such a study would be the only way to tell if a treatment really can reduce the number of fractures as you reach the age when such fractures are most likely to occur. (Merck has launched such a study on Fosamax.)

Lest you think that these issues are of scientific interest only, it's important to remember that there's a lot of money riding on the diagnosis of a "treatable" disease. As I said earlier, Premarin is the biggest-selling drug in America. The gynecology literature recommends that women who are reluctant to go on long-term estrogen be given a bone-density test to help convince them of its necessity.[34] Merck has gotten into the business of bone-density screening, hoping to spur the gynecologists to give more tests and prescribe more Fosamax.[35]

The Good News: Estrogen Does Prevent Fractures

Large long-term observational studies have demonstrated that women who took Premarin for more than seven years had 50 percent fewer fractures of the spine.[36] The Study of Osteoporotic Fractures (SOF) followed a cohort of 9,704 women over sixty-five for at least seven years. These researchers found that *current* users of estrogen had 60 percent fewer wrist fractures, 40 percent fewer hip fractures, and 35 percent fewer nonspinal fractures when compared with women who had never taken estrogen. Current users who started estrogen within five years of menopause showed an even larger effect: all nonspinal fractures decreased by 50 percent, and hip fractures went down 70 percent, as did wrist fractures, in comparison with women who had never been on estrogen. And women on estrogen and progestin showed the same effect. Notice the emphasis on "current users." Unfortunately, women who had taken estrogen and then stopped, even if they'd taken it for ten years, had no decrease in their risk of fractures. This was also true for those who started estrogen more than five years after menopause.

These data are quite consistent, and impressive, although they're from observational studies with all of the biases we outlined in Chapter 4. It's likely that estrogen therapy reduces the risk of fracture, even if it isn't yet clear exactly how much. Moreover, this effect makes sense: animal and human studies have found that estrogen can halt the decrease in bone density and add 5 percent to total bone mass.[37]

Still, don't get too excited—this figure of 5 percent is somewhat of an illusion. Estrogen appears to halt or slow bone resorption, rather than actually building bone: thus the 5 percent represents a filling in of resorption pits rather than a development of new bone. Returning to our metaphor of the "bone house," it's as though estrogen finishes off the job of building new rooms that have already been started but doesn't help you build any more rooms after those. On the other hand, this beats having half-finished rooms. Also, estrogen may improve the microarchitecture of bone, making fracture less likely, and some studies have shown that estrogen increases your body's ability to absorb calcium from the intestine and increases calcitonin production from the thyroid.

Progesterone and progestins have also been shown to decrease osteoporosis in animals, possibly through their androgenic effects. Small nonrandomized longitudinal studies have shown an increase in the bone mass of women on "natural" progesterone.[38] It's possible that estrogen and progesterone in combination may complement each other in helping to prevent bone loss. Nonetheless, we don't have randomized controlled studies to confirm this hypothesis.

When Should You Start Taking Estrogen to Prevent Fractures?

If you have personal risk factors for osteoporosis—very low bone density, a high rate of bone loss—and no contraindications for using hormones (see page 264), then you may well want to take estrogen, with or without progestin, starting at menopause. The more difficult question is what to do if that is not the case.

On the basis of their data, the SOF researchers recommended that women who want protection against fractures should start taking estrogen soon after menopause and continue indefinitely. The problem with this, as they point out, is that it would mean taking estrogen for thirty years or more. We know some of the risks that ten years of estrogen can entail. We know none of the risks that longer use might bring.

Because it's unclear which women would actually benefit from long-term estrogen therapy for protection against osteoporosis, some enthusiasts suggest that *all* women should take estrogen beginning at menopause. I find that a disturbing approach. We don't know which of these women would have any fractures, let alone severely disabling fractures, and meanwhile we're exposing them all to the diseases we know estrogen can cause. You might end up trading a broken wrist for breast cancer.

Another approach would be to screen and treat women beginning at age sixty-five or seventy.[39] This is based on the recent findings that bone loss at menopause is less accelerated than had been previously believed and that the period of high loss is briefer than had been feared.[40,41] In addition, there's some evidence that an eighty-year-old woman who's taken hormones since menopause has only slightly higher bone mass than a woman of the same age who began treatment at age sixty-five. One researcher has estimated that if estrogen therapy prevented future bone loss and was administered to all sixty-five-year-old women, the incidence of hip fractures would be reduced by 73 percent.[42] And when a woman is sixty-five, we can more precisely estimate her risk of hip fracture and target her treatment more accurately. It's beginning to appear that, at sites other than the spine, bone loss continues unabated into very old age and probably accelerates at the hip—the most important region for predicting hip fractures.[43] Finally, there's a growing body of evidence that hormone therapy can reduce fractures in the elderly.

Furthermore, new studies of other drugs such as Fosamax[44] (see Chapter 14) suggest that women who had already suffered at least one spinal fracture and were treated with Fosamax reduced their risk of breaking a hip by 51 percent and of breaking a wrist by 44 percent. Fractures of the spine were 46 percent lower for women who took this drug than for those who took only calcium. The women on Fosamax also lost less height than women who didn't take it.

This suggests that there's an alternative to thirty years on estrogen.[45] Have a bone-density study at age fifty. If it's very low (more than 2.5 standard deviations below that of a thirty-five-year-old), consider lifestyle changes and possibly drugs (see Chapter 14). If your bone density is moderately low (1 to 2.5 standard deviations below that of a thirty-five-year-old) you could take dietary calcium and vitamin D, change your diet, begin an exercise program (see page 209), and then repeat the test in five years. If your bone density is high or normal, wait and have another test at age sixty-five, when you can better estimate the risk of hip fracture, since by that time the process of loss is starting to be visible. At fifty, when you're just starting to lose density, there's no way to tell if you're going to be a high or a low loser. If the second bone scan at sixty-five reveals high bone loss, you can start estrogen or Fosamax then, and perhaps still reduce fractures, while lessening the danger of breast cancer from the estrogen itself.

NEW TREATMENTS FOR OSTEOPOROSIS: IS PREVENTION NECESSARY?

Finally, it's important to remember that the study of osteoporosis is continuing. There's a lot of research going on about how osteoporosis happens. In addition, new drugs are being developed all the time. We may soon be able to test for microarchitecture as well as bone density, and to determine genetically who is actually going to be a fast loser or a slower one. We're likely to have drugs that will allow us not only to prevent bone resorption but actually to build bone. It's naive to think that the way we approach osteoporosis today is the way we'll approach it twenty or even ten years from now. My guess is that this disease, which has been such a hot topic in recent years, will become less important as new treatments make drugs that promise a shaky sort of "prevention" unnecessary and obsolete.

CHAPTER 6

Heart Disease:
What's Your Real Risk?

The image of heart disease has undergone a transformation in recent years. Once perceived as an almost exclusively male concern, it's now recognized as a major problem for women as well. We're assaulted with the fact that almost half of all women in the United States die from cardiovascular disease—disease of the heart and blood vessels.

This can sound alarming, and the pharmaceutical companies have used it to frighten women into taking hormones as a preventive. However, there are problems with this approach. One problem is that, as we'll discuss shortly, it's not clear that hormone therapy can prevent heart disease. A second problem is that the death rates aren't as dire as they sound. Ultimately, everyone dies of "heart failure": your heart ceases to beat, and you die. Many deaths from heart disease occur in elderly people whose bodies have been weakened by other diseases. Death certificates rarely record "old age" as the official cause of death. So to some extent the dire statistics simply mean that you have to die of something, and your risk of cardiovascular disease increases with age.

Heart disease is not a "symptom" of menopause. Heart disease is heart disease. It's more common in postmenopausal women than in premenopausal women, but that's because postmenopausal women are older than premenopausal women. It's like gray hair: you're more likely to have gray hair after menopause than before it, but menopause doesn't cause gray hair—rather, they both tend to happen in later life.

The standard line has always been that women are protected from heart disease as long as their bodies make estrogen, and then after menopause they lose that protection and the rates of heart disease for men and women become equal. But in fact, the rates *never* become equal. In this country, women in their sixties and seventies have 45 percent less heart disease than men in the same age bracket. Women develop heart disease much later than men—seven or eight years later. Women's risk rises continuously as they get older, but there's no sudden increase with menopause.[1] We never catch up.

WHAT IS HEART DISEASE?

Heart Disease and Cardiovascular Disease

I should clarify what I mean by *heart disease.* I'm not talking here about congenital heart disease, which you're born with, or the kind caused by rheumatic fever. No one has ever claimed that these are connected to estrogen or to menopause. In fact, these fairly rare conditions can even hit very young adults, like the athletes who have been in the news in recent years. The kind of heart problems at issue here are the kind caused by atherosclerosis, the narrowing of the arteries that feed the heart.

Cardiovascular disease is a broader term, which usually includes both heart disease and stroke. Stroke, like heart disease, is a vascular disease: a disease of blood vessels. In both cases, the blood vessels become narrow, either through spasm or through atherosclerosis, and not enough blood gets to a critical place: to the heart in the case of heart disease, and to the brain in the case of stroke. Cardiovascular disease also encompasses high blood pressure and coronary artery disease.

Arteries and Cholesterol

We're really only beginning to understand some of the mechanisms of atherosclerosis and arterial blockage (see Figure 6.1). J. A. Berliner and his group at UCLA stated in 1995 that "atherosclerosis is a chronic inflammatory condition that's converted to an acute clinical event by the induction of plaque rupture, which in turn leads to thrombosis."[2] But what does that mean in English?

I've been trying to figure out a good analogy for this process. Since I live in Los Angeles, a freeway came to mind. In Chapter 5, I talked about the "bone house," so for this chapter let's move outdoors. Imagine a three-lane freeway that has a chronic problem of litter thrown into the ditch on the side of the road (see Figure 6.2). That's similar to chronic inflammation and plaque formation. (A plaque is a thickened area in the lining of the artery.)

Cholesterol deposited
in middle layer of artery

Inflammatory cells, foam cells,
and calcium in thickened plaque

Plaque ruptures and causes
clot that clogs artery

FIGURE 6.1   The atherosclerotic process.

The first step involves a buildup of cholesterol. Cholesterol is a type of fat made by the liver. People often think of "fat" as either the stuff in your food or the body fat that shows up in your hips and tummy. But there are numerous kinds of fat in your body. Just as fat you eat can take the form of butter, lard, or olive oil, fat in your body can take the form of cholesterol and triglycerides, as well as the fatty tissue that makes you appear chubby. You always have cholesterol circulating in your blood. It's a building block for many of the hormones the body makes. Estrogen, vitamin D, and testosterone all start out as cholesterol.

Our bodies make lots of cholesterol—nearly all that we require. So we really don't need to eat any. Unfortunately, though, we do eat it. Meat and dairy products, which figure strongly in the American diet, are full of cholesterol.

It used to be thought that there was just one kind of cholesterol, but then scientists discovered that it's broken down into two types: "good" HDL (high-density lipoprotein) and "bad" LDL (low-density lipoprotein). What makes these "good" and "bad" is what happens within the blood vessels.

An artery has three layers. The smooth inner lining (the endothelium) is like the highway. The middle layer, which is a latticework (the media), is like the drainage ditch on the side of the road, and the outer layer (the adventitia) is like the outer wall that blocks access to the highway. LDL can pass through the lining of the artery and sit in the middle layer. Let's say the LDL is represented by the garbage that's being thrown out of the cars into the drainage ditch. The more LDL there is in your blood, the more of it gets into the middle layer of the blood vessels. After a while, the cells in the artery secrete materials that can oxidize LDL—chemically change it into a more dangerous form (the garbage becomes rotten). This process ends up creating cholesterol-loaded cells that form a fatty streak in the artery wall. These can actually be seen in the lining of the arteries. HDL (good cholesterol) has been found to protect against LDL oxidation (like a street sweeper who cleans up garbage before it has time to rot).

The next step toward atherosclerosis is an inflammatory reaction. Certain white blood cells, part of the body's immune system, are attracted to the arteries that have been damaged by LDL and get trapped there, forming a plaque. The reaction feeds on itself, like rats attracted to the garbage piling up in the ditch; finally, the pile gets so big that it starts to encroach on the slow lane of the highway, causing traffic (blood flow) to start slowing down.

FIGURE 6.2   A metaphor for atherosclerosis.

The inflammatory plaque then causes calcium to be formed, and this in turn causes the arteries to harden—and to constrict. (The pile of rotten, rat-infested garbage is by now blocking the slow lane and narrowing the middle lane.) Then the heart gets less and less blood to feed its own muscle. When the heart is deprived of too much of its blood supply, there is severe pain. This pain, which is called *angina*, frequently follows strenuous activity that increases your need for blood. Often it gets better when you rest. (This is like a rush-hour traffic jam; the narrowing of the highway will make it hellish at rush hour, but the flow of traffic is better during the rest of the day.)

Angina is always a serious warning signal. If the underlying problem isn't taken care of, eventually the soft inflammatory plaque ruptures into the vessel, forming a clot that blocks the blood vessel and stops the blood flow. The heart muscle fed by that artery dies. This is a heart attack. (The pile of garbage spills into the middle lane, blocking traffic completely.)

I've gone into this much detail because it's important to understand that there are different things you can do at each step along the way to help minimize the likelihood of getting a heart attack. The earlier you start, the better your chances: get that litter off the road the first time it shows up. I'll talk about that more in Chapters 12 to 14.

WHAT PUTS YOU AT RISK OF A HEART ATTACK?

Family History

As with almost every other disease, family history is important in coronary artery disease. It can indicate whether you've inherited genes that make you more susceptible to the atherosclerotic process, whether you're more likely to have high LDL, and whether you're more likely to oxidize LDL or to develop an inflammatory reaction. Research is now going on to determine the precise ways in which genetic factors contribute to coronary artery disease.

Lipid Levels

The fats and fatty substances in your body are called *lipids.* These include HDL, LDL, cholesterol, and triglycerides. Your lipid "profile" can determine your risk for a heart attack. In general, you want high HDL and low LDL, cholesterol, and triglycerides. The ratio of HDL and LDL is also important (see Table 6.1).

Many factors influence the levels of LDL and HDL. Insulin, diet, exercise, obesity, age, and hormones all affect the way fat is metabolized.

TABLE 6.1   Cholesterol Levels

	Total cholesterol	HDL	LDL	Triglycerides
Good	<200	>70	<130	50–250
Borderline	200–240	35–70	130–159	250–500
Bad	>240	<35	>160	>500

Key: < = less than; > = greater than

One factor that's clearly controlled by genes is how you metabolize dietary fat (see Chapter 12 for a discussion of dietary fat). This can be partly measured by testing your blood cholesterol. Across cultures, men with high cholesterol have a higher death rate from coronary heart disease than men with low cholesterol. Women are also affected by cholesterol, but it turns out that we're less affected than men are. Don't get too cheery, though: women are *more* susceptible to problems that result from a bad ratio of HDL to LDL. Remember, overall cholesterol isn't all that matters. You really need to know your LDL and HDL as well, and you need to have your triglycerides measured after an overnight fast.

In women, the level of HDL is usually higher than it is in men. An increase in HDL cholesterol of 1 milligram per deciliter (mg/dl), the units in which cholesterol is usually measured in the United States, is associated with a 3.2 percent decrease in the risk of heart disease in women (compared with 1.9 to 2.35 percent in men). In fact, HDL trumps total cholesterol.

Most of these levels are a result of a combination of genes and diet. Some lucky people can eat a whole cheesecake and still have low cholesterol, while others just look at a cheesecake through the bakery window and their cholesterol shoots up to 400. The lucky ones have genes that make it easier to metabolize cholesterol.

Other factors affect lipid levels as well. As you age, your good HDLs fall and your bad LDLs rise. Some of that change may be related to menopause. After menopause, particularly if you gain weight, your LDL increases. Exercise increases HDL and lowers cholesterol levels. Moderate alcohol intake raises HDL levels. (Remember, that's *moderate* alcohol; too many three-martini lunches are likely to give you a heart attack, not prevent one.)

Personality Type

There are other factors related to cholesterol levels that are less well publicized (maybe because they don't fit our biases). For example, there is some relationship between personality, the mind, and cholesterol levels. We've all heard of the type A personality. Recent research by Redford Williams has found that the factors that really increase heart disease are self-involvement, hostility, and cynicism.[3] A researcher from the University of California in San Francisco who taped conversations[4] found that the more frequently people referred to themselves, the greater the likelihood that they would develop heart disease and die from it. There are also many studies supporting the concept that social isolation is an important risk factor for heart disease; but although this is an important finding, it's less relevant to women, who by and large tend to be more social. Problems with women come more when they lose control over their lives.

Some fascinating observational studies of monkeys demonstrate biologically how that works. In a group of female monkeys, one is dominant; the others are subordinate. When monkeys were fed a high-fat diet, the HDL levels of the subordinate ones went down and their lipids changed, far more than was the case with the dominant monkeys. The subordinate monkeys had a risk of heart disease three times greater than the dominant ones.[5]

Recent studies on humans parallel this. One study[6] noted that working women had more risk factors for heart disease than housewives—they were more likely to smoke, less likely to exercise, and more likely to drink alcohol and coffee. Nonetheless they still had higher HDL levels than the housewives. If they quit working and became housewives, their HDL levels went down. A similar study[7] hypothesized that women with high-powered jobs would have the most heart disease because they were under the most stress. What they actually found was that the career women had less heart disease. It turned out that the more control a woman had over her life, the less likely she was to have heart disease. So cholesterol levels may relate to being in a role where you perceive that you have less control over your life—like a housewife who spends twenty-four hours a day at the beck and call of her children and spouse. It shows an interesting mind-body connection.

I'm not necessarily advising that you lower your cholesterol by getting a job—a particular woman may in fact have more control over her life as a housewife than she would in an outside job. What is much more significant about these studies is that they demonstrate that diet is not the only factor determining your cholesterol level.

Diabetes

Diabetes is a disease of sugar metabolism. There are two kinds of diabetes. The first, which usually occurs in childhood, is called *insulin-dependent* (formerly *juvenile*) diabetes. It's caused by the body's failure to produce enough insulin, the hormone that regulates sugar metabolism. People with this form of diabetes take daily insulin injections to compensate. The second, more common, form of the disease is called *adult-onset, non-insulin-dependent*, diabetes. This occurs when the body makes insulin but for some reason is unable to use it. Adult-onset diabetes is most likely to develop in people who are obese, come from families with diabetes, and have high blood pressure. It can often be controlled by diet, weight loss, and exercise.

Uncontrolled diabetes of either type has a treacherous effect on the very small arteries throughout the body. Diabetes doubles a woman's risk of coronary heart disease. When you've got diabetes on top of high blood pressure, obesity, high cholesterol, and high triglycerides, it quadruples the risk of heart disease. In fact, 80 percent of diabetics die of heart attacks. This is a particular problem for women. When a diabetic woman has a heart attack, she's more likely to die from it than either a diabetic man or a nondiabetic woman.

Smoking

Smoking at least triples the risk of coronary heart disease, probably chiefly because it increases the oxidation of LDL and secondarily because it increases vessel spasm—and spastic vessels don't transport blood very well. The more you smoke, the more effect smoking has. Further, it increases the risk of adult-onset diabetes—which as we've just seen, is a risk factor for heart disease.

Overweight

Obesity—defined as being more than 20 percent over the target weight (see page 203) for your height—is a strong risk factor for coronary heart disease in women. Forty percent of coronary heart disease found among all women is related to excess weight. Even women of average weight have about a 30 percent higher risk than thin women.

High Blood Pressure

High blood pressure, like cholesterol, can lead to heart attacks. It increases the stress on the blood vessels and thus increases the chance of artery narrowing and plaque rupture.

In part, obese people tend to have high blood pressure because they have more blood vessels, which the body creates to bring blood to all that fat. Weight loss is more likely to control high blood pressure (hypertension) in women that in men. However, women get less benefit from antihypertensive drugs. All women over forty should have their blood pressure checked regularly. Doctors call it the "silent killer" because it's asymptomatic.

Blood Clots

If your blood clots easily, you're more prone to heart disease. There's a balance between factors in your blood that make clots and factors that break them up. If you have more of the factors that make clots and fewer of those that break them up, you're at a greater risk for a heart attack. This is why doctors advise many men to take an aspirin a day: aspirin thins blood so that it won't clot as much. Once the doctors started studying women and heart disease, they discovered that we need less aspirin than men do—half a tablet a day. If you think you're at risk of heart disease, though, don't just start popping aspirin. Get a medical workup from your doctor. Aspirin is a drug, and like all drugs it has side effects, so don't take it regularly without checking with your doctor.

THE NATURAL HISTORY OF HEART DISEASE

Heart disease in women doesn't usually occur until their seventies or eighties. A fifty-year-old white woman has a 46 percent lifetime probability of developing heart disease and a 31 percent probability of dying of it. Death from coronary heart disease occurs at a median age of seventy-four years.[8] Smokers have three times as much heart disease as nonsmokers and account for most of the early deaths from heart disease.

Some women will experience angina (chest pain) as a symptom of heart disease before they have a heart attack, but about a third of women with heart disease never have any warning symptoms—they have a sudden, massive heart attack and die instantly. (Although this is often described in the medical literature as a terrible event, it may actually be a better way to die than a lingering, painful illness—particularly if you're at an advanced age in which death in the near future is inevitable.)

What is it like to have a heart attack? A heart attack is usually accompanied by crushing chest pain. (Any new chest pain should be evaluated by your doctor.) However, women often have other patterns of pain—such as pain in the arm, neck, jaw, teeth, or back—usually associated with physical exertion or emotional stress and lasting longer than two minutes. You may also feel dizzy, faint, sweaty, nauseated, short of breath, or weak. If you think you're having a heart attack, stop what you're doing and lie down immediately. Get help: call 911 to get an ambulance or have someone take you to a hospital. If you can get to a hospital within four to six hours after the first hint of a problem, emergency treatment may be able to dissolve the clot that caused the attack.

After the initial treatment, you'll go to a coronary care unit (CCU) where the rhythm of your heart can be monitored. Once the acute event is over, you'll be moved to an intermediate care unit and rehabilitation will begin. This usually means evaluating your risk factors and lifestyle and starting you on a low-fat diet and exercise program. Six weeks later you'll undergo further studies to see whether you need surgery or angioplasty (a method to open up narrowed arteries). You may need to take drugs such as beta blockers, aspirin, and ACE inhibitors (see Chapter 14) to decrease the chance of another attack.

Women have a higher probability of dying in the year following heart attacks than men do (45 percent of women compared with 10 percent of men);[9] and 40 percent of women, compared with 13 percent of men, have a second heart attack within that year. Some of this is due to the fact that, by and large, women who have had heart attacks are older, have more high blood pressure and diabetes, and have more severe or unstable angina than their male counterparts. Women are more likely than men to suffer psychological consequences of a heart attack. They're less likely to return to work, and if they do return, they tend to return later than men do. They have more frequent depression and are less likely to return to their previous activities. This may be in part because they are more likely to be older and widowed. However, with good rehabilitation, psychological and social support, and lifestyle changes, women can recover from heart attacks and resume their lives.

ESTROGEN AND HEART DISEASE

Natural Estrogen: Not a Factor?

The claims that estrogen therapy can prevent heart disease are interesting but problematical. For one thing, levels of women's own natural estrogen seemed to have little or no effect on their rate of heart disease. There's something mysterious in this. In osteoporosis, breast cancer, and endometrial cancer, factors associated with the body's own estrogens correlate with the risk of the disease. For example, the larger your lifetime supply of estrogen—whether because you started menstruating early, took certain medications, or never became pregnant—the greater your risk of breast cancer and the lower your risk of osteoporosis. After menopause, women who are obese and have more of their own estrogen have less osteoporosis and more breast and endometrial cancer. Estrogen, whether it's your own or you get it from medication, has a consistent effect on risk for these conditions. But there's no clear relationship between heart disease and your body's own estrogen. The amount of estrogen your body makes over your lifetime doesn't appear to have any effect on your risk of heart disease. Onset of menstruation doesn't seem to affect risk, nor does anorexia or amenorrhea (lack of periods).

In 1995, Elizabeth Barrett-Connor did studies to see if levels of hormones in the blood affected heart disease.[10] She measured testosterone, estrone, and androstenedione. She found no relationship between the blood levels of these sex hormones and heart disease in postmenopausal women, or in men. Nor did she find any relationship between blood levels of estrogen and cholesterol levels, LDH, and triglycerides. Other studies have confirmed this finding. Although obesity increases blood levels of estrogen, it certainly doesn't decrease heart disease in the way it decreases osteoporosis. On the contrary, as we all know, obesity is one of the greatest contributors to heart disease.

So we're left with the paradox that your body's own estrogen doesn't protect you from heart disease, while chemical forms of estrogen apparently do.

Estrogen Therapy and Heart Disease

As we mentioned in Chapter 1, the first clinical study on estrogen and heart disease took place with men and showed that giving them estrogen increased their risk of heart attack.[11] The only prospective randomized controlled clinical study of estrogen and heart disease in women was published in 1979 by Lila Nachtigall.[12] The subjects were eighty-four pairs of randomly chosen postmenopausal women. Half received high-dose Premarin with a progestin. The other half were given no therapy. Although there was no difference in the number of heart attacks, the lipids of the women on hormones were better. This study was, of course, too small to allow any generalized conclusions.

Later observational studies suggested that giving estrogen to postmenopausal women seemed to decrease their risk of heart disease.[13] In 1991, Meir Stampfer and Graham Colditz did a review of all of the observational studies that had looked at the connection between estrogen therapy and heart disease. They found that women on estrogen therapy alone had a 50 percent lower risk of heart disease than women who weren't on estrogen.[14] In a second review they found that women on both estrogen and progestin had a similar decrease in their risk of heart disease.[15]

One of the largest studies included in Stampfer and Colditz's review was the Nurses' Health Study, a prospective study of nurses who were followed for ten years.[16] This study showed that the women who had taken estrogen postmenopausally had only half the risk of coronary heart disease experienced by those who hadn't. However, few women in the study were over sixty-five, so we don't know how many will get heart disease in their seventies, when it's more likely to strike them.

The question of age was addressed in another of the large prospective studies. This study followed 7,610 women in a retirement village called Leisure World.[17] The average age of these women was seventy-three. In this group, estrogen therapy appeared to offer the oldest women the greatest protection against both fatal and nonfatal heart attacks. Those currently on estrogen had only half as many fatal heart attacks as those who had never been on estrogen therapy.

Although all of the observational studies have been consistent, the fact that they are observational means that the question remains whether estrogen lessens the risk of heart disease, or whether women with generally good health were more likely to be on estrogen in the first place.[18] This is where all the biases we mentioned in Chapter 4 come in. None of these were large, randomized, controlled blinded studies. In all of them, the women who took estrogen were of higher socioeconomic status, better educated, thinner, more likely to be nonsmokers, and more likely to have had a hysterectomy (60 to 80 percent).[19] These women were more likely to go to doctors (that's how they got their hormones in the first place) and therefore more likely to have had overall preventative care, such as having their blood pressure checked and their cholesterol monitored. Finally, the women who stayed on hormones were more likely to be compliant (see Chapter 4).[20]

Remember that all of these other factors can themselves affect vulnerability to heart attack. Cardiovascular disease in people over sixty-five is 80 percent higher among those who are least educated than among those who are college-educated—and in people under sixty-five, it's at least twice as high. Also, the least educated people have twice the risk of people with a high school education.[21] Since better-educated people tend to get better-paying jobs, the fact that women who take hormones have a higher socioeconomic status and more education is really significant. Remember the monkeys—the dominant ones had higher HDL levels.

In the Nurses' Health Study, the researchers didn't take the women's social class into consideration, assuming that nurses would all be from the same class. They neglected to consider, however, that a woman's social class is usually a function of her husband's or father's class rather than of her own occupation. As in the other studies, then, the women on hormones in this study may well have been of a higher social class than those who didn't take hormones.

Compliance is also an issue. Only one fourth of all women who are prescribed estrogen take it for an extended period of time, as their doctors recommend. The other three fourths decide for themselves at some point not to take it or to stop taking it.[22] As you'll recall from Chapter 4, there is some evidence that compliant patients in general, regardless of what they're complying with, have a significantly reduced risk of heart disease.

Even taking all this into account, though, there are still possible biological explanations for at least some of the apparent effect of estrogen on heart disease. The first to be identified was the effect of estrogen on cholesterol. Estrogen increases HDL and decreases LDL. This can have a marked effect on subsequent heart disease. In one randomized study on rabbits whose ovaries had been removed, estrogen proved as good as a low-cholesterol diet in lowering cholesterol, and the two together were even better.[23]

Hormones and Heart Disease: The PEPI Study

If you have a uterus and opt for postmenopausal hormone therapy, you need to take progesterone to help prevent the endometrial cancer that "unopposed" estrogen can promote (see Chapter 8). Does progesterone cancel out any of estrogen's good effects on heart disease? After all, progesterone has many of the effects of male hormones, and male hormones are bad for lipids.

The first randomized controlled study to investigate estrogen and progesterone therapy and its effects on lipids in women was the three-year PEPI study.[24]

The PEPI study randomly divided 875 women into five groups. Group 1 got placebos. Group 2 got 0.625 milligram of Premarin daily. Group 3 got 0.625 milligram Premarin plus 10 milligrams of Provera twelve days a month (this is one of the standard ways it's given). Group 4 got Premarin and Provera continuously (an attempt to decrease the bleeding seen with the twelve-day regimen). Group 5 got Premarin plus cyclical micronized progesterone (twelve days a month).

Let me clarify some terminology before I continue. A *progestin* is a drug that has some of the same effects as progesterone, but other effects as well. *Provera* is a progestin commonly used with estrogen therapy. *Micronized progesterone* is formulated in a laboratory to be exactly like the hormone progesterone we make in our bodies. (See Chapter 15 for a discussion of the uses and misuses of the word *natural* in regard to hormones.) "Micronized" means simply that it's broken up into very small pieces so you can absorb it better. Some preliminary data indicate that micronized progesterone might be less likely to interfere with estrogen's effect on cholesterol.

The results of the PEPI study were reported in 1995.[25] Since it had lasted only three years, the researchers couldn't study the effects of estrogen-progesterone on heart attacks; thus they focused on changes in HDL. They found that the group for which the results were most positive—that is, their levels of HDL went up—was group 2, on estrogen alone. This group was followed very closely by group 5, on estrogen plus micronized progesterone. Next came groups 3 and 4, on estrogen and Provera, which reduced somewhat the positive effects of estrogen on HDL. Not surprisingly, group 1, on the placebo, showed the least effect on HDL levels. Interestingly, however, the placebo had some effect: LDL went down a little, and HDL went up a little.

So the average increase in HDL was similar for Premarin alone (group 2) and Premarin with micronized progesterone (group 5). (In addition, micronized progesterone was able to protect the uterus, as the researchers discovered by doing endometrial biopsies.) Groups 2 and 5 both had significantly higher HDL levels than the groups who got Provera either cyclically (group 3) or continuously (group 4). In all groups, HDL levels gradually fell after the first six to twelve months, although they didn't fall all the way down to the original baseline. LDL fell to its lowest levels in the same time period, but it remained stable thereafter. Adding Provera to Premarin did counteract some of the beneficial effects of Premarin on cholesterol. Triglyceride levels increased in every group except the one that got the placebo.

Assessing the Findings

Direct Effects of Estrogen

Impressive as the PEPI study is, the changes it found in cholesterol don't account for all of the decrease in deaths from heart disease found in the observational studies (if we assume that these are all valid). Five or ten years of improving cholesterol levels should put hardening of the arteries off for an equivalent five or ten years. But it doesn't. If you've been off estrogen for a while, your risk of heart attack returns to what it was before you took estrogen. When this is teased out in the large studies, it appears that only one fourth to one third of the reduction in heart disease results from improving cholesterol levels. The additional reduction may result from direct effects of estrogen on the blood vessels themselves.

Let's go back to our garbage-filled highway. Results of coronary arteriography studies[26]—X-ray studies in which dye is injected into the coronary arteries to see how narrowed they are—show that women who are on estrogen have less heart disease than those who aren't. (The piles of garbage aren't as high.) In addition, if we inject high doses of estrogen directly into a woman's coronary arteries, they dilate (a man's don't). In other words, even if an artery is narrowed by plaque, it still has some stretch in it and will dilate when treated with estrogen. (It is, I must admit, hard to dilate a highway; but I never promised my analogy would carry all the way through.

Maybe we could picture a cop motioning drivers into the service lane.) Although we know estrogen can dilate your arteries when it's dripped directly onto an artery, we don't know if taking estrogen every day will have the same effect when you're having a heart attack. But it's possible.

Estrogen may also have an antioxidant effect, preventing the oxidation of LDL when it's trapped in the blood vessel wall. (Remember, oxidation is analogous to our pile of garbage becoming rotten.)

Some of these direct effects may be more important in women who already have coronary artery disease. If your arteries are wide open, it doesn't really matter if you can dilate them. On the other hand, if they're narrowed it can be critical. This may be why we see estrogen having a stronger effect in older women (who are more likely to have coronary artery disease) and on women who are currently taking estrogen than on women who took estrogen for a time and then stopped. For estrogen to work in this direct way, you must be on it when you have a heart attack.

Effects of Progestins and Progesterone

Though the PEPI study showed that adding progestins and progesterone to estrogen had an effect on cholesterol, it didn't address whether they block the direct dilating effects of estrogen on the blood vessels of the heart. Arterial walls contain progesterone receptors as well as estrogen receptors. Other studies, on both humans and animals, do address this.

At Bowman Gray Medical School, monkeys are used to study post-menopausal heart disease. The monkeys' ovaries are removed to make them menopausal, and then various drugs and diets are applied to see what the effects will be.[27] (This isn't exactly a good model for women who have their ovaries when they go into menopause, but we have to use what we have.) In one study, some of the monkeys were put on Premarin alone, some on Premarin and Provera, and (interestingly, as we'll see in Chapter 12) some on a high soy-protein diet.[28] The researchers did angiography on the animals and dripped onto their coronary arteries a substance designed to make the arteries constrict. The arteries of the monkeys on Premarin and those on a high soy diet didn't constrict, while those of the animals on Premarin and Provera did. Again, Provera was blocking a positive effect of Premarin. In one study of monkeys whose ovaries were removed, cyclical progesterone blocked some of the dilation of blood vessels, and continuous Provera completely obliterated it. Another study, with women, showed that Provera caused the blood vessels to constrict.[29] No one to my knowledge has actually tried these experiments using progesterone rather than a progestin. As we saw in the PEPI study, there may well be a difference.

Most recently, the Nurses' Health Study looked at whether progestins blocked the positive effects of estrogen in women taking them over a period of time. Contrary to what you might expect from the animal studies, the researchers found that the addition of progestin did *not* markedly affect the benefits of current use of estrogen postmenopausally.[30]

Effects of Other Hormone Additives

Needless to say, if we're unsure about the effects of progestin in coronary heart disease protection, we're completely in the dark regarding other hormonal additives such as testosterone. One small study on women showed no difference in lipid levels in the women taking androgens along with estrogen. No direct effects on blood vessels were studied.[31] One study on monkeys showed that their lipid profiles did not deteriorate when testosterone was added. This does not, however, shed any light on possible long-term effects. I think it's naive not to recognize that estrogen can have so many varied effects while maintaining that male hormones like testosterone will affect only libido. Although there are as yet no long-term studies, the fact that heart disease is so much more common in men than women is enough to give one pause.

Directions for Further Research

Almost all the studies done in the United States on estrogen and heart disease have used Premarin, which is taken by mouth and broken down by the liver. In this process it affects the production of the lipids that pose such a risk factor for heart disease. Other estrogens—especially those that are absorbed through the skin, by injection, or vaginally—may not have the same effect on lipids, although their direct effect on the blood vessels should be the same. But again, we can't be certain until further studies are done, using these other forms.

What we need is a randomized controlled study of different forms of estrogen and progestins and progesterone in postmenopausal women. At least, though, we now have the Women's Health Initiative, which will address some questions about Premarin and Provera and make the results available in 2008. Another study, which may turn out to be even more important, is looking at whether hormones can prevent a second heart attack; it is aptly named HERS (Heart and Estrogen-Progestin Replacement Study). HERS is investigating the use of estrogen, progesterone, or both in women who already have coronary heart disease. To be eligible, a woman must have had a heart attack, coronary bypass surgery, or angioplasty, or must have greater than 50 percent narrowing of one or more major coronary vessels. Ten years before the Women's Health Initiative, this study will provide an answer to at least part of the question about hormones and heart disease—whether hormones help prevent second heart attacks.

What You Really Want to Know: Should You Take Estrogen to Prevent or Treat Heart Disease?

Meanwhile, should you take estrogen—with or without other accompanying hormones—to prevent heart disease or to treat existing heart disease? The PEPI study concludes that we need a randomized controlled study to really know the effects of hormone therapy on heart disease. So for now, this must be a personal decision based on inadequate information.

I think the situation appears to be similar to that with osteoporosis. Although at the moment we lack data proving that secondary prevention works, more data will come from the HERS study. The strongest effect on heart disease is seen with women who are currently taking estrogen ("currently" means at the time when a heart attack would be likely to occur). I think you need to evaluate your own risk factors and cholesterol levels. If you are at very high risk (cholesterol over 300, high blood pressure, and a family history of heart disease), you might consider taking hormones. On the other hand, if you have only moderately elevated cholesterol, you might consider a diet and exercise program; then at age sixty-five you can reevaluate the situation.

If you are going to take hormones in an attempt to prevent heart disease, it seems logical that you should take the regimen that is safest and has the best effects. If you have no uterus, you should take estrogen alone. If you have a uterus, you should take estrogen and micronized progesterone (see Chapter 15).

But not everyone needs to take hormones. Elizabeth Barrett-Connor is the epidemiologist and family physician in San Diego who wrote the first paper showing a relationship between hormone therapy and heart disease. In a paper written in 1993, she said: "No other prescription drug has been given on such a large scale to prevent disease in healthy women without proof of efficacy by a randomized clinical trial. . . . It is also important to remember that estrogen replacement is drug treatment, not really replacement therapy; the dose and route are unphysiologic and the level of circulating estrone is higher than that sustained by premenopausal women."[32]

I must admit, even more than with osteoporosis, I lean toward caution here. To give all women drugs to prevent heart disease when we don't have randomized controlled data to show that they work seems crazy to me. These drugs all have side effects and long-term problems—and we know of other ways to prevent heart disease that are less dangerous.

CHAPTER 7

Breast Cancer:
Every Woman's Fear?

Advocates of estrogen therapy like to focus on the diseases it seems to protect against. Unfortunately, there are also life-threatening diseases it can promote. Perhaps the most alarming of these, because it's already an epidemic, is breast cancer.

HOW BREAST CANCER BEGINS

In order to understand the relationship between estrogen and breast cancer, we need first to understand what is known about how and why breast cancer develops (see Figure 7.1). Breast cancer starts in the lining of the milk ducts. First, extra cells begin to form in this lining—a condition called hyperplasia (*hyper* means "too many," and *plasia* means "cells"). These cells then become odd-looking (atypical hyperplasia) and start filling the duct. Most of the time, neither hyperplasia nor atypical hyperplasia leads to cancer. When the cells start to look bizarre, like cancer cells, and are filling the duct but are still totally contained within it, they are called ductal carcinoma *in situ*, DCIS. DCIS is also called precancer. About 30 percent of the time, the cells develop the ability to break out of the duct into the surrounding fat—this is called invasion—and at that stage, you have cancer. These same cells can then gain access to a blood vessel and head out to the rest of the body. This process is termed *metastasis*. And it is metastasis that eventually kills you.

What starts this process? Cell growth, division, and invasion are all programmed by our genes. Cancers are started by faulty genes. You can inherit

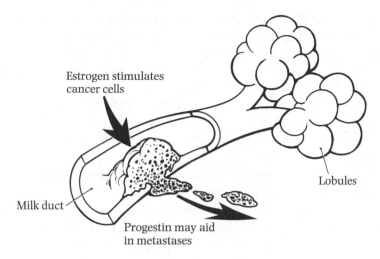

Estrogen stimulates
cancer cells

Lobules

Milk duct

Progestin may aid
in metastases

FIGURE 7.1   Hormones and breast cancer.

a faulty gene from your father or mother (or both), or you can inherit normal genes but something in the environment can come along and damage one of them. Actually, even an inherited gene needs something in the environment to cause the final mutation needed to lead to breast cancer—so breast cancer, like other cancers, is caused by a combination of abnormal genes and carcinogens in the environment.

Over the past several years, many discoveries have been made about breast cancer genes. For example, BRCA 1 (which stands for "breast cancer" 1) is a gene prevalent in families that have a lot of breast and ovarian cancer; BRCA 2 is a gene prevalent in families with a lot of male and female breast cancer. However, BRCA 1 and BRCA 2, important as they are, explain only 5 to 10 percent of breast cancer; they are not responsible for the vast number of cases.

More important for the average woman are the factors in her life that can cause a mutation in a normal breast gene or cause a mutated gene to grow and propagate. In this regard, the most common culprits are estrogen and progesterone.

RISK FACTORS IN BREAST CANCER: ESTROGEN AND PROGESTERONE

Are estrogen and progesterone a deadly duo? Estrogen was once thought to be the only hormone involved in starting and causing the progression of breast cancer. This idea came about because researchers believed that the breast responded to hormones in the same way as the uterus. In the uterus, estrogen causes cancer and progesterone protects against it. But the breast isn't the uterus; the breast responds to hormones quite differently.

Most hormones work through receptors on the outside surface of a cell. A receptor is like a lock that a specific hormone fits into, allowing the hormone to enter a cell or at least cause something to happen in a cell. Researchers initially assumed that all of the locks were the same; if progesterone blocked the effects of estrogen in one place, it would block them everywhere. We are now finding that this isn't entirely true. The researcher Katherine Horwitz has shown that the progesterone receptor in the uterus is completely different from the progesterone receptor in the breast.[1] For example, in the uterus, the drug RU 486 will block progesterone (that's how it causes a miscarriage); in the breast, it will act like progesterone and stimulate tissue to grow. This has been a source of confusion. In addition, as with the heart, we can't assume that progesterone and progestins have the same effect in the breast.

Malcolm Pike, a researcher from the University of Southern California, has theorized that unlike cancer of the uterus, which is caused by estrogen alone, breast cancer is caused by estrogen and progesterone together.[2] Examining the risk factors for breast cancer provides some evidence that gives weight to Pike's hypothesis.

Your Own Estrogen and Progesterone as Risk Factors

One of the first studies done on the connection between hormones and breast cancer looked at 6,908 women who had had hysterectomies between 1920 and 1940, and compared them with 1,479 women who had gone through natural menopause.[3] Women who had had both the uterus and the ovaries removed before age forty had a remarkably lower incidence of breast cancer—75 percent lower. But there was no such decrease among the women who had kept their ovaries. This was the first study to suggest that early surgical menopause protected women from breast cancer, and that hormones had something to do with the disease.

Since then, many other risk factors point to the effect of your own estrogen and progesterone on the risk of breast cancer. We know, for example, that the younger you are when you start your period and the older you are when you enter menopause, the higher your risk of getting breast cancer will be. In other words, the more exposure you have to your own hormones, the more you are at risk. If you become pregnant before age thirty, you decrease your risk of breast cancer; and if you have no children, your risk increases. If you exercise more than three times a week in the years before menopause, your risk of breast cancer decreases, presumably because you've altered the length of your cycle and decreased your levels of estrogen and progesterone. Postmenopausal obesity increases the risk of breast cancer, presumably because it raises the level of estrogen. Alcohol consumption also raises estrogen levels and increases the risk of breast cancer.

Of course, there are also risk factors for breast cancer that aren't hormonally related. But having more than one risk factor can compound the risk—and this often involves an interaction between hormonal and non-hormonal factors.

Radiation, for example, especially at an early age, appears to increase the risk of breast cancer. In the 1950s, doctors were radiating people for a variety of problems, believing that radiation was completely safe. As a result, a large number of women who were treated for various conditions with radiation as girls and young adults in the 1950s have developed breast cancer.[4] Researchers theorize that breast tissue doesn't develop fully until you've gone through a full-term pregnancy and are capable of making milk, and immature breast tissue is thought to be more sensitive than mature breast tissue to carcinogens such as radiation. Because of this, radiation in younger women is more dangerous than the same radiation later on. To take another example, in the 1950s, HCG (human choriogonadotrophic hormone)—the hormone that rises during pregnancy, inhibiting estrogen and progesterone—decreased the risk of breast cancer when it was given to women for weight loss.[5] Perhaps this caused the breast tissue to be more mature.

Many other external environmental pollutants are carcinogenic because they mimic estrogen. The pesticide DDT is metabolized into DDE, which is a form of estrogen. Some researchers believe that such environmental pesticides are contributing to the increased incidence of breast cancer.[6] Some studies have shown that the average sperm count has declined in men; this is also thought to be related to higher environmental estrogens.

At the same time, plant estrogens (phytoestrogens), such as those found in soy, seem to protect against breast cancer.[7] This, again, may result because different receptors react differently, or the same receptor reacts differently, to different compounds. As with the varying effects of progesterone versus progestins, natural estrogen may stimulate the breast and phytoestrogens may react with the receptor in a different way.[8] Substances in soy appear to block estrogen in the breast while acting like estrogen in other organs, such as the bones (see Chapter 12).

What you eat may affect the amount of endogenous estrogens you have. For example, vegetarians have lower levels of estrogen in their urine than meat eaters. Several studies have even shown that women who develop breast cancer have higher blood levels of estrogen and testosterone.[9]

Hormones as Drugs and the Risk of Breast Cancer

Since your body's own hormones can cause breast cancer, it makes sense to conclude that hormones taken as drugs will also increase your risk. DES, a form of estrogen that was given to pregnant women to prevent miscarriages in the 1950s, increased their risk of breast cancer.[10] Birth control pills taken for over ten years increase the risk of breast cancer in those women still taking them.[11] (We don't know about the current low-dose pills, as they haven't been used long enough.) It should come as no surprise that estrogen taken for more than five years postmenopausally also increases the risk—in fact, most studies find that it increases the risk by about 30 percent.[12] The real surprise, to me, is that we haven't seen more of an effect from hormone therapy.

In fact, there are several reasons for believing that the effects are even worse than the studies suggest. First, as we discussed in Chapter 4, the women on estrogen in most studies of hormones have a lower risk of breast cancer to start with, are more likely to have had a hysterectomy (including removal of their ovaries), and are healthier. And they are more likely to have mammograms than women not on estrogen, because they are going to a doctor regularly.

Second, although there have been a lot of observational studies on estrogen and the risk of breast cancer, they're hard to compare because they're not always studying the same thing. For example, it's reasonable to assume that your risk of breast cancer is probably related to how long you take the hormones; but unfortunately, not all the studies take that into consideration. Many studies only compare women who have never taken hormones to women who have, without considering how long the hormones were taken. Some studies have looked at the risk of breast cancer in women *currently* on hormones versus women who took them in the past. But even these studies don't take duration of use into account—and it's the studies looking at women who are currently taking hormones and have been taking them for at least five years that show the biggest increase in risk of breast cancer.[13] (In studies of osteoporosis and heart disease, by contrast, current users of hormones have the lowest risk.) With all these different ways of looking for an effect, it's not surprising that the results are often said to be inconsistent.

Third—again as we discussed in Chapter 4—the size of a study is critical as well. Many of these studies are not large enough to demonstrate an increased risk unless it's doubled or tripled. Yet when a disease as common as breast cancer increases by even 20 or 30 percent, a lot of women are affected.

Fourth, the first data we have about the effects of postmenopausal hormone therapy on breast cancer are based on the first "wave" of users—

women who were given only estrogen and no progestin. Doctors didn't start adding progestin to estrogen prescriptions until the late 1970s, when women on estrogen alone had begun to show a higher incidence of endometrial cancer. Only now, when enough women have been on both hormones for a long enough time, are we beginning to see any results for estrogen and progestin together.

A study by C. Schairer looked at women in the Breast Cancer Detection Demonstration Project (BCDDP), a nonrandomized screening program.[14] It compared women on estrogen and progestins with those who weren't, and found that women on estrogen and progestins had a slightly increased (20 percent higher) risk of breast cancer.

One of the biggest studies we have to date, the Nurses' Health Study, which we discussed in Chapter 6, showed in June 1995 that adding progestin to estrogen not only failed to reduce women's incidence of breast cancer, but actually increased it—as Malcolm Pike's model (discussed earlier) would suggest. This wasn't a huge increase, but it's an effect nonetheless. Women taking estrogen alone had a 36 percent increase in their risk of breast cancer; those on estrogen plus progestin had a 50 percent increase; those on progestins alone had a 240 percent increase. However, the number of women on progestins alone was small, so it is important to repeat the study before we give the findings too much credence. This study also looked at women who were taking estrogen and testosterone, which had been added to their regimen in the hope that it would restore libido. These women's risk of breast cancer was increased by 78 percent.[15]

Another important finding of the Nurses' Health Study had to do with the effects of duration of use and age. Women who at the time of the study had been taking estrogen and progesterone for five to ten years had a 46 percent increase in their risk of breast cancer. Also, the older a woman was, the higher her risk. Women between ages sixty and sixty-four who had been taking hormones for five years or more had an increase in risk of 71 percent. This is important when you look at the way hormones are being marketed to prevent osteoporosis and heart disease. To prevent these two diseases, women are told to start taking the hormones at age fifty and continue them for the rest of their lives. This means that by the time a woman is sixty-five, she'll have been taking hormones for fifteen years, considerably raising her vulnerability to breast cancer.

Thus the Nurses' Health Study provided important new information, especially on the combination of progesterone and estrogen. As I mentioned in Chapter 4, the media reported these findings widely. A week later, however, a study from Seattle appeared to contradict the Nurses' Health Study.[16] The Seattle study found no effect on the risk of breast cancer from either estrogen alone or estrogen and progesterone together. The media and the pharmaceutical companies used this to discredit the Nurses' Health Study (though it was also suggested by some that the scientists were simply unable to make up their minds). But the Seattle study included only about 1,000 women (the Nurses' Health Study follows almost 122,000 women). This means the Seattle study would not have been able to find any increase smaller than 250 percent. The Seattle study wasn't exactly wrong; it just said that, with the number of patients it looked at, no increased risk was found. It couldn't have found one—there weren't enough women in the study to catch an increase the size of the one the Nurses' Health Study revealed.

To me the conclusion is clear: there's an increased risk of breast cancer for women who take Premarin or Premarin and Provera postmenopausally for five or more years.

As with heart disease, though, we haven't really distinguished between progestins and progesterone. Some evidence does indicate that progestins cause breast cancer in rats and mice. But here it's harder to draw conclusions. In one recent study, women who were scheduled for breast reduction applied progesterone cream to their breasts for two weeks before the operation.[17] Researchers then looked at the cells in the breast tissue that had been removed to see if the progesterone had stimulated them to multiply. They found that there was *less* cell division. Their conclusion was that progesterone directly applied to the breast might even help prevent breast cancer. This study is very like the ones we discussed in Chapter 6 regarding the direct application of estrogen into coronary arteries. It is hard to know if a high dose applied directly has the same effect as a lower dose taken by mouth for a long time. Nonetheless, this result is interesting and needs to be studied further.

One crucial question is whether cancers caused by postmenopausal hormone therapy are the same as cancers that occur on their own. There's a continuing tendency to extrapolate from what we know about the uterus, and so some researchers have theorized that hormonally promoted cancers might be less aggressive. The endometrial cancers caused by estrogen tend to be fairly nonaggressive and treatable, as you'll read in Chapter 8. This led some early researchers to assume that the same would be true of breast cancer: if you got breast cancer from taking hormones too long, perhaps it would be easier to cure because it would be less aggressive than other breast cancers.

Two studies have seemed to confirm this,[18] as did data from my own research at UCLA. The percentage was not large, but there was a slightly higher proportion of low-grade cancers among women on hormones. We can't be sure why this is. One possible explanation, though, is that women on hormones, as we've noted before, tend to be people who get better med-

ical care than others, so they're more likely to get regular mammograms—
and the kind of breast cancers that mammograms are best at finding are
precisely those cancers that respond best to "early detection."

Still, these aren't the only findings that have come up. The Nurses'
Health Study showed a 45 percent increase in the risk of death from breast
cancer in women who took hormones for more than five years. So it isn't
just relatively harmless *in situ* cancers that women get from hormones.[19]

If You're Already at Risk

Some studies have looked at whether women already at risk for breast cancer will compound their risk if they use estrogen. This question is not clear-
cut, because risk factors don't always add up: it's somewhat like a prisoner
who's committed two crimes getting concurrent sentences rather than
consecutive sentences. There are no good studies on whether estrogen and
progestins increase the risks for women already at risk for breast cancer,
but the few studies looking at the use of estrogen in women with a family
history of breast cancer have found an increase in risk of 70 percent, the
same as for women without a family history. There have been no randomized controlled studies, though.

Recently, there have been disturbing studies about still another possible
effect of hormone therapy on the risk of breast cancer. This has to do with
detection of breast cancer. Young women have dense breast tissue. Usually,
breast tissue in postmenopausal women is less dense and thus doesn't hide
cancers as well. But taking hormones can stimulate breast tissue, causing
it to become denser. Cancer and breast tissue are the same density, so the
effect on a mammogram is like looking at a polar bear in the snow.

This problem of detection appears to be worse when women take combined estrogen and progestins. One study reported that 30 percent of
women on estrogen and progestins will show an increase in dense tissue.[20]
A report from the *Journal of the National Cancer Institute* said that the mammograms of women on hormone therapy were more difficult to read.[21] I
used to see this in my own breast surgery practice all the time: I'd look at a
patient's mammogram and think, "She must have started hormones,"
because suddenly her breast tissue was dense, which it hadn't been in previous mammograms. Then, if the woman stopped her hormones, within
six months her mammogram would be back to normal.

There are at least two serious implications here. First, controlled randomized studies have shown a decrease of 30 percent in the death rate from
breast cancer of women over fifty who get regular mammograms.[22] Postmenopausal hormone therapy may wipe out some of that benefit. Second,
retrospective studies have demonstrated that women with dense breasts in

general have more breast cancer.[23] Density may represent hormones stimulating the tissue, which in turn could cause more cancer. These two implications create a frightening double jeopardy: you're more likely to get breast cancer, and less likely to catch it in time to save your life.

If hormone therapy not only increases the incidence of breast cancer but also makes it harder to diagnose, we may find the current epidemic mushrooming as more women take estrogen and progestins for longer periods of time.

BREAST CANCER AND YOU

Early Detection

With all the media hype about mammography and breast self-examination, you may be tempted to dismiss concerns about the increased risk of breast cancer on the assumption that if you're diligent about your health care, your cancer can be detected early and cured. I wish this were true, but as I've seen so often and so tragically in my practice, it's not something you can count on. Even apart from the obscuring effect hormones have on breast tissue, mammography at its best is far from a guarantee that breast cancer will be caught at an early, curable stage. A mammogram isn't the equivalent of a Pap smear, and the concept of "early detection" is somewhat misleading. It works only about 30 percent of the time. Women can still get small cancers that have already spread by the time they're diagnosed.

What You Really Want to Know: What Is It Like to Have Breast Cancer?

Breast cancer often takes a woman by surprise. Seventy to 80 percent of women with breast cancer have no risk factors. No one in their family has ever had it, and they did everything right. The first sign is usually a lump you find while showering, rolling over in bed, or making love, or an abnormal routine mammogram.

When a biopsy reveals cancer, you'll need to have the tumor removed by either a lumpectomy or a mastectomy. During the surgery, a few lymph nodes will be removed from under your arm and examined for cancer cells. If there is cancer in the nodes or if there's another reason to believe that there might be microscopic cancer cells elsewhere in the body, you'll receive chemotherapy for four to six months, tamoxifen (an estrogen blocker) for five years, or both. (Which of these systemic treatments is best depends on a number of factors.) If the nodes are negative and there's no reason to believe that there are cancer cells elsewhere in the body, you'll probably have only local treatment: lumpectomy and six weeks or so of radiation therapy; or mastectomy, with the option of breast reconstruction.

The median age for breast cancer is sixty-nine. Approximately one third of the women diagnosed with breast cancer will die of it. A fifty-year-old woman has a 10 percent lifetime probability of getting breast cancer and a 3 percent chance of dying of the disease.[24] Most women who develop breast cancer tolerate their therapy while continuing their normal lives. Neither the treatment nor the disease is physically disabling unless the disease spreads. Once this spread (metastasis) develops, the course is usually fairly rapid, with most women dead within two to three and a half years.

What You Really Want to Know:
When You've Already Had Breast Cancer

Women who have already had breast cancer may increase their risk of a recurrence of the original cancer or of a second breast cancer if they take hormones. Yet ironically, these are sometimes the very women who strongly feel the need for something like hormone therapy. They're dealing very directly with their fear of death, and they can get excited by the hype about hormone therapy—it will keep them from getting heart disease; it will keep them from getting a fractured hip.

Further, women who have undergone chemotherapy for breast cancer often go into an abrupt menopause similar to that experienced by women who have had a hysterectomy and had their ovaries removed. This can lead to severe symptoms. The idea of hormone therapy can be particularly enticing to a younger woman who has been put into this premature menopause. Her youth has been taken away from her, and here's this wonder drug that will give it back. Sadly, it may end up shortening her life instead.

Some research is beginning to confirm the danger. Studies looking at the basic biology of estrogen and progesterone suggest that progestins actually help cancers to become more invasive.[25] As we have discussed, to be dangerous, cancer cells have to be able to invade tissue outside of their normal territory. Progestins make it easier for cancers to invade and spread. So giving progestins to women with breast cancer may make the difference between an *in situ* cancer and a metastatic cancer.

Another worrisome study followed four women who were taking both estrogen and progesterone after treatment for breast cancer.[26] They all developed metastasis. When they were taken off their hormones, however, the metastasis temporarily disappeared. This suggests that the hormones were fueling the metastases. Limited as this study is, it does give one pause.

Finally, it's important to realize that a woman who's had cancer in one breast has an increased risk of developing cancer in the other breast. Post-menopausal hormone therapy increases this risk. The risk of a new breast cancer overwhelms any possible benefit of hormone therapy in preventing osteoporosis or heart disease.[27]

As we've noted, at one time doctors—recognizing the likelihood of a con-nection between hormone therapy and breast cancer—were reluctant to give hormones to women who had had the disease. Now, however, with all the marketing of hormone "replacement" therapy, there's been a disturb-ing turnaround: since there's no solid proof of danger, many doctors have decided that it's fine.

To me, that's appalling. Logic suggests that it's dangerous to give hor-mones to women whose disease is already related to hormones. There's no proof that the hormones *don't* increase the risk of recurrence, and these are human lives we're dealing with.

Maybe I'm being unfair. Perhaps the doctors are just unwilling to tell these women their prognosis. Lord knows, it isn't easy to confront a patient with the fact that her chance of living long enough to get osteoporosis or heart disease is far less than her chance of dying from her breast cancer. But even if that's the case, doctors owe it to these women to give them the best shot at a longer life. Maybe I've just been too close to it. I've seen too many of my own patients die before they should have died; I'd have been so grateful if some of them could have lived into their seventies or eighties, even if they did end up with broken hips or heart attacks. Most women with breast cancer agree with me. A recent survey of women with breast cancer found that they weren't willing to accept hormone therapy if it meant even a very small risk of a recurrence.[28]

Doctors who are promoting the use of hormone therapy for women with breast cancer cite the fact that both estrogen and progestins are given to treat metastatic breast cancer. This is true, but the doses are much higher. And, paradoxically, high doses kill cancer even though low doses may cause it.

Another argument used to support estrogen therapy for women with breast cancer is the fact that limited observational studies have suggested that women who become pregnant after treatment for breast cancer, despite all the hormones pregnancy creates, have no higher mortality rates than women who don't become pregnant.[29] But new, larger observational studies show that women who get breast cancer while pregnant—with the same proliferation of estrogen going on in their bodies—have an increased risk of recurrence.[30,31]

Furthermore, a recent overview of all the studies of treatment for breast cancer reported that removing the ovaries of a premenopausal woman (a treatment for breast cancer that was used before the development of chemotherapy) is as effective as chemotherapy in preventing recurrence.[32] When you remove a woman's ovaries, of course, you remove most of her body's own estrogen and all of its progesterone. This would certainly make you think: if removing estrogen and progesterone helps prevent recurrence, then how can adding estrogen and progestins be good?

Finally, the use of tamoxifen, with its estrogen-blocking effects in the breast, has been important in controlling postmenopausal breast cancer— again leading me to believe that adding estrogen is likely to be dangerous.

Several small, nonrandomized studies of the use of hormones for postmenopausal women with breast cancer show no increase in recurrence.[33,34] The follow-up, however, has been short, and the studies were of women who were already at low risk of recurrence, so they're hard to evaluate. Until we have a lot more evidence that it's safe, I feel that *preventive* hormone therapy for women who have had breast cancer is a bad idea. Certainly the twenty or thirty years of hormones that clinicians are currently pushing seems unreasonable.

Once in a while, I've had a breast cancer patient who, knowing the risks, still wants to be on short-term hormone therapy to relieve menopausal symptoms. A study of women with breast cancer done at Johns Hopkins showed that 49 percent of women experienced a physical or emotional problem related to menopause after the diagnosis of breast cancer. Half of these women felt they were in need of treatment.[35] Obviously, we need to develop appropriate treatments for this group of women. Meanwhile, though, if a woman has severe symptoms that are interfering with the quality of her life, I think she would be wise to investigate many of the alternative methods for relieving symptoms before settling on hormone therapy. (We discuss some of these in Chapter 11.) At the very least, if she feels she must take hormones, she should do so for the shortest possible time.

As I've said before, there's no free lunch.

CHAPTER 8

Endometrial Cancer: The First Problem with Estrogen

The one danger from long-term estrogen therapy that isn't disputed is its link with cancer of the endometrium—the lining of the uterus. (Because cancer of the actual uterine wall is very uncommon, the term *uterine cancer* almost always refers to endometrial cancer.) I described in Chapter 1 the complicated hormonal dance that occurs monthly in your body between puberty and menopause. As part of that dance, the endometrium is first built, then sloughed off with your period, and then rebuilt.

UNDERSTANDING ENDOMETRIAL CANCER

The endometrial lining is meant to be replaced monthly unless it's needed to support a pregnancy. If it's not shed regularly, it can become cancerous. Endometrial cancer is genetic, just as breast cancer is. It starts with flawed genes that are either inherited or acquired through exposure to carcinogens. Estrogen may cause some mutations, but we believe that its main role in endometrial cancer is to increase cell division, giving any mutations already there the opportunity to multiply. Progesterone can block this process if it causes the lining of the uterus to shed (see Figure 8.1). All the mutated cells, even the cancerous ones, flow out during your period. Because of this, endometrial cancer is unusual in a woman who is menstruating normally, since she's regularly shedding her endometrium.

After menopause, unless you've had a hysterectomy, you still have an endometrium—a uterine lining. Usually, if your own levels of estrogen production aren't too high, this lining atrophies or becomes inactive. So even if

Estrogen stimulates endometrial lining growth

A drop in progesterone stimulates sloughing of endometrial lining

FIGURE 8.1   Effects of hormones on the uterine lining.

precancerous cells are present, they lie dormant. If for some reason the cells are stimulated to divide, however, the precancerous or cancerous mutations will have a chance to increase, and they won't be automatically shed at the end of the month in a period. This is how women get endometrial cancer.

Once endometrial cancer develops, it can invade the blood vessels (just as breast cancer can) and spread to other organs. So, like any cancer, it can kill you.

But unlike breast cancer, endometrial cancer gives you early warning signs. As the uterine lining builds up, it causes spotting or bleeding. Spontaneous bleeding in a woman who hasn't had a period in a year always needs to be checked out. So does persistent heavy menstrual bleeding. (As we said in Chapter 3, the problem isn't always cancer; there are a number of more likely possibilities.) Fortunately, the uterine lining is readily accessible and can be easily biopsied in a doctor's office.

Sometimes the biopsy will find signs that the endometrium is precancerous. Though precancer is a frightening idea, it's a far cry from cancer itself, especially when it's in the short-lived endometrium rather than a permanent, critical organ. Still, you want to be careful with it.

The first indication that there may be a problem is if the biopsy finds an increased number of cells. This is called simple or adenomatous hyperplasia (*adenomatous* means in a gland-forming organ; *hyper,* as we saw in Chapter 7, means "too many"; *plasia* means "cells"). Hyperplasia is often a cause of irregular or heavy bleeding in perimenopausal women (see Chapter 3). This is thought to arise because some women have cycles in which they don't ovulate and therefore don't produce progesterone to help them shed the endometrium. You may have several such cycles, and then, when you do ovulate, end up with a period in which the blood just seems to gush—"your basic flooder," as one of my friends calls it.

If you have such cells and they're abnormal-looking, they're called atypical (see Figure 8.2). Atypical hyperplasia can be simple or complex, depending on whether the increased cells are also interfering with the normal architecture of the uterine lining. Complex hyperplasia is more ominous than simple hyperplasia.

The next step after atypia is thought to be cancer. But this is far from an inevitable progression. In 1985, the researcher Robert Kurman showed that only 1 percent of women with untreated simple hyperplasia went on to develop uterine cancer; and even with complex atypical hyperplasia, only 29 percent of women developed cancer.[1]

Hyperplasia can be treated with a progestin. It's given for twelve days to balance the estrogen, and then when it's stopped, it causes the lining of the uterus to slough off, thereby eliminating any precancerous cells that may be there.

What Is It Like to Have Endometrial Cancer?

Actual endometrial cancer is usually a disease of older women. The median age of endometrial cancer is sixty-eight years. This cancer is very curable.

If the problem is precancer, as just noted, it can be treated with progestin. But if the problem is cancer, you'll usually need a hysterectomy. (See Chapter 11 for a description of what to expect with a hysterectomy.) When endometrial cancers are detected at an early stage—as most are—this is all the treatment necessary. Women with more advanced disease usually need radiation therapy as well. Although early-stage endometrial cancer is 93

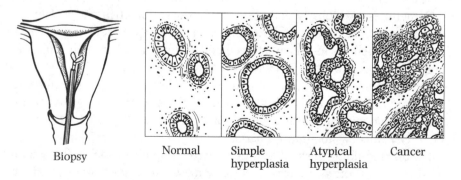

| Biopsy | Normal | Simple hyperplasia | Atypical hyperplasia | Cancer |

FIGURE 8.2   Uterine cancer development.

percent curable, there are still some women who are diagnosed at a later stage, and women do die of this disease.

RISK FACTORS IN ENDOMETRIAL CANCER

All of the risk factors for endometrial cancer have to do with increased estrogen that isn't balanced by progesterone—so-called unopposed estrogen. So women who take estrogen are obviously at risk.

Weight is also a major risk factor because, as I said earlier, fat has an enzyme called aromatase that produces estrogen in postmenopausal women. Postmenopausal women who are between twenty and fifty pounds overweight have three times the normal risk of endometrial cancer; if you're more than fifty pounds overweight, you have nineteen times the risk of endometrial cancer. In fact, the best way to prevent endometrial cancer is to keep your weight down with exercise and a healthy diet.

Diabetes triples your risk of endometrial cancer. So does high blood pressure. It's not clear, however, whether these are independent risk factors or are related to being overweight. (Both adult-onset diabetes and high blood pressure are often associated with obesity.)

The breast cancer drug tamoxifen, since it blocks estrogen in the breast but acts like estrogen in the uterus, has also been shown to cause endometrial cancer.

At the same time, there are some factors that *decrease* the risk of endometrial cancer. Premenopausal women who take birth control pills have a lower incidence of endometrial cancer, and the protection lasts for at least fifteen years after they've stopped taking the pills. This is probably because the balanced estrogen and progesterone in the pill prevent abnormal buildups in the lining of the uterus. Regular exercise decreases the risk of endometrial cancer by lengthening your menstrual cycle and thus lessening the amount of both hormones you're exposed to in your lifetime. Eating a diet high in soy protein will have a similar effect. Smoking, which does so much harm in other ways, decreases the risk of endometrial cancer because it reduces the amount of estrogen you have naturally. (I need hardly add that I don't advise taking up smoking as a preventive measure—lung cancer is a ghastly alternative to endometrial cancer.)

Estrogen as a Risk Factor

It isn't surprising that estrogen given alone (unopposed by progesterone) to postmenopausal women increases their risk of endometrial cancer significantly. The researcher Deborah Grady published a meta-analysis of endometrial cancer in 1995.[2] (A meta-analysis takes a large group of studies and combines their results.) Women who had used estrogen at any point in their lives, whether for one year or thirty years, had 2.3 times the normal risk of endometrial cancer. Those who took it for less than a year had 1.4 times the normal risk. Those who took it for more than ten years had almost 10 times the normal risk. Those who took it for twenty years had 20 times the risk.

Interestingly, women who took Premarin had a greater risk than those who took synthetic estrogens. Users of Premarin were 2.5 times more likely to get endometrial cancer than nonusers, while women who used synthetic estrogens like Estrace were only 1.3 times more likely to get it than nonusers.

Women who used unopposed estrogen were 4 times more likely to get an early-stage cancer than a late-stage one. Women on estrogen had 6 times as many noninvasive cancers (precancers) and 4 times as many invasive cancers as nonusers. This finding has been interpreted to mean that estrogen is much more likely to stimulate an *in situ* or noninvasive cancer and is said to support the theory that the kind of endometrial cancer caused by unopposed estrogen is a "better"—or at least slower-growing—kind of cancer. As with all the diseases we've been discussing, though, we have to consider the "healthy woman" effect. These women were going to the doctor to get their hormones and were thus more likely than women who were not on hormones to have their cancer detected at an early stage. But even at that, these women weren't completely out of the woods. Their death rate from endometrial cancer was almost three times that of women who had never taken hormones.

If you take estrogen, your risk of endometrial cancer is worse if you smoke cigarettes or are thin. Obese women have a lot of their own estrogen, and one would think that would make their risk of endometrial cancer worse. But it seems to be the opposite. It's the women who don't have that much of their own estrogen and who then supplement it who are more at risk.

It's important to remember that for a fifty-year-old woman the lifetime risk of developing endometrial cancer is 3 percent. So doubling your risk by taking estrogen would raise it to 6 percent.[3] As we've pointed out before, an increase in risk can be less important if a disease is less common but more important if a disease is more common. It may or may not be worth it to you to take that increased risk.

Progestins as a Risk Factor

You'll remember from Chapter 7 that the first wave of postmenopausal women who took hormone therapy in the United States received only estrogen. When the reports came out about increased rates of both endometrial hyperplasia and endometrial cancers in women who had taken unopposed Premarin, the drug companies and doctors had to do something. The risk was related to the fact that with estrogen the lining of the uterus built up continuously and unnaturally, without being shed. So doctors began adding progestin to the estrogen regimen for a few days in each cycle. When the progestin was stopped, the uterine lining would shed and eliminate the risk. This combined hormone therapy caused a prompt decrease in the incidence of both hyperplasia and cancer of the endometrium in women taking it (and a prompt increase in sales of tampons and sanitary napkins, since they all started bleeding again).

However, there are still no good long-term studies of progestin and how it affects cancer. Some cancers take many years to develop, so we can't tell to what extent the combined therapy really results in fewer cancers and to what extent late-developing cancers will prove the benefits illusory. In addition, since many postmenopausal women are encouraged to take hormones all their lives, we need long-term studies to see the effect of twenty or thirty years of hormone use.

There are other unanswered questions about progestins. It isn't clear how much progestin is necessary to prevent uterine cancer. In one study, women who took estrogen with progestin for ten days of the cycle had a 50 percent increased risk of uterine cancer, while those who took the added progestin for twelve days had no increase in uterine cancer.[4] Some doctors are doing research to see whether taking progesterone only every three or four months to shed any uterine buildup might not be enough to protect against endometrial cancer. Intrauterine progesterone, which is inserted by a doctor like an IUD, is also being studied. In the PEPI study, discussed in Chapter 6, 100 milligrams of micronized progesterone daily for twelve days appeared to be enough to protect the uterus without counteracting the positive effects of estrogen on lipid levels.[5]

Then there's our other recurrent problem: we don't yet have data on the long-term safety of the combination of estrogen and progestins. In fact, the FDA has approved the use of progestins alone only for short-term treatment of women with uterine bleeding problems, *not* for long-term prevention. (A pill combining Premarin and Provera was approved in 1996—see Chapter 15—but the indications for Provera have not been changed.) This often comes as a shock to women whose doctors have prescribed progestins for prevention. What many people don't realize is that once having approved a drug for any use, the FDA can't control the other uses that doctors put it to. In other words, since the progestin Provera is approved for bleeding problems, doctors can decide to prescribe it for virtually anything, such as the prevention of osteoporosis—or ingrown toenails, for that matter. But the FDA's approval for a certain use implies that the agency thinks there's enough benefit, and low enough risk, to support that use—and only that use.

I agree with the FDA's decision not to approve progestins for long-term use. I think we need more data about progestins and progesterone before we get carried away. But most of the medical community has taken a different approach to progestins and progesterone, an approach characterized by tunnel vision: it is simply assumed that the drugs protect the uterus and have no other effects. This is unlikely to be the case with any hormone.

In fact, many of the symptoms of perimenopause and menopause become worse when you take progestins and progesterone (see Chapter 15); women complain especially of bloating and depression. The biggest problem, however, is that you start bleeding again. Women who are menopausal will get periods again, and those who are perimenopausal may have heavy, irregular bleeding. Needless to say, this hasn't pleased women. In fact, it's the reason most women stop taking postmenopausal hormone therapy.

In an effort to prevent this bleeding, doctors began giving the progestins in a different way: continuously. The idea was that taking a smaller dose every day might counteract the stimulating effect of the estrogen and allow the uterus to become inactive. If you take progestins this way, you'll still bleed at first, but after six months to a year, the bleeding will peter out. (Of course, you'll need a few biopsies along the way to make sure that there's no cancer—see Chapter 4.) This solves the bleeding problem, but once again, it's changed the picture. We can't simply extrapolate the data from cyclical estrogen and progestin therapy to continuous therapy. As we discussed in Chapter 6, continuous progestins have a different effect on the heart from cyclical progestins, which means that they might have different effects in many other areas. I'm amazed that doctors continue to prescribe drugs and combinations of drugs for which we have no actual data on long-term safety, and no proof that they're effective for anything but short-term symptoms.

As we noted in Chapter 7, in the process of helping to prevent endometrial cancer, progestin may well increase the risk of breast cancer, and breast cancer is already far more common than endometrial cancer. Remember also that progestin dilutes some of the positive effects of estrogen on lipid profiles, as well as some of the direct effects on the heart. So we're using progestin for one single purpose, to protect the uterus, and ignoring the wide-ranging damage it can do.

A Cautionary Tale

The story of endometrial cancer and the long-term use of estrogen is a cautionary tale indeed. As we've discussed in Chapter 2, Robert Wilson's book *Feminine Forever* set off a mania for long-term estrogen therapy for every woman. At the time, there were no studies documenting the alleged beneficial effects, nor were there studies on the safety of this approach. That, of course, didn't stop anyone. Here was the fountain of youth, and both women and their doctors enthusiastically ran toward it. It made sense, after all, according to the dogma of postmenopausal "ovarian failure" and "estrogen deficiency." And women had estrogen in their bodies naturally before menopause, so how could it be dangerous?

As we now know, nothing is that simple. The uterus is controlled by a bevy of hormones, not just estrogen, and supplementing only one of them throws off the choreography of the hormonal dance. Women have died from endometrial cancer caused by the estrogen they were taking to keep them young. Yet here we go again, repeating this scenario. We have limited data on long-term use of estrogen and progesterone and no good studies about the benefits or risks. But we're plunging ahead with widespread use because "it makes sense." I hope we can be wiser this time and demand adequate data about safety and firm evidence of benefit before we jump onto a bandwagon that may again sacrifice women's lives to the pharmaceutical fad of the day.

CHAPTER 9

For Better or Worse: Hormone Therapy and Other Diseases

In chapters 5, 6, and 7 we discussed the diseases most commonly linked with hormone therapy. The newspapers are also chock-full of other potential associations—some positive, some negative. In this chapter I'll review the data we have for them. We'll start with the disorders that hormones are thought to help; these include Alzheimer's disease, stroke, and colon cancer. We'll then go on to areas of potential harm: ovarian cancer, gallbladder disease, thromboembolic disease, fibroids, endometriosis, and a few others.

THE GOOD NEWS?

Alzheimer's Disease

As we mention later, there are some data suggesting that estrogen might affect thinking and memory (see Chapter 11). Because of this possibility, some people have wondered whether estrogen might also protect against Alzheimer's disease, the best-known form of dementia—and a form that's more common in women than men.

Risk Factors for Alzheimer's Disease

We know that Alzheimer's disease runs in families and therefore is caused in part by genetic defects, but we don't yet know what its other causes are. Women have 1.5 to 3 times more risk of getting Alzheimer's disease than men. This may, in part, be simply because women live longer. But there's also a greater risk if you're thin or if you've had a heart attack—and both of these factors, as you've seen, are related to estrogen levels.

Natural History of Alzheimer's Disease

Although many of us fear dementia more than most other diseases, Alzheimer's actually isn't all that common. Also, it's most likely to happen when you're very old. It's fourteen times more common in people over age eighty-five than in those between sixty and sixty-five. A recent study of a community in Boston[1] found that the probability of getting Alzheimer's disease is 0.6 percent in people between sixty-five and sixty-nine; 1 percent in those between seventy and seventy-four; 2 percent in those between seventy-five and seventy-nine; 3.3 percent in those between eighty and eighty-four; and 8.4 percent in people eighty-five and older. Senile dementia, which includes Alzheimer's as well as other dementias, levels off at 40 percent at age ninety-five. Few of us live to be ninety-five, however.

What Is It Like to Have Alzheimer's Disease?

The earliest symptom of Alzheimer's disease is an inability to learn or recall new information. Patients have trouble finding words, become disoriented, or have a tendency to get lost. They may have behavioral problems such as depression, irritability, suspiciousness, or delusions. Deterioration continues inexorably over a period of up to a decade or longer. Eventually, many patients lose the ability to communicate or even to recognize their closest relatives. Although there's some difference in the symptoms in men and women, the course of the disease and its severity are the same.

Estrogen and Alzheimer's Disease

A study of postmenopausal women in a retirement community called Leisure World found that women who took estrogen had a 30 percent lower incidence of Alzheimer's disease. This finding, of course, is subject to all of the "healthy women" biases we've mentioned several times before. The authors of the study believe that it hints at a possible connection, but research is far from conclusive.[2] Another, smaller observational study compared 143 women with Alzheimer's disease and 92 without it.[3] The women with Alzheimer's disease were less likely to be on estrogen than those in the control group, but the study was too small for its results to be even remotely conclusive. A population-based study done in Seattle was unable to find any association between Alzheimer's disease and use of estrogen.[4]

There are also several small, short observational studies (involving fewer than 15 women) in which estrogen was shown to improve symptoms of women with Alzheimer's disease.[5] The jury is still out here.

As this book was going to press, a larger observational study of 1,124 women in New York found that 5 percent of the women taking estrogen developed Alzheimer's disease, while 16 percent of the women who weren't on estrogen developed the disease.[6] Though the study was praised for including Hispanic and African-American subjects, it was still subject to the healthy woman bias—perhaps even more than other studies have been. As we discussed in earlier chapters, the "healthy woman bias" exists because the women who take menopausal hormones tend to come from a higher socioeconomic background, have a higher level of education, and get better overall health care than those in the general population. In our culture, black and Hispanic women have disproportionately low incomes, poor health care, and low levels of education. Thus the women in these communities who are taking menopausal hormones are likely to be an even more select group than are white women on hormones.

More interesting is a report by Roberta Benton, a molecular pharmacologist at the University of Southern California. She reported at an international Alzheimer's meeting at Osaka, Japan, that equilin, one of the horse hormones in Premarin, may be more effective than estrogen in stimulating nerve growth.[7] So we need to be careful about assuming that estrogen is always responsible for effects that result from a medication that includes other hormones as well.

Although Alzheimer's disease is rare and occurs late in life, it's extremely frightening, and the pharmaceutical companies have noted how scared women are. One representative of Wyeth-Ayerst, the makers of Premarin, said, at a conference on hormones in Philadelphia, that "cognition can provide the gut-level response to breast cancer."[8] The implication was that if the makers of Premarin could show that estrogen prevents Alzheimer's disease, it would be enough of a benefit to counteract women's fear of getting breast cancer from taking estrogen: fear of Alzheimer's trumps fear of breast cancer. Not surprisingly, Wyeth-Ayerst is conducting a large randomized controlled study to see if estrogen does have an effect on Alzheimer's disease. If the researchers do find a connection, though, there will still be questions. Is it worth endangering your life to avoid a disease you probably won't live long enough to get in the first place? And given the advanced ages of people with Alzheimer's, would it be wiser, if you do take hormones to prevent it, to start when you're seventy rather than when you're fifty?

The FDA has approved the first drug designed to address the cognitive deficits of Alzheimer's disease. Tacrine increases the levels of acetylcholine, a neurotransmitter in the brain. Unfortunately, its benefits are modest at best, and many people experience side effects. Although it wasn't directly studied, there's some evidence that women on estrogen as well as Tacrine had a better effect than either drug alone or placebo.[9]

Stroke

Two contradictory factors have led researchers to look at a possible connection between stroke and hormone therapy. The first is that the early formulations of birth control pills increased the rate of stroke in women over thirty who took them. These pills had higher doses of hormones, and some of the risk showed up only in smokers, who are already at risk for stroke. Nonetheless, we do know that high-dose estrogen increases blood clots, so there's been a concern that hormone therapy would increase strokes. At the same time, since estrogen appears to lower the risk of cardiovascular disease, researchers have looked for a similar benefit with stroke.

What Is a Stroke?

There are several types of strokes. The most common, the *thrombotic* stroke, occurs when a clot forms in a narrowed artery and blocks the flow of blood. This is similar to the way a heart attack occurs. An *embolic* stroke occurs when a clot travels from another area (usually the heart) or a particle of plaque breaks off from a hardened artery (usually the carotid) and is carried through the bloodstream into a narrow vessel, which it blocks. There's a third type of stroke called a *hemorrhagic* stroke, which happens when a blood vessel breaks and bleeds into the brain. This type has no relationship to estrogen.

"Stroke" is really a word for any condition in which blood is kept from flowing into an area of the brain served by a blocked or damaged blood vessel. That section of the brain dies, and the area of the body that it controls becomes nonfunctional. If you're lucky, the surrounding areas of the brain compensate for the dead part, and you'll recover some function. But if the area is too big, the stroke can cause significant disability, or even death.

Risk Factors for Stroke

Strokes are more common in older people. They occur in men more frequently than women, and in African Americans more frequently than Caucasians. A family history of stroke increases your risk, as do high blood pressure, heart disease, smoking, obesity, and high levels of red blood cells. A diet high in salt or a sedentary lifestyle can also increase your risk of stroke, by increasing your risk of high blood pressure.

Hormones and Stroke

What does all of this have to do with estrogen? In fact, none of these risk factors appears to have any relationship to estrogen or progesterone. Not surprisingly, the studies that have looked at the risk of stroke in women who have taken hormones postmenopausally have shown mixed results. Some have found a small decrease in the rate of stroke,[10] while others find no effect.[11] A meta-analysis of all of the studies revealed no effect on stroke.[12]

Because there have been no randomized controlled studies, we can't completely rule out a link between stroke and hormones. Better studies are needed, and the Women's Health Initiative will be monitoring stroke in its large randomized controlled study. Until there's further evidence, though, it seems unwise to take hormones to prevent stroke.

Colon Cancer

Colon cancer is the second most common cancer in women (after breast cancer). Some observational data suggest that women on hormone therapy have lower rates of fatal colon cancer.[13]

Colon cancer begins in the lining of the large intestine and grows to a size that can bleed or obstruct the large bowel. Most colon cancers are thought to arise in adenomatous polyps—outgrowths of the lining of the colon. These polyps occur in 30 percent of men and women, without any symptoms. Only about 1 percent or less of these polyps ever turn cancerous, however.

Risk Factors for Colon Cancer

Polyps are one risk factor. The biggest risk factor is a family history of the disease, which increases your risk by 50 percent. There is an inherited disease called familial polyposis coli in which the colon is studded with polyps, many of which turn into cancer when you're young. This cancer also occurs more often in people who have had ulcerative colitis, a chronic bowel disease characterized by bloody diarrhea.

If you eat a meat-based diet, you have twice as high a chance of getting colon cancer than if you eat meat less than once a month. Obesity increases the risk of colon cancer by 30 percent. Finally, constipation increases the rate of colon cancer. A diet high in fiber and fruits and vegetables decreases the risk of colon cancer. So does an aspirin a day.[14] (Don't take aspirin for this purpose without checking with your doctor.)

In retrospective studies, colon cancer appears to be more common among women who have had breast, ovarian, or endometrial cancer.[15] This implies a genetic or hormonal link.

Some characteristics of colon cancer suggest that hormones may have an influence. For example, the fact that pregnancy affects bile salt metabolism, which has long been believed to be a factor in the development of colon cancer, has led some researchers to investigate whether pregnancy protects against colon cancer. To date, these studies have been contradictory. Some studies have suggested that the more children a woman has and the earlier she has them, the lower her risk,[16] but others have shown no connection.[17] One study found that both men and women with many children had a lower rate of colon cancer than those with few or none—which suggests that if there is a connection, it's related more to lifestyle than to biology.[18] So the link between hormones and colon cancer is neither consistent nor simple.

Estrogen and Colon Cancer

Observational studies in recent years have found an almost 50 percent lower risk of colon cancer among women on estrogen therapy.[19] All of these studies, however, have the limitations of the healthy woman effect we've discussed elsewhere. Women who take hormones appear to be healthier than women who don't, and they have a decreased incidence of a number of diseases, unrelated to the hormones themselves. One study of postmenopausal women noted that those on estrogen were 16 percent more likely to get screening tests for colon cancer than other women. A meta-analysis of all of the studies found that hormone therapy had no effect on colon cancer.[20] But as the authors of that analysis noted, there hasn't been the kind of randomized controlled study that's needed to answer the question. Again, the jury is still out.

Osteoarthritis

Preliminary studies suggest that estrogen therapy may lower the risk of osteoarthritis, a form of arthritis that affects 16 million Americans, mostly women over age forty-five. A large observational study[21] of 4,366 white women age sixty-five and older showed that women taking estrogen had the lowest incidence of osteoarthritis. More studies need to be done to see if ERT can actually prevent osteoarthritis, but this finding is promising.

THE BAD NEWS

Of course, for every preliminary study of the good estrogen therapy might do, there's another story about potential harm. The potential damage is an increase in your risk of ovarian cancer, lung cancer, gallbladder problems, and thromboembolic disease (disease caused by blood clots)—and possibly other disorders.

Ovarian Cancer

Ovarian cancer isn't very common, but it's deadly and therefore very frightening. Ever since the comedian Gilda Radner died from ovarian cancer, women have been especially aware of this potential killer. One in eighty women (1.4 percent) will develop ovarian cancer. Like breast cancer, ovarian cancer is more common among older people. The median age for ovarian cancer is fifty-nine.

The major problem with ovarian cancer is that we don't have a good way to detect it early. Because the ovaries are hidden deep in the abdomen, ovarian cancer is often far advanced by the time it's detected. Thus the treatments aren't very effective; only 38 percent of women with the disease live for five years after it's been diagnosed.

It's not clear what causes ovarian cancer, but as you might expect with an organ whose job is to create hormones, there seems to be a hormonal link.

Risk Factors for Ovarian Cancer

Ovarian cancer is most common in women whose families have a history of it. The lifetime probability of ovarian cancer increases from about 1.6 percent in a thirty-five-year-old woman who has no family history of ovarian cancer to about 5 percent if she has one first-degree relative (a mother, sister, or daughter) with it and 7 percent if she has two affected first-degree relatives. Women who have the BRCA 1 gene (see Chapter 7) have a 50 percent risk of ovarian cancer over a lifetime.[22]

The risk for ovarian cancer increases the more you ovulate. So the younger you are when you get your first period and the older you are when you reach menopause, the higher your risk. There have been several observational studies of a possible link between fertility drugs (which increase ovulation) and ovarian cancer. Although there seems to be an increased risk, these studies were too small to allow certainty. Several large studies are now looking into the issue.[23]

Birth control pills, on the other hand, decrease the risk of ovarian cancer, probably because they decrease ovulation. The thirty-five-year-old with two relatives who have ovarian cancer could reduce her risk to about between 3 and 4 percent by taking birth control pills for five to nine years.

One retrospective observational study found that women who had hysterectomies reduced their chances of getting ovarian cancer by about 30 percent.[24] But this study is a bit shaky because among the women who had hysterectomies, it wasn't always clear how many still had one or both ovaries. In some cases, the surgeons had taken out one ovary and left the other. In some cases, part of an ovary was removed. In others, the ovaries were left intact. That could well account for some of the apparent reduction of risk. Some critics of the study have also pointed out that the surgeon doing the hysterectomy had a chance to look at the ovaries and was likely to leave them in only if they looked healthy.

Estrogen and Ovarian Cancer

Large observational studies have suggested that estrogen therapy may actually increase the chance of getting ovarian cancer. One study found that women on estrogen replacement therapy had higher death rates from ovarian cancer.[25] Between 1982 and 1989, the researchers observed 240,073 peri- and postmenopausal women who hadn't had either a hysterectomy or ovarian surgery. In those seven years, 436 women died of ovarian cancer. The incidence was higher in women who took hormones postmenopausally for more than six years; their risk increased by 72 percent. The women who took hormones for a time and then stopped had a 48 percent increase in risk.

This study looked only at use of estrogen. So far, we have no way of knowing whether progestins and progesterone increase the risk, decrease it, or have no effect at all. Progestin increases the risk of breast cancer and decreases the risk of endometrial cancer, so we can't make any assumptions about what it does to the ovaries.

So far, again, the studies are inconclusive. We need more and better studies. But they're hard to do, because with such a rare cancer, only studies on very large numbers of women will give us any significant data.

Gallbladder Disease

Estrogen affects the way bile is metabolized, and thus it can lead to gallstones. Because of this, gallbladder disease is more common in women than in men. Women on Premarin have two and a half times as many gallbladder operations as other women.[26] The risk is higher if you're currently taking hormones, and it decreases five years after you stop. There's a theory that this risk doesn't occur in women who take hormones through a patch rather than as a pill, since the patch doesn't require breakdown in the liver, but there haven't been enough studies yet to prove this.

Although gallstones are rarely fatal, they often require surgery, with all of its risks and complications. Gallbladder removal can now often be done with a laparoscope and so entails less time in the hospital; still, it's an operation and it's not a lot of fun.

Risk factors for gallbladder disease include being overweight, eating a high-fat diet, having a family history of the disease, and high fertility. Generally it's a disease of middle-aged women. When I was in medical school, the teachers said that the risks for gallbladder disease were being female, fat, fertile, and forty.

Thromboembolic Disease

The term *thromboembolic disease* refers to conditions in which the body is more likely to form blood clots. It includes thrombophlebitis (clots in the veins), pulmonary embolus (blood clots that have traveled to the lungs), and clots that form in arteries in the legs. Strokes and heart attacks can also be considered thromboembolic if they're caused by a clot traveling to and then blocking an already narrowed artery.

The early high-dose birth control pills increased the risk of blood clots, especially in older women who were smokers. As a result, there has been a lingering concern that estrogen therapy would do the same.

There are experimental data showing that estrogen increases clotting factors. This appears to be related to dose: the higher the dose of estrogen, the higher the risk of clotting. If you smoke, the risk is even higher. In one study of oral contraceptives, smokers on the pill had 4 times more clotting episodes than women who weren't on the pill, while nonsmokers had only 1.7 times the risk of women who weren't on the pill.[27] Another study of postmenopausal women on estrogen, however, found no effect.[28]

But in October 1996, three studies increased the concern about thromboembolic disease caused by hormone therapy. Each of the three studies[29,30,31] showed a two- to fourfold increase in phlebitis in the veins of the legs, whether the women took estrogen alone or combined with a progestin. In addition, there was a doubling of the risk of pulmonary embolus, a potentially fatal condition that occurs when one of the clots travels to the lungs. The increase in phlebitis occurred soon after the women started hormone therapy, which means that if you're prone to phlebitis, you should be careful about taking hormones even for a short time to relieve your symptoms. It's interesting that these findings got almost no press attention, while the findings that hormone therapy had a favorable effect on osteoarthritis (see page 139), which was published at almost the same time, was widely reported.

The final answer on this issue isn't in. Some clinicians feel that if you have any history of clotting problems such as thrombophlebitis, you shouldn't be on estrogen therapy. Others feel that only repeated episodes of clotting represent a contraindication. These might indicate a genetic propensity to clot, but if you had one episode of thrombophlebitis after a broken leg (a situation likely to cause temporary clotting), that wouldn't count. Most doctors agree that women shouldn't be on estrogen therapy immediately following a heart attack or a stroke because of the risk of further clot formation. (I know we said it was probably good to be on estrogen at the moment you have a heart attack, but this is after.) Since most of the effects of the clotting factors come from having estrogen pass through the liver, women who have a propensity for clotting should use the patch or some other parenteral route (see page 260) if they really want to be on estrogen.

Fibroids

As we mention in Chapter 3, fibroids tend to shrink with menopause. This would lead you to believe that fibroids will bloom again if you start hormone therapy. And you are probably right. One study showed that much of the bleeding problems of postmenopausal women on estrogen came from submucosal fibroids that were reactivated by the hormones.[32] Another study found an increase in size of fibroids in women using the patch and a progestin, but not in those taking estrogen and a progestin by mouth.[33]

Endometriosis

Endometriosis is a condition in which some of the lining of the uterus travels to other areas, usually in the abdomen. Patches of uterine tissue can end up on the bladder, the large intestine, or the lining of the abdomen. This wouldn't be a problem except for the fact that these patches can respond to your cyclical hormones and bleed or swell, causing pain. The treatment is often with hormone blockers such as Luprin. If that doesn't work, you might need a total hysterectomy and removal of both ovaries. If you are then started on estrogen therapy and there are any patches left over somewhere, you may still have problems.[34,35] This may be one reason to either forgo hormones or add a progestin to estrogen even though you have had a hysterectomy.

Lupus

Lupus is an autoimmune disease that attacks almost every organ of the body. It can be fatal. It's more common in African-American women than in white women. The Nurses' Health Study has found women on hormone therapy double their risk of lupus.[36] We have no idea why this might be, but women with autoimmune diseases or with a family history of lupus should be cautious about hormone therapy.

Other Diseases

Small observational studies have linked estrogen therapy with an increase in risk for several other diseases. One is *asthma*,[37] but the data are so preliminary it's hard to know how to interpret them. Some studies suggest that estrogen therapy can increase the risk of *melanoma*, a severe kind of skin cancer that's often fatal if not caught early. Melanomas[38] are known to be sensitive to hormones, and any woman with a history of melanoma should be cautious about hormone therapy.

In the spring of 1996, a report came out showing that women have a higher death rate from *lung cancer* than men and have more lung cancers even when they don't smoke.[39] This preliminary study suggested that estrogen therapy could increase the risk of lung cancer. Again, more study is needed to confirm this.

None of this means that you shouldn't consider taking hormones, especially if you really need them to relieve short-term symptoms. But you should certainly factor all these possibilities into your decision. Taking hormones may be worth the risks; then again, it may not. The next few chapters will help you make that decision.

CHAPTER 10

What Are My Options for Feeling Better Right Now?

So far we've been talking about what causes perimenopausal and menopausal symptoms, what diseases you're more vulnerable to as you get older, how hormones affect them, and what the drug companies want you to think about all of this. And you've probably been sitting there thinking, "Well, yes—but what am I supposed to do *right now?*" Preventing life-threatening diseases is ultimately more important to your health than dealing with current symptoms, but it's also less immediate. You can decide next month, next year, or later than that if you want to take steps to prevent osteoporosis or heart disease. But if you're experiencing unpleasant symptoms right now, even next month can be a long time away. You want to know how to get a good night's sleep *tonight.* You need your hot flashes gone by next week when you have to speak at a convention. You need a solution for vaginal dryness before your two-week vacation in Hawaii.

In chapters 12 to 15 we'll talk in more detail about lifestyle changes, alternative approaches, drugs, and surgery as they relate to a healthy life and to prevention of disease. Chapter 16 will offer suggestions about how you can incorporate all the information in the book into a personalized formula to help you determine what, if anything, you want to do about menopause. But in the present chapter and Chapter 11, I want to focus on different options for what you're feeling right now. If you're one of the lucky 10 percent of women who have no perimenopausal or menopausal symptoms, you can just skip ahead.

The first step is to let you know that *there are different options.* This is something your doctor may not tell you. Too often, doctors act as though you have only one choice—hormones. You've got hot flashes? Take hormones. You're nervous about vaginal dryness? Take hormones. You don't have hot flashes and you're not nervous about vaginal dryness? Take hormones anyway—you never know what might happen.

Well, there *are* other approaches besides hormones; there are even other drugs. And you should know about all of them before you decide what to do—or what not to do.

The second step is to remind you that *you may not want, or need, to do anything.* I'm always struck by the absurdity of a doctor telling a symptom-free woman with a spry ninety-year-old mother that she must do something to "treat" her menopause or dire things will happen. Your symptoms may be so mild that you'd rather just put up with them for a while and not change your habits or risk your health to control them. For many women, the best way to "manage menopause" is to just go about your life and let it happen.

My goal here is not to give you a prescription but rather to present a menu from which you can choose what seems most reasonable to you. What you choose to do may depend on how much your symptoms are bothering you or how fast you feel you need to relieve them—or on a number of other factors, which we'll discuss in depth in Chapter 16.

Since nothing exists in a vacuum, you'll soon see that some of the options for addressing short-term symptoms also help prevent disease. The exercise you do to help you deal with hot flashes and insomnia may have the "side effect" of adding years to your life. The estrogen you use for vaginal dryness may help prevent osteoporosis. Therefore, you'll probably want to read all of Chapters 11 to 16 before you decide on a course of action.

OPTIONS FOR TREATING SYMPTOMS: THREE LEVELS OF APPROACHES

The strategy I'm always most comfortable with is one that starts with the least risky approaches and goes on to riskier approaches only if necessary. Unless you're in an emergency situation, I always think it's worth trying the lowest-level, safest approach first, and moving up to the next level or levels only if that fails. And I find it useful to categorize the levels as (1) lifestyle approaches, (2) alternative approaches, and (3) drugs and surgical approaches.

The first level is lifestyle approaches—making changes in the way you eat, exercise, or otherwise go about your life. Level 1 involves little or no risk. Some of the interventions at this level are simply common sense: if you have hot flashes, dress in layers. Some are less familiar: eat more tofu to decrease hot flashes. The second level I call *alternative* approaches. Unlike the lifestyle options, all of the interventions at level 2 require you to buy something (such as herbs or supplements) or to go to a practitioner (such as an acupuncturist). But they're still approaches that, if embarked on carefully, involve little or no risk. The third level is *drugs and surgery.* Interventions at level 3 involve the highest risk, and often the highest cost.

Some approaches, or treatments, are specific for a particular symptom, while others are good for many symptoms. I'll discuss each approach in general first, in this chapter, and then discuss their applications for specific symptoms in Chapter 11.

LEVEL 1: LIFESTYLE APPROACHES

Surprisingly, there has been less research on how changing your lifestyle can affect symptoms of perimenopause and menopause than on how it can help prevent disease. Nonetheless, a healthy diet, exercise, and stress reduction are important tools for combating many of the symptoms you may have. Becoming more fit, as we discuss in Chapter 12, will help you feel better in general, and that certainly will affect your short-term symptoms. What you eat is important; as we have discussed in Chapter 2, Japanese women have few menopausal symptoms and no word for hot flashes. This has been attributed to their lifestyle, including a diet that is very high in soy, which contains plant estrogens (phytoestrogens). And techniques for reducing stress can lessen or even eliminate some symptoms.

LEVEL 2: ALTERNATIVE APPROACHES

Alternative medicine, including herbal remedies and acupuncture, has been getting increasing attention as we begin to realize that Western medicine may not have all the answers. Still, the United States is behind most of the world in accepting them. Only one third of Americans are now seeking complementary therapies, compared with 50 percent of Europeans and 80 percent of the world's population as a whole.[1] Also, unfortunately, alternative methods can sometimes be more expensive than hormone therapy and other Western medicine, because most insurance plans won't cover them. This is changing, however, and some managed care plans do cover alternative practitioners.

What you most want to know, of course, is how effective alternative approaches are. Ideally, we should have a lot of solid, long-term scientific studies to turn to. Sadly, we don't. Some alternative remedies have been tested scientifically and some haven't. (Of course, as we have seen, we don't have many scientific studies on hormone therapy either.) Many Western scientists, with their proprietary attachment to our own allopathic, or traditional Western medical, approach, have ridiculed or ignored alternative approaches. American researchers in this country are now starting to remedy this, however. Growing interest in this area has given rise to the recently created Office of Alternative Medicine at the National Institutes of Health. Columbia University in New York City has a study looking at Chinese herbs for treating hot flashes, and Tufts University in Boston has two studies looking at soy protein for treating several menopausal symptoms. Still, in my own search of the literature, I've found that most of the good studies on herbs have been done by the Chinese; and none of them specifically addressed symptoms of perimenopause and menopause, probably because Chinese women usually don't have the symptoms Western women complain of.

Dr. Rosemary Duda[2] of Harvard did a small survey of 201 postmenopausal women. Some of these women had had breast cancer, which meant that they weren't considered candidates for hormone treatment. Duda found that 35 percent of the women were using nontraditional therapies—including chiropractic, acupuncture, massage, spiritual approaches, and meditation—to treat perimenopausal and menopausal symptoms. Ninety-six percent of those women got relief from their menopausal symptoms; and although only 3 percent of the postmenopausal women and 12 percent of the postmenopausal women with breast cancer used herbal remedies for relief of symptoms, 74 percent of them found these remedies highly effective.

As with hormone therapy, though, many of the studies we do have on alternative treatments were not randomized or controlled (see Chapter 4), and so the value of the treatments studied is still in doubt. And—again as with hormone therapy—until we have these gold standard studies, we can't say with absolute assurance that these methods work all the time, or that they don't have any side effects. This doesn't mean that you might not want to try something, even if it isn't proven—you just should know that it isn't. Committed as I am to vigorous scientific research, I don't believe that the comparative lack of studies on most of these alternatives should keep you from considering them, any more than it should keep you from considering hormone therapy. Most of these approaches come out of centuries-old traditions and have worked for millions of people.

Unfortunately, in the eternal quest for easy answers, some people now deify alternative methods as they once deified Western medicine. But just as we're learning to insist on proof that what the M.D.s tell us is really accurate, we need to demand as much proof as possible for every alternative mode. In the same way that we can't say with certainty that the combination of estrogen and progesterone is effective and safe for long-term use, we can't say with certainty that homeopathy or Chinese herbs are effective or safe. People tend to be in one of two camps: either they feel that since these methods haven't been studied for years in a Western laboratory setting, they must be quackery; or they believe that since these methods don't involve *drugs* in the commonly used sense of the word, they're safe and natural. Neither belief is wholly accurate. As with Western drugs, we need to look at each alternative therapy to see what is known about its long-term safety or efficacy, and how that knowledge has been acquired. In both situations you have to consider all the information available and make your own choices. When you've acquired enough information, or at least understood the limits of the information you have, then you can decide which approach or combination of approaches is best for you.

Indeed, a combination of approaches is often the most useful route to take. An either/or mentality toward conventional and alternative approaches can deprive you of the best solutions for your health issues. My coauthor, who has had severe chronic asthma for many years and was taking large amounts of medication daily, has been working with an acupuncturist since 1995. Now she sees the acupuncturist about once a month and continues to take her medications. But she takes a quarter of the medication she used to take, and her asthma is far better controlled than it was by the drugs alone.

Just as you should shop around until you find a gynecologist or primary care physician whose skill you trust and who you feel shares your philosophy of health and life, you need to find an alternative practitioner who meets your standards. Some forms of medicine (such as Chinese medicine) are associated with philosophical or religious points of view. They are based on a belief that spiritual, emotional, and physical harmony or balance is the key to health. Other traditions, such as homeopathy, have a different theory of treatment. Some disciplines, such as naturopathy, include several differing schools of thought, some of which you may feel more comfortable with than others.

I think we need to approach every practitioner and practice the same way—with a critical and questioning mind. Throughout this book, I've been asking you to question the standard Western approach to menopause as a disease that requires drug treatment, and we need to be equally questioning of, for example, the Chinese theory that menopause is a diminishing of *jing* energy. By "questioning," I don't mean "dismissing." As you question, you come up with answers, and they aren't always the answers you might have expected before you started asking your questions. The theory behind any practice is important, but it isn't the only thing that matters. You may not believe that menopause is a disease, but you can still get relief from your hot flashes with hormones. Nor do you have to believe in *jing* energy to get relief from acupuncture or Chinese herbs.

Some practitioners, such as those who practice acupuncture, are licensed by the state. Others, such as herbalists, are not. In Appendix 1, I list various governing or licensing bodies for some of the different disciplines and ways to find an appropriate practitioner. Even if they're not actually licensed, however, all reputable practitioners have some kind of training, and it's worth your while to find out what that training is when you're thinking of working with any health care practitioner. (Like M.D.s, most alternative practitioners are likely to display their accreditation certificates on their walls, so if you're too shy to ask, you can start from there.)

As with Western doctors, making sure practitioners have the appropriate credentials or training is only a first step. You also have to make sure you're comfortable with and confident about their approach to your problem. The relationship between practitioner and patient is one of the most important aspects of any healing tradition. Practitioners of alternative healing are as varied in their personalities and approaches to patients as are medical doctors.

Some of the more relevant alternative approaches for perimenopausal and menopausal symptoms—herbs, biofeedback, acupuncture, and homeopathy—are worth reviewing generally before we get specific.

Herbs

An *herb*, as I'm using the term here, is basically a plant used for a medicinal purpose. In this country, their use is now considered alternative, though in France and Germany 30 to 40 percent of medical doctors use herbal remedies as their primary approach. Many drugs currently used in the United States are based on herbs, but because a plant can't be patented, American pharmaceutical companies sometimes isolate the active ingredient of an herb and then patent that as a drug. In addition, the FDA requires that any herb marketed for a medical purpose must meet the same standards as a drug—an expensive and time-consuming process that many manufacturers don't want to undertake. As a result, most herbs are sold as food supplements rather than as medications. Many Americans thus have the impression that herbal preparations are weak and ineffective. This has been a double-edged sword. People often either dismiss the healing properties of herbs or underrate the potential dangers. (I read a report of digitalis poisoning that occurred because an inexperienced consumer mistakenly used foxglove to make tea.)[3]

In Europe, herbal products can be marketed as drugs only if they have been proven safe and effective. In countries such as Japan and Germany, herbs are better-regulated, dispensed only by licensed pharmacists, and covered by insurance when a doctor has prescribed them. Because all this is lacking in the United States, there is no regulation of herbs, and thus there's a great variation in quality. There have been recent reports of "ginseng tea" with no ginseng. And, as we discuss in Chapter 13, there have been rare but serious problems with contaminated traditional Chinese herbal formulas.

Many factors go into making an herb effective. The plant must be properly identified, and it has to be harvested at the right time of year, when it's most potent. The best way to ensure the quality of any herb you use is to collect and process it yourself. This, of course, requires a certain degree of expertise—not to mention time and energy. If you pick the wrong herb, you may harm instead of help yourself. For those of you who are interested, I recommend Susun Weed's books, which show pictures and give recipes for processing.[4]

If you don't want to grow or collect your own herbs, you can order them by mail (see Appendix 2) or buy them in a local health food store, a Chinese pharmacy, or sometimes even in a local grocery. I suggest that you carefully read the label on any herb you buy; it should include the amount of the active ingredient in each capsule. If you're getting herbs off the shelf rather than through a qualified practitioner, you might be wise to get a recognized brand. Identify the herb you're buying by its botanical name, to avoid confusion.

Another concern is always whether herbs are safe. It's one thing to make sure an herb has the right active ingredient—but can that ingredient do any harm? Reports from the American Association of Poison Control Centers and the Center for Disease Control show that most herbs are perfectly safe. They found no substantial evidence that herbal products are a major source of toxic reactions.[5] Nonetheless, this doesn't mean that you should use herbs without learning all you can about them. And keep in mind that *natural* does not mean "safe." You can walk into your local health food store and easily buy herbs capable of causing miscarriage, heavy menstrual bleeding, or worse. Recently a supplement called ephedra was banned in several states when reports surfaced linking it with several fatalities.

This makes it very important for you to know the source of your medications. Not all herbs are equal. As with drugs, some can counteract others. You need to read up on the subject and work with a reliable practitioner who can guide you. I suggest that you seek the advice of an herbalist, a traditional Chinese doctor, or a naturopath—just as you would consult with your doctor before taking a new medication. This is also the best way to ensure that if you take an herbal pill, it will be effective and safe. Further, working with a qualified practitioner gives you the benefit of someone who will take your whole medical history into consideration, just as a principled M.D. will do. And always tell your primary care doctor if you're taking any herbs. Both of your practitioners can help you determine if the herbs could interfere with any other medications you're on or could aggravate any medical condition. For example, some herbs can be dangerous for people with high blood pressure. Marie Cargill, an herbalist and acupuncturist, notes that many Americans have very disturbed, dysfunctional digestive systems, resulting from the birth control pill, antibiotics, or various and sundry other drugs. "This changes the whole flora of your stomach and gastrointestinal tract," she says, adding that since many herbs need to be digested, this change in flora can affect their absorption and make you ill.[6]

Herbs can be taken in a number of forms. Sometimes you prepare them as a tea. This is usually a small amount of herb brewed in hot water for a short time. It's a good way to deliver some herbs but is relatively weak. A very strong tea—a lot of herbs brewed for a long time—is called an infusion. Tinctures or fluid extracts are made by soaking the herb in alcohol. Tinctures are generally the most effective method of taking herbs. Pills are a grab bag—many are good, but others contain so little active herb that they're virtually worthless. Nonetheless, pills are the most popular for Americans—we're accustomed to taking our medications in pill form rather than taking the time to brew or soak them. And we tend to dislike the taste of many herbs, though some, like chamomile, have become fairly popular. If you're taking an herb in capsule form and it appears to be having no effect, consider trying a tincture or tea before abandoning it entirely.

Everyone has an individual reaction to herbs, just as to foods and drugs—and this includes allergic reactions. I suggest that you stick to one herb at a time, or wait until you have used one herb for a period of time before adding a second. Side effects from herbs are usually milder than those from drugs, but they can happen. If you find that an herb is affecting your digestion, stick with it for a few days to see if your body is simply adjusting to it. An herb that really doesn't agree with you may cause nausea, dizziness, stomach pains, diarrhea, headache, or blurred vision, and these effects generally come on quite quickly. If you experience any of these reactions, stop taking the herb immediately—or decrease the dose drastically—and report the reaction to your practitioner or doctor. Trust your body. If something makes you feel worse, don't take it. And never assume that if a little is good, more is better—any more than with Western medication. One aspirin will make your headache go away; twenty will land you in the hospital.

Herbs used specifically for menopausal symptoms are those that appear to have plant hormones or hormone precursors in them, or those that stimulate the formation of these hormones. These plant estrogens, called phytoestrogens, can bind with the estrogen receptors in your body and compete (by trying to fill the same receptor) with your natural estrogen.

They have the interesting ability to raise a low level of estrogen but lower a high level (by replacing a strong estrogen with a weaker one). Because of this, they're often known as "balancers." In a premenopausal woman, they decrease estrogen; in a postmenopausal woman, they increase it.

Women who have had breast cancer are often concerned about using herbs that are phytoestrogens. Will such herbs cause a recurrence, or a new breast cancer? The answers are really not in yet. The level of estrogen in these plants is very low; their activity is at most only 2 percent as strong as estradiol.[7] In addition, some of the phytoestrogens, such as the genestein in soy (see Chapter 12), block tyrosine kinase, an important enzyme for cancer growth, and also block the development of new blood vessels in tumors. These antitumor effects seem to outweigh any slight estrogenic stimulation they might have. There is also a theory that some phytoestrogens might act like tamoxifen (a drug used to treat women with breast cancer), blocking estrogen in the breast and acting like it in other organs. But we're not certain of this. In the absence of data, I think it's probably better to use the herbs that aren't directly thought to be estrogenic to treat symptoms of perimenopause and menopause (see Table 10.1). Nonetheless, if it's a choice between herbs and medications like Premarin, I think you're better off going with the herbs.

TABLE 10.1   Natural Agents that Affect Hormones

Agent	Effect
Agents that reduce estrogen in women	
Camellia sinensis (green tea)	Inhibits interaction between estrogen and estrogen receptors in estrogen-responsive tumors in vitro.[8]
Dang gui shao yao san (formula)	Suppresses estradiol secretion by rat ovarian follicles in vitro.[9]
Dietary fat reduction	Decreases estrogen production and increases estrogen metabolism.[10,11]
Fiber	Binds estrogen in human feces and facilitates estrogen elimination.[12,13]
Genistein (isoflavone)	Increases production of sex-hormone-binding globulin in vitro.[14,15]
Gui zhi fu ling wan (formula)	Acts as weak antiestrogen agent in female rats by inhibiting ovarian DNA synthesis. Reduced plasma estradiol levels by 50 percent when given orally to female rats. Suppresses estradiol secretion by rat ovarian follicles in vitro.[16]

TABLE 10.1   *(Continued)*

Agent	Effect
Humulus lupulus (hops)	Prevented estrogen production in female rats stimulated with gonadotropins. Gonadotropins are hormones produced by the pituitary gland and placenta that stimulate the male or female sex organs.[17]
Lignans	Although lignans, such as those found in flaxseed (*Linun usitatissimum*), possess weak estrogen activity, they may produce weak antiestrogen effects by competing for estrogen receptor sites, especially in premenopausal women.[18]
Phytoestrogens	Phytoestrogens, such as those found in soy, compete with estrogen for binding to receptor sites. Phytoestrogens also act as weak estrogens and appear to produce estrogen effects in postmenopausal women and antiestrogen effects in premenopausal women.[19,20]
Xiao yao san and *er chen tang* (formulas)	Markedly decreased saliva estradiol levels in women with proliferative breast disease.[21]
Agents that increase estrogen	
Foeniculum vulgare (fennel)	Stimulated estrogen production in animals. Active ingredients are thought to be in the essential oils.[22]
Glycyrrhiza uralensis (*gan cao*) and *Paeonia lactiflora* (*bai shao* and *chi shao*)	These herbs stimulate the activity of aromatase, an enzyme that converts testosterone to estrogen. Paeoniflorin (from *P. lactiflora*), and glycyrrhizin and glycyrrhetinic acid (from *G. uralensis*) stimulated aromatase activity in the rat ovary to promote estradiol synthesis. Formulas containing *P. lactiflora* increased estradiol secretion from cultured rat ovarian follicles. A formula consisting of *P. lactiflora* and *G. uralensis* increased DHEA-S, a precursor of estrogen, and increased serum estrogen concentrations in rats whose ovaries were surgically removed. This formula lowered serum testosterone levels in sterilized female rats by stimulating aromatase activity. When the formula was administered to women with polycystic ovarian disease, serum testosterone levels decreased and the ratio of estrogen to testosterone increased. In conventional medicine, inhibitors of aromatase have been used in the treatment of breast cancer.[23]
Liu wei di huang tang (formula)	This formula increased plasma estradiol levels and increased estrogen receptors on leukocytes in menopausal women. In contrast, the formula increased plasma testosterone and lowered plasma estradiol in patients with *kidney yin vacuity*, a disease pattern in Chinese medicine that is common in menopausal women.[24]

TABLE 10.1   *(Continued)*

Agent	Effect
Pimpinella anisum (anise)	Stimulated estrogen production in animals. The active ingredients are thought to be in the essential oils.[25]
Salvia miltiorrhiza (dan shen)	Increased the level of plasma estradiol in female rats.[26]

Biofeedback

Biofeedback uses physical measurements to help you to learn to regulate certain bodily functions. This technique can be helpful for people who have trouble being aware of their bodies. It's also useful in influencing or controlling other symptoms such as headaches, chronic pain, asthma, and muscle disorders. Biofeedback has been effectively used to treat urinary incontinence, which is discussed in Chapter 11.

Acupuncture

Acupuncture, which is the form of Chinese medicine most familiar to Americans, has been used for many of the symptoms of menopause. It's based on the premise that acupuncture needles can be placed in the body so as to affect *chi,* the life force energy, which travels through paths known as meridians. Along the meridian are many points. Each meridian and each point are involved in a number of problems—or imbalances. For example, point 6 in the spleen meridian is considered the origin of many menstrual problems, and an acupuncturist treating heavy bleeding would include this point in the needling process. Fibroids, uterine cysts, and migraines also belong in part to this point. The kidney meridian is also involved in most of these problems.[27]

An acupuncture treatment targets several points along one or more meridians. Today the needles are usually disposable, since patients fear AIDS. Some practitioners prefer to use nondisposable needles, which they sterilize, but you can always insist on disposable needles. Sometimes a needle can sting very slightly, but usually you don't even feel it going in.

Many acupuncturists prefer to work with a combination of acupuncture and Chinese herbs, both of which are components of traditional Chinese medicine. Not all acupuncturists are practitioners of Chinese herbal medicine, but almost all practitioners of Chinese herbal medicine are also acupuncturists. So if you're interested in combining the two—which may be the most effective use of Chinese medicine—it's important to ask if an acupuncturist has studied Chinese herbal medicine when you're seeking out a practitioner.

There are more than thirty American schools and colleges of acupuncture and Chinese medicine. In addition, there is a national Council of Acupuncturist Schools and Colleges, which oversees the training and education of practitioners, and the National Commission for the Certification of Acupuncturists, which helps to ensure competence. There are also national associations. To date, acupuncture has been legalized as a form of health care in over twenty states; several other states are in the process of legalizing it. Some insurers will even pay for acupuncture for certain conditions. In states where acupuncture is licensed and regulated, you can find the names of practitioners by contacting the state department of health or department of licensing. In other states, make sure that an acupuncturist is board certified. This usually means that "Dipl. Ac."—for "diplomate of acupuncture"—appears after the practitioner's name.

Homeopathy

Homeopathy claims that its roots go back to Hippocrates. It was formally organized by Samuel Hahneman in the 1790s. He proposed the law of similars, or "Like cures like." This means that a substance that can produce a set of symptoms in a healthy person can be used in greatly diluted portions to treat someone who suffers from those symptoms. This isn't as odd as it might first sound. It's similar to what we do with vaccines, in which we use a small, modified virus to enable the body to develop immunity to the disease caused by the virus. It's also similar to desensitization methods used in treating allergies.

Underlying this principle is the concept of vital energy, which is similar to *chi* in traditional Chinese medicine. When you're healthy, the theory goes, you're in a state of balance and harmony. When the balance is destroyed, symptoms are the body's way of trying to restore it. Therefore you should never simply suppress symptoms. Allopathic (traditional Western) medicine tries to help the body get well by destroying the pathogens that cause a disease, while Chinese medicine seeks to strengthen the body's ability to deal with disease. Homeopathy tries to provoke the body in order to strengthen its vital force so that it can heal itself. Homeopathic practitioners feel that the pharmaceutical approach of Western medicine doesn't strengthen the body but may actually weaken and disrupt it further. There are homeopathic remedies intended for acute and chronic symptoms, as well as some intended to strengthen the constitution so that the symptoms won't recur. A homeopathic practitioner carefully studies the symptoms and then chooses the remedy that will most closely mimic them.

Homeopathy can be helpful with many of the symptoms of menopause, since it's an individualized approach and each woman's symptoms manifest themselves differently. The exact match of remedy and symptom is important for the success of homeopathy. (Since homeopathy focuses on symptoms, it isn't used for prevention.)

There have been some studies and clinical trials of homeopathy, including double-blind prospective studies, and they've found that it often has an effect. (Unfortunately, though, none of the studies looked at the treatment of menopausal symptoms.) Some researchers feel that results achieved with homeopathy are simply the placebo effect—that the amount of the active ingredient is too small to have any real effect. Nonetheless, one randomized, controlled double-blind crossover study of homeopathic belladonna showed that healthy volunteers did notice a difference between the homeopathic belladonna and a placebo. (The study was not trying to treat anything, but rather trying to demonstrate that a homeopathic remedy had more than a placebo effect.)[28] Despite such data, many doctors are uncomfortable about encouraging homeopathy because they can't explain how it works. I find this prejudice rather ludicrous; there's much in Western medicine that we still don't fully understand but that we use anyway because we know it works—aspirin, for example.

There is currently no licensing in homeopathy. Most practitioners are licensed providers from another discipline, and they include practitioners of other healing arts. Many are M.D.s, chiropractors, naturopaths, acupuncturists, nurses, nurse practitioners, physician's assistants, pharmacists, or dentists. You should ask about the training of any practitioner you're considering working with. Several organizations have tried to establish a certifying exam, but the exams are relatively new, so lack of certification doesn't necessarily mean that a practitioner is no good. (A list of training institutions and certifying groups is given in Appendix 1.)

You'll see many over-the-counter homeopathic remedies at health stores and even supermarkets, but because of the highly individualized nature of the practice, they're probably a waste of money. The one you pick off the shelf may or may not match your symptoms well enough to benefit you. I suggest consulting a trained homeopath first, to direct you to the right remedy. Nevertheless, for your information, we'll point out some of the most commonly used remedies for menopausal symptoms in Chapter 11.

LEVEL 3: DRUGS AND SURGICAL APPROACHES

We can talk all day about the benefits of a healthy lifestyle and the advantages of herbs and other alternative approaches, but there will always be women who need or want to go to the third level of treatment, which includes drugs (hormones and others) and surgical procedures, both major and minor. Side effects are inevitable with this approach, and they run the gamut from mildly irritating to devastating. Often, however, the side effects are well worth the relief or the protection that this approach provides. The risk may well be worthwhile in your individual case, but you need to know exactly what you are risking. I'll discuss all the combinations and permutations of hormonal drugs in Chapter 15.

Remember that these three levels of approaches aren't mutually exclusive. You can use different approaches at different times or combine several at the same time. There are all kinds of possibilities, depending on what you need at any given moment.

CHAPTER 11

From Flashes to Fuzzy Thinking: What You Can Do Right Now

Let's look now at the most common short-term perimenopausal symptoms and the ways they can be treated. I'll tell you where we have data and where we don't. If you have a symptom not covered here, you may still want to try one of these approaches by seeing a practitioner who can fashion a treatment just for you.

HOT FLASHES AND NIGHT SWEATS

Hot flashes and night sweats can be extremely variable. You can get them every day for two weeks, and then they're gone for a month or two. This can make it difficult to know whether a treatment is having an effect. It seems to work, you breathe a sigh of relief—and a few weeks later you're flashing again. With hot flashes, you really need a lot of patience. Try something, see what happens, and if it works, stick with it for a while. Then, after a few months or a year, stop what you're doing and see if the flashes are gone for good.

Approaches for Hot Flashes

Lifestyle: *dress in layers, avoid caffeine and alcohol, exercise, eat a high-soy (50 g/day) diet; try meditation, stress reduction, visualization, affirmations*
Supplements: *vitamin E (800 mg/day); B vitamins; bioflavinoids (250 mg 5–6 times a day); herbs such as black cohosh, dong quai, fennel, anise, sarsaparilla, wild yam root, motherwort*

Treatments: *acupuncture, paced respiration, homeopathy*
Drugs: *clonidine, natural progesterone, Megace, estrogen therapy or hormone
   therapy*

Lifestyle Changes

Keep It Cool

The first steps in dealing with hot flashes are the obvious ones. Dress in layers so that you can adapt your attire to your temperature at any given time.
Keep the temperature of the room cooler. Although this may sound too
simple, there's actually scientific evidence that it works. One study found
that women who stayed in a cool room (68 degrees F, or 19 degrees C) had
significantly fewer and less intense hot flashes than women in a warmer
room (86 degrees F, or 31 degrees C).[1] The researcher in this study reported
that a woman whose drenching hot flashes woke her up hourly at home
slept through the night when she stayed in the cooler laboratory overnight
as part of the study.[2]

Exercise

Only two studies, both observational, have looked at whether exercise can
affect hot flashes. In one, women who belonged to a fitness club reported
less severe hot flashes than those who did not.[3] Unfortunately, this study
didn't examine how much physical activity the women performed. The second study[4] found that only 6 percent of physically active women have hot
flashes, compared with 25 percent of women who don't exercise regularly.
Many woman have suggested that they "walked their way through menopause," and I'd certainly recommend trying exercise—it's got so many benefits to offer and little downside (see Chapter 12).

Pinpoint Your Triggers

Some women can pinpoint what will trigger their flashes—a hot cup of tea,
for instance, or a stressful family battle. Some triggers are more avoidable
than others. You can forgo tea, but unless your teenager transforms herself
into Mother Teresa, family battles may be inescapable. Nonetheless, you
might find it helpful to keep a "hot flash diary" for a few days to help you
identify what your triggers are and which you *can* avoid. Even if you can't
circumvent triggers completely, just knowing ahead of time that a certain
situation is likely to cause a flash will help you feel more prepared for it.
(Not all flashes have identifiable triggers, unfortunately.) Many women find

that eliminating spicy foods, caffeine, and alcohol can reduce their flashes. Drinking lots of cool water can help as well.

Eat Soy Protein

Soy protein appears to decrease hot flashes. (Remember those Japanese women who have no word for hot flash?) A randomized controlled study in Australia compared the effects of soy flour and unbleached wheat flour in forty-seven women with hot flashes. Women who ate an additional 40 grams of soy flour a day showed a rapid and significant decrease in hot flashes. The number of flashes and their intensity decreased by 40 percent within six weeks and continued to decrease over the next six weeks. The group who ate wheat flour, which was meant to be the placebo group, had no change in flashes for the first six weeks. But then, interestingly, their hot flashes decreased by 25 percent in rate and intensity in the second six weeks. (Wheat flour probably wasn't the best choice for a placebo, because it too contains phytoestrogens, although weaker ones than soy. Still, that's good to know: if you eat a lot of wheat, it can lessen your hot flashes.[5])

Two centers are currently conducting randomized double-blind controlled studies of soy for treating menopausal symptoms. In one study, 240 women who have hot flashes or night sweats will all drink a soy-rich beverage every day for two years. Although the individual women won't know which soy drink they have, one group will get less than 1 milligram of isoflavone (the phytoestrogen in soy), a second group will get 34 milligrams, and a third group will get 50 milligrams. Their hot flashes and other perimenopausal symptoms will be tracked. Another study will track the effects of soy on hot flashes for women at high risk for breast cancer or with breast cancer.

Clearly, you'll have even more data about soy in the near future. In Chapter 12, I'll discuss more about soy and different ways to add it to your diet. To date, there are no studies of flaxseed and hot flashes, but its high plant estrogen content makes it worth a try.

Although there's some epidemiological evidence that dietary soy actually helps prevent breast cancer, there are no direct studies. My gut feeling is that eating more soy is probably okay, but we'll need to watch for the results of studies going on right now. Since our data are on *dietary* soy only, I would avoid pills and powders for the time being.

Reduce Your Stress

Most women with hot flashes say that stress exacerbates them. It should therefore come as no surprise that reducing stress and using certain behavioral techniques can have an effect on hot flashes.

The best study on this[6] randomly divided women with hot flashes into three groups. The first group received training in paced respiration, the second received training in progressive muscular relaxation, and the third group—the control group—received training in biofeedback. The "paced respiration" group had 40 percent fewer hot flashes over twenty-four hours, compared with the other two groups. Paced respiration is quite easy. You breathe from deep inside your abdomen, slowing down to six times a minute (the normal rate is about ten to fifteen breaths a minute). Try breathing in for five seconds and then breathing out for five seconds, and you'll have the right timing. To get the right feel, put one hand on your abdomen and the other on your chest, and let the hand on the abdomen rise and fall with your breath, making sure that the hand on the chest *doesn't* rise and fall. Practice this every day for fifteen minutes. Then whenever you feel a flash coming on, slow down your breathing.

In another study, women were randomly assigned to one of three tasks: (1) perform the relaxation response (see Chapter 12) daily for seven weeks, (2) read a book every day for seven weeks, or (3) do nothing. The women practicing relaxation reported a 28 percent drop in the intensity of their flashes and a smaller decrease in the number of flashes.[7] In another study, four women trained in several stress-reduction techniques reduced their hot flashes by 41 to 90 percent.

Though they haven't been studied in any formal way, meditation (see page 162), prayer, visualization, and affirmation (autosuggestion) have been used by many women to reduce symptoms. Visualization, which I'll discuss in more detail in Chapter 12, involves imagining that the changes you want to happen in your body (or in your life) are actually happening. For example, you might imagine that the hot flashes are leaving your body through your feet. Or you can imagine your discomfort metaphorically—as a fire, for example. Then, visualize your immune system as a force attacking it—a firefighter putting out the blaze. In affirmation, or autosuggestion, you use a verbal rather than a visual approach. You tell yourself, over and over, that you're in the state you wish to be in—for example, "My body is cool and comfortable." As we explain later, you shouldn't phrase this negatively—if you say, "I don't have hot flashes," you embed the idea of hot flashes even more in your mind. Also, you want to conceptualize in the present, not the future.

Alternative Approaches to Hot Flashes

Acupuncture

Acupuncture has also proven helpful in treating hot flashes in many women. A randomized controlled study in Sweden[8] compared two groups of women. One group received acupuncture with superficial needles at twelve points (this was as close to a placebo as the investigators could come), and the other received "classical acupuncture" at eight points and electroacupuncture (in which a very low electric current is applied to the needles) at four points. Both groups had less than half their usual number of hot flashes. In the placebo group, flashes increased again during the three months after treatment; in the electroacupuncture groups, the levels remained lower. This suggests that acupuncture may be a good, safe approach to hot flashes.

Vitamin E

Vitamin E has been suggested as a treatment for hot flashes in many popular books. Most of the clinical studies of vitamin E for hot flashes were actually done in the 1940s and were not placebo-controlled, but they did find that vitamin E was helpful. The one double-blind placebo-controlled study I could find lumped hot flashes together with eleven other menopausal symptoms. This study[9] compared vitamin E with estrogen and a placebo and found that vitamin E was no more effective than the placebo. Although this study has been used to discredit vitamin E as a treatment for hot flashes, it's hard to draw that conclusion because the study didn't focus on this one symptom. What we need is a randomized controlled study of the effect of vitamin E alone on hot flashes.

In a survey (not a study) of 438 women, 57 percent who had hot flashes reported taking vitamin E for them and 27 percent felt that it had helped.[10]

In the absence of data, those who suggest taking vitamin E advise that you start at 400 milligrams daily and increase the dose to 800 milligrams if necessary. You should not take more than 1,000 milligrams a day. One recent report has suggested that women with breast cancer should not take vitamin E supplements at all: this was a study in Stockholm, which found that women with breast cancer who took supplemental vitamin E had a higher rate of treatment failures than women who did not take it.[11] This report doesn't prove that supplemental vitamin E is bad for women with breast cancer, but with such a deadly disease, it's wise to heed any danger signals. I'd suggest that if you've had breast cancer, you should stay away from it.

Bioflavinoids

Bioflavinoids have an estrogenic effect about 1/50,000 that of estrogen. They've been used to treat hot flashes as well as vaginal dryness, bladder problems, and water retention. The richest source of bioflavinoids is the inner peel of citrus fruits. They're also found in many other sources, from buckwheat greens to bourbon. (I learned about this in a delightful way: one of my patients from Kentucky brought me a bottle of bourbon labeled "Kentucky bioflavinoids.") They're often taken with vitamin C. The dosage is one 250-milligram capsule five to six times a day.

Other supplements, including B vitamins, have been suggested for hot flashes but have not been studied in any formal way.

Herbs

A number of native herbs are commonly recommended by naturopaths and herbalists to treat hot flashes. Each woman reacts individually to herbs, so you may need to try a few under the guidance of an herbalist. Susun Weed told me she found that hormone-rich herbs aggravated her hot flashes and sleeplessness and that the best herbs for her were "cooling" herbs such as chickweed and elder, and "liver helpers" such as milk thistle and dandelion.[12] Other women I've talked to swear by black cohosh, vitex, or dong quai. One size doesn't fit all, so do your own research and find what works for you.

Black cohosh (Cimicifuga racemosa)   This plant is a member of the buttercup family and is also known as black snakeroot, bugbane (because its flowers repel insects), and squawroot. The root supplies estrogenic sterols (the building blocks for the steroid hormones such as estrogen, progesterone, and testosterone) and was used for menopausal symptoms by Native Americans and the colonists. It has been studied actively in Germany. In a randomized controlled double-blind study, eighty women were selected to take Remifemin (a capsule form of black cohosh), Premarin, or a placebo. After twelve weeks the women who took the herb reduced their menopausal symptoms as much as the women who took Premarin; both did better than the placebo group.[13] Another randomized controlled study compared Remifemin, estriol, and Premarin plus progestin in women who had just had hysterectomies that included removal of the ovaries. This study found no difference in symptoms among the three groups.[14] Researchers have found that black cohosh appears to work by decreasing levels of luteinizing hormone, which is associated with hot flashes.[15] According to herbalists, black cohosh also strengthens the pelvic muscles, improves digestion, lessens water retention, and calms the nerves, although there are less scientific data to support these claims.

According to Susun Weed, the dosage for hot flashes is ten to fifteen drops of tincture once or twice a day. If you're taking the dry powdered extract, you'd take 250 to 500 milligrams a day.

Black cohosh does have some side effects. Because it's estrogenic, it can stimulate the uterus and exacerbate heavy menstrual bleeding, which must be checked out with an endometrial biopsy. It can also cause headache, dizziness, visual disturbance, and nausea. These effects are more common in preparations from the dried or powdered root. Remifemin is being marketed as the "natural answer for women experiencing normal midlife changes." In Germany, it's the most popular natural alternative to estrogen. However, the German Commission, a governmental regulatory group, limits the use of any black cohosh product to six months, since data on long-term safety are lacking. Its estrogenic effects make it a poor choice for women with breast cancer. One tablet contains 1 milligram of 27 deoxyacteine (the active ingredient), and you take two tablets twice a day. It's readily available in health food stores.

***Garden sage* (Salvia offincinalis)**   Herbalists recommend sage to treat excessive sweating, night sweats, mood swings, headaches, and digestive problems. I could find no scientific studies on it related to menopause; but, like other plants we've mentioned, it contains bioflavinoids and phytosterols, so it both acts as a weak estrogen and has some progestogenic effects. In one study it relaxed smooth muscles and tended to decrease blood pressure; maybe this mechanism helps with hot flashes.[16] A relative of sage, *Salvia miltiorrhiza* (in Chinese, *dan shen*), increased the level of estradiol in female rats.[17] For this reason, it should probably be avoided by women with breast cancer. It can be used in cooking as a condiment or drunk in a tea. The dosage, according to Weed, is one to two spoonfuls of dried leaf infusion one to eight times daily, or fifteen to forty drops of fresh leaf tincture one to three times daily. Doses that exceed this have the potential to harm your kidneys and liver.

***Motherwort* (Leonurus cardiaca)**   Although it hasn't been formally studied, motherwort is used to relieve hot flashes and night sweats. Weed says you can take it to stop a hot flash after it's started or to help you get back to sleep after being awakened by a night sweat. Motherwort may have some estrogenic effects. There's one report in the literature of motherwort stimulating pregnancy-dependent breast cancers in mice (though inhibiting spontaneous tumors); thus I'd err on the side of caution and avoid it if you have or are at risk of breast cancer. It's bitter and so is best taken as a tincture. The dosage is fifteen to twenty-five drops tincture of fresh flowering plant one to six times a day. But don't use motherwort if you have heavy menstrual bleeding, since it may increase bleeding.

***Dong quai* (Angelica sinensis)**   This drug (also spelled *dang quai*) is used in the East to equalize high and low levels of estrogen. Its phytoestrogens are highly active, though still only 1/400 as potent as estrogen. Dong quai may also have some beneficial cardiovascular effects, especially in dilating coronary blood vessels and preventing spasm in them. Most of its benefits are thought to result from the fact that it's a coumarin, which is a type of compound that decreases blood clotting.

Herbalists recommend dong quai to eliminate hot flashes very quickly. If you feel hot all the time, however, it may make you flash even more. The usual dose is ten to forty drops of the fresh root tincture one to three times a day or four to eight ounces of dried root infusion or tea daily. Dong quai can sensitize your skin to the sun, causing a rash or sunburn. You should avoid it if you have heavy menstrual bleeding, take blood-thinning drugs (it has been shown to interfere with coumadin), have fibroids, are bloated, or have diarrhea, as it can exacerbate these problems.

I was able to find one study of *dang gui shao yao san*, a Chinese herbal formula that includes dong quai, which found that it suppressed estradiol secretion by rat ovarian follicles in a test tube.[18] This would lend some credence to the claim that dong quai acts to reduce estrogen, which could mean that it's safe for women with breast cancer.

Other herbs and combinations of herbs   Some herbs are used to help counteract hot flashes by cooling the body's temperature. I could find no research on them, nor could I find any reports of ill effects. *Chickweed (Stellaria media)* is one such herb. The dose is twenty-five to forty drops of fresh plant tincture taken once or twice a day. Herbalists say you'll get results in a week or two. *Elder flower (Sambucus species)* tincture is used to set the body's thermostat. When hot flashes are driving you crazy, try twenty-five to fifty drops of fresh elder blossom tincture several times a day, and you should see results within a few days. *Violet (Viola species)* leaves are used to cool perimenopausal women who feel hot. Use dried leaves to make an infusion and drink at least a cup a day. *Dandelion (Taraxacum oficiniale)*—yes the very same dandelion you destroy in your garden—is also a traditional Chinese herb (*pu gong ying*). It is taken in doses up to 30 milligrams to "clear heat toxins." The dosage is 1,000 to 3,000 milligrams in capsule form, two to three cups of tea daily, or one to two teaspoonful of dandelion tincture three times a day. Tell your doctor if you try these herbs.

Susun Weed suggests that women with hot flashes include plants that cool the system, such as chickweed, elder, and violet; plants that "nourish the liver," such as dandelion; and plants rich in phytosterols, such as black cohosh. She suggests that you choose one from each group and make your own special blend. Other blends have been suggested by various herbalists. If you work with an herbalist, she or he can help you design the right combination for your needs.

Although many Chinese herbs in addition to those listed above have been used for hot flashes, I couldn't find any specific recommendations for them and very little in the way of scientific study. Most traditional Chinese herbs are given in combinations or formulas that have been developed by trial and error over the centuries. They often include *dang gui, gan cao (Glycyrrhiza uralensis,* otherwise known as licorice), and *bai shao* and *chi shao* (*Paeonia lactiforai,* or peony). Both licorice and peony raise estrogen levels by increasing the aromatase enzyme that converts testosterone to estrogen.[19,20] Licorice can also raise levels of cortisol and other adrenal-gland hormones.[21] In large amounts (over 100 grams daily), it can cause low blood potassium and high blood pressure.[22] These effects appear to be exaggerated in women who are taking oral contraceptives.[23] Therefore, if you have heart problems or high blood pressure or are taking hormones, you should avoid licorice. Be sure to tell your doctor if you're trying licorice. (Fortunately, the herb has no relation to the candy, so you don't have to give up your Good 'n' Plenty!)

Chinese herbal formulas used for hot flashes include *liu wei di huang wan* ("quiet contemplative"), which raises estrogen levels in menopausal women,[24] and *xiao yao tang* ("relaxed wanderer"), which lowers the level of estrogen in women with benign breast disease and therefore may be safer if you've had breast cancer.[25]

I suggest that you see a traditional Chinese practitioner to help you sort through these various formulas, make up specific prescriptions for you, and suggest safe places to get other herbs.

Homeopathy

I could find no randomized controlled studies of homeopathic remedies, nor are there any reports of harm. Again, you'll do better to see a practitioner to help you identify the best remedy for you. As you read the following descriptions, you'll realize how individualized these remedies are. Some of the homeopathic remedies recommended for hot flashes are:

- Lachesis—especially for flashes that start from the top of your head, are worse just before sleep and immediately upon awakening, and are accompanied by sweating and headaches.
- Pulsatila—especially for flashes that occur around the face and are accompanied by mood changes and tearfulness.
- Kresotun—for burning heat and sweats that attack your whole body.
- Belladonna—useful when you experience waves of overwhelming heat, a flushed face, and throbbing.

Drugs for Hot Flashes

Nonhormonal Drugs

A few nonhormonal drugs have been used for hot flashes, with varying success. These are especially important for women who have been treated for breast cancer and are experiencing chemotherapy-induced meno-pause. Such women often suffer from severe hot flashes, made even worse by the addition of tamoxifen, and shouldn't take estrogen. (See Chapter 14 for a discussion of the use of estrogen for women who have had breast cancer.) Before describing these drugs, I should point out that many of the studies of hot flashes and drugs (including estrogen as well as non-hormal drugs) have shown a significant placebo effect—in some studies up to a 40 percent reduction in rate and intensity of flashes. That's not to say that hot flashes are all in our heads, but that the mind-body component is real.[26]

The oldest drug used for hot flashes is Bellergal—a combination of bel-ladonna alkaloids, ergotamine (which constricts blood vessels and is com-monly used for migraines), and phenobarbital. It has never been quite clear to me whether Bellergal really stops hot flashes or whether the phenobar-bital in it simply makes you stop caring about them. One double-blind study[27] found that women on Bellergal had 60 percent fewer hot flashes than women on placebo. It's still prescribed occasionally today, but the sedative effects of the phenobarbital limit its use somewhat. Bellergal may be worth a try if you're truly suffering over the short haul, but exercise cau-tion; since it contains a barbiturate, it could become addictive.

More recently, researchers have been studying clonidine (Catapres) for hot flashes. This drug was originally used for high blood pressure because it affects the responsiveness of blood vessels (remember that hot flashes cause the blood vessels to dilate) and blocks norepinephrine (which goes up with hot flashes).[28] A double-blind crossover study found that clonidine reduced the number and frequency of hot flashes. (It also found that a placebo decreased hot flashes, although not as much.) Studies of women taking clonidine by mouth, vein, or patch have reported fewer hot flashes, although interestingly, their skin temperature and levels of leutinizing hor-mone were unchanged.[29] Whether clonidine changed the women's percep-tion of these symptoms or whether this was a placebo effect was unclear. It *was* clear, though, that the women felt better.

The side effects of clonidine include dry mouth, nausea, fatigue, head-aches, and dizziness. The usual dosage is 0.05 to 0.4 milligram. Unfortu-nately, you get both the best effect and the worst side effects with the highest dose.

Lofexidene is another nonhormonal drug used for hot flashes. In a double-blind placebo-controlled study, this drug decreased hot flashes by 74 percent with a dose of from 0.1 to 1.6 milligrams.[30] Since lofexidene is the same type of drug as clonidine, it has similar side effects: dry mouth, fatigue, and headache.

Hormones and Hot Flashes

Generally speaking, estrogen therapy in any form is good for eliminating or at least decreasing hot flashes and night sweats, as many studies have shown. If you need a reliable result rather quickly (in about two weeks), estrogen is probably your best choice. I think it's important for women who choose estrogen therapy for relief of hot flashes or night sweats *not* to feel that this is a bad choice. No studies have found that short-term use of estrogen is dangerous, and it certainly can improve the quality of your life. (But in the case of women who have had or are at risk of breast cancer, we can't say it's safe, so it's wise to be cautious.) In Chapter 15, we discuss the various ways you can take estrogen therapy, any of which will work to quell hot flashes.

Adding progestin to the estrogen doesn't seem to change the response. In fact, estrogen and progestin have each been used individually to treat hot flashes. Megace (or megesterol) is a progestin that has been used to treat breast cancer that has spread. In an effort to find a reasonable alternative to estrogen therapy for women who've had breast cancer, a randomized controlled study was done to see if lower doses of Megace could be used to treat hot flashes.[31] The study, which included ninety-seven women who had had breast cancer, and, interestingly, sixty-six men with prostate cancer who developed hot flashes from testosterone-blocking therapy, found that the hot flashes were reduced in frequency and intensity by 21 percent in the group receiving a placebo and by 85 percent in the group receiving megesterol. This important study suggests a new choice for treating hot flashes in women who have had breast cancer.

I've heard and read that some gynecologists are prescribing the birth control pill for perimenopausal women who are still menstruating and are having hot flashes. Certainly the pill should help hot flashes by balancing out your hormone shifts, although I have been unable to find any studies on this approach. Smokers and women with high blood pressure should not take the pill because of the possible increased risk of stroke. My other concern is the risk of breast cancer. An analysis[32] of the effect of birth control pills on the risk of breast cancer found no increased risk among women age twenty-four to thirty-nine but did find a risk for both younger and older women who were currently taking the pill. Specifically, women age forty-six to fifty-four had just about double the risk of breast cancer. If they stopped the pill, the additional risk disappeared after three years. This would suggest that women should approach this therapy with the same caution as for menopausal estrogen therapy.

Some of you may decide to take estrogen and stop there. Others may want to combine estrogen with some of the other approaches we've discussed here. One observational study looked at the use of black cohosh by women who were withdrawing from estrogen and testosterone given by injection. It found that women who took black cohosh were able to withdraw more easily with fewer additional shots of drugs.[33] You might want to start on estrogen while increasing the soy in your diet or beginning an exercise plan. Or you could start on estrogen and take it for a year or two and then try tapering off with the help of herbs. Hot flashes are often the reason women start on estrogen, but they shouldn't be the reason for long-term use. Generally, your hot flashes would naturally stop after three and a half years, and at that point you should be able to taper off your estrogen. (In Chapter 15, we'll discuss how to taper off.)

HEAVY BLEEDING

The symptom that sends many perimenopausal women to the doctor is bleeding. As I mentioned in Chapter 3, neither irregular bleeding nor heavy bleeding is uncommon. But both can be a real nuisance, and heavy bleeding can be frightening. Most of the time, heavy bleeding is transient and needs no treatment. But if it continues for more than a month or two, or if the bleeding is more than just slightly heavier than usual, you need to check it out (see page 46).

Approaches for Bleeding and Fibroids

Lifestyle: *exercise*
Homeopathic remedies: *lachesis, sepia*
Supplements: *Chinese herbs, bioflavinoids, flaxseed, vitex, wild yam root (the wild yam root is taken two weeks before you expect your period)*
Drugs: *natural progesterone, Provera, Lupron*
Treatments: *D and C, or Chinese herbs, acupuncture*
Surgery: *hysteroscopy, myomectomy, hysterectomy*

Lifestyle Changes for Heavy Bleeding

Getting enough iron is important, as is drinking a lot of fluid. This won't end the bleeding, but it will replace these nutrients, which are lost with the blood. Many practitioners support a low-fat diet high in fruits and vegetables; but while good diet is important for many reasons, I haven't found any evidence that it will specifically address bleeding.

Alternative Approaches for Heavy Bleeding

Acupuncture is said to be very effective for erratic bleeding or flooding, although I could find no specific studies in the literature supporting this claim.

I couldn't find any good randomized controlled studies of the use of herbs or homeopathy for bleeding problems either. Nonetheless, certain herbal and homeopathic remedies are commonly recommended.

Herbs to Treat Heavy Bleeding

The herbs thought to be most helpful for heavy bleeding are those that act like or increase progesterone: vitex, lady's mantle, flaxseed, and wild yam root. As with all approaches, let your health care provider know what you are doing.

***Vitex or Chaste Tree* (Vitex agnus-castii)**   I did find one randomized, controlled double-blind study of women with low progesterone levels caused by too much prolactin. Vitex was shown to normalize the cycles and raise levels of progesterone and estrogen.[34] It's therefore worth trying as a way to regulate your periods if you're bleeding too much or too frequently. This is especially helpful if you have high prolactin levels (sometimes manifested by a milky nipple discharge).[35] Herbalists also consider it good for shrinking fibroids. It's a slow-acting tonic, so you might need to use it daily for two or three months before you feel its effects. Susun Weed recommends twenty drops of the tincture once or twice daily, three capsules of freshly powdered berries daily, or one cup of tea. In general, this should be an amount equivalent to 30–40 milligrams. The study cited above reported no side effects, but tell your doctor if you plan to try Vitex.

***Lady's Mantle* (Alchemilla vulgaris)**   Lady's mantle is used in Germany to control bleeding. When taken for one to two weeks before your period, it will prevent flooding. The usual dosage is five to ten drops of the fresh plant tincture three times a day for up to two weeks out of the month. If you've already begun flooding, it can still help, though it will take three to five days to be effective. Let your doctor know.

***Flaxseed* (Linum usitatissimum)**   Flaxseed contains prostaglandins that are important for preventing flooding, but be careful—too many can cause cramping, so you'll want to keep your doctor informed. These prosta-glandins are made from gammalinoleic acid (GLA), which can be found in the oil of flaxseed. The oil is good only if it is fresh, so buy it in small quantities, store it in your refrigerator, and use it before it goes rancid. You can take one to three teaspoons of flaxseed oil in the morning or grind the seeds and sprinkle them on your cereal. Or you can soak the seeds overnight and drink the whole thing, seeds and all, for breakfast.

Wild Yam Root   Most commonly prescribed synthetic hormones are made from the wild yam, including all of the estrogens except Premarin, as well as progesterone, progestin, and testosterone. Wild yam contains diosgenin, which is the laboratory precursor of all of these drugs. Unfortunately, there's no evidence that the human body converts diosgenin to hormones. So wild yam or wild yam extract is not the same as natural progesterone, which we'll discuss in Chapter 12. It does, however, have some effects and has been suggested to help balance the cycle. A tincture of twenty to thirty drops taken daily for the two weeks before your period may help decrease bleeding from hormonal imbalance. Tell your doctor if you're thinking of trying this.

There are also herbs you should *avoid* if you're bleeding heavily or irregularly, such as black cohosh, dong quai, and motherwort, which, as we said earlier, can exacerbate such bleeding.

Homeopathic Remedies for Heavy Bleeding

As with hot flashes, none of these homeopathic remedies have been studied in randomized controlled studies.

Homeopaths recommend lachesis if your blood is dark and thick and if you're experiencing a lot of anger. Sepia is used for heavy, frequent, painful bleeding accompanied by backache or depression. Belladonna is used for flooding with clots; secale is used for flooding without clots. There are many other remedies. They should be tailored to your particular situation by a homeopathic practitioner.

Drugs for Heavy Bleeding

The only drugs commonly used to treat heavy or irregular bleeding are hormones, which are given in an attempt to rebalance the hormonal shifts that often cause the bleeding. Sometimes they work, but at other times they simply intensify the problem, since creating the right balance in a hormonal environment characterized by constant change is extremely difficult.

The first step—after making sure you don't have a fibroid or a polyp—is to try a progestin. This will balance the estrogen and at the end of the cycle will cause your endometrium to slough so that you will get a period. You might be given Provera for three months in an attempt to stabilize the endometrium. Oral micronized progesterone could also be used for this purpose, although it has never been studied. "Natural" progesterone (see Chapter 14) might also be useful, although the amount found in the specially compounded skin creams is variable and there have been no studies on its efficacy.

If some type of progestin or progesterone doesn't seem to control bleeding, your doctor might prescribe Lupron. Lupron inhibits the hormones from the hypothalamus and puts you into a reversible menopause with all the attendant symptoms. It's sometimes used for two to three months to stave off bleeding until scheduled surgery. Although it usually will stop the bleeding, it doesn't work for everyone.

Surgery for Heavy Bleeding

Surgery is the ultimate "breaking and entering." As a surgeon, I know there's a time and a place for it. Nonetheless, the number of unnecessary operations that take place in this country is alarming. Hysterectomy is the most common major nonobstetrical surgical procedure in the United States. This is certainly the choice with the highest risk—not only short-term risk but also, often, long-term consequences. You can stop taking a drug if it turns out to be the wrong choice. You can't put your organs back in if you find you didn't need that hysterectomy.

Actually, however, surgery is more often the cause of menopause than a treatment for its symptoms. One third of the women in this country have had a surgical menopause before age sixty—a hysterectomy that includes removal of the ovaries. In Europe, the proportion is only one seventh, perhaps because medicine is socialized in several European countries and there is less of a profit motive.

Even if surgery is the best option for you, hysterectomy isn't the only possibility, and it may not be the best one. As we've mentioned in Chapter 3, there are several operations used to diagnose and deal with bleeding perimenopausally.

You can have a polyp or a fibroid removed without losing your uterus. A polyp can be removed by a hysteroscope (see page 47). Fibroids can be removed by a myomectomy. There are two ways a myomectomy can be done. One is to go through the cervix into the uterus if the fibroids are in the inner lining of the uterus (this is more common with bleeding fibroids); the other is to surgically remove the fibroids through an abdominal incision.

FIGURE 11.1   Uterine ablation.

Hormonal bleeding that doesn't respond to progestins can sometimes be treated by dilation and curetage (D and C), though this is less common now than it was in the past. As the lining of the uterus is scraped away, it gets a chance to start anew. If your hormones are now balanced, you won't bleed again.

If a D and C doesn't work and there's no sign of cancer, you can have an endometrial ablation (see Figure 11.1). Using an electrical cautery, the doctor burns and destroys the lining of the uterus. This is more thorough than a D and C, and the uterine lining scars down as a result. Fifty percent of women who have this procedure will never have a period again. In 40 percent of women, a few lining cells will be left and they'll have a light period. Ten percent will have no relief. This procedure should be performed only if you don't want to have more children. The scarring and lack of adequate lining cells would make it hard to sustain a pregnancy. A recent prospective study from London followed 525 women for five years after endometrial ablation. For over 85 percent of the women, heavy bleeding was controlled by this simple office procedure; 79 to 87 percent were satisfied with the procedure. For 80 percent of these women, no further surgery was required. Only 9 percent needed a hysterectomy during the five years after the procedure.[36] Of course, no operation is without some complication. This study reported that 2 percent of the women had a perforation of the uterus, which was then sutured. Other problems included infection and bleeding. No one had to undergo an emergency hysterectomy, however.

A new procedure is being tested in which a balloon is inserted into the uterus and then filled to compress the lining. An electric current is then applied to cauterize the endometrium. If it proves safe and effective, this procedure could be done in the health care provider's office.

Clearly, a hysterectomy should be your last resort for treating bleeding. If your gynecologist suggests it first, you need to get a second opinion. Nonetheless, many women with severe bleeding report that they are happy with having chosen surgery. I'm not antisurgery. After all, I am a surgeon. I'm just trying to counteract the current overuse of surgery, and to encourage you to consider other options.

One survey of women who had had hysterectomies did find that they experienced marked improvement in a range of symptoms, including pelvic pain, urinary symptoms, fatigue, and sexual dysfunction.[37] One of my own patients called me while I was writing this book because she'd been having problems with bleeding. She'd had an endometrial biopsy and then a D and C and had some atypical hyperplasia, which can be a precursor to cancer. She wanted to talk about hormones after surgery. I had a long talk with her about whether she really wanted to have surgery. After exploring all of the options and discussing all of the risks, she told me: "I still think that a hysterectomy is right for me; when I had precancer of the breast I really didn't want a mastectomy and did fine with conservative surgery, but this time I feel that the right thing is to have my uterus out." (She did decide to keep her ovaries, however.) I was happy that she had made an informed decision.

A hysterectomy is major surgery, usually done in a hospital under general anesthesia. Depending on the reason for the hysterectomy, it can sometimes be done through a long flexible tube called a laparoscope (so-called Band-Aid surgery). In a total hysterectomy, the uterus and part of the cervix are removed (see Figure 11.2). Sometimes this can be done through

Total hysterectomy

Total hysterectomy with oophorectomy

FIGURE 11.2   Hysterectomy.

the vagina, a less risky surgery that spares you an abdominal incision. In a total hysterectomy and bilateral oophorectomy, the uterus, cervix, both ovaries, and both fallopian tubes are removed. The vagina is retained. Sometimes the cervix is also retained, since some women feel that they have better orgasms when they have some cervical stimulation. (Sparing the cervix makes the operation easier from a surgical standpoint. Nonetheless, if you retain your cervix, some uterine tissue may be retained as well, and you should then consider adding a progestin to your estrogen therapy if you elect to take it.) You usually have a catheter in your bladder during surgery, and often postoperatively for a few days.

As I've mentioned, women who have hysterectomies and retain their ovaries typically go through menopause two years earlier than other women. But when the ovaries are removed, the effects are far more dramatic. Few women are clearly told that having their ovaries removed will plunge them into menopause. The effect is so immediate that some doctors put an estrogen patch on the patient while she's still in the operating room. Many women will have severe hot flashes within two hours after surgery. Unfortunately, estrogen therapy doesn't always compensate for the missing hormones. As I said in Chapter 1, the ovary makes more than just estrogen; when you lose your ovaries, you also lose progesterone and some of your testosterone and androstenedione—as well as any other hormone the uterus and ovary might make that we are as yet unaware of. The medical profession is becoming more conscious of this, and as a result we are reappraising the casual removal of ovaries in the course of a hysterectomy. A colleague of mine, the gynecologist Marcie Richardson, says that the only reason she would suggest that a woman have her ovaries removed is if she has severe endometriosis. Endometriosis can spread to other organs, so you can still have it after your uterus has been removed. Reoperating to treat endometriosis after you have had a hysterectomy can be very difficult because of the scarring.

It's important to know that, contrary to popular belief, you still have some risk of ovarian cancer even if your ovaries are removed. There is ovarian tissue in the areas around the ovary, so that the danger of ovarian cancer, unlike that of uterine cancer, can never be completely eliminated. In one study, twenty-eight women in sixteen high-risk families all had their ovaries removed to prevent ovarian cancer. Three of these women subsequently developed the disease.[38]

Also, removal of the ovaries can produce its own set of problems. Women who undergo surgical menopause have worse symptoms of menopause and, as I've mentioned, having your ovaries removed, whether or not you take hormone therapy, makes you far more vulnerable to osteoporosis and heart disease than women who experience natural menopause, probably because our bodies need more than just estrogen.

Furthermore, the idea that estrogen therapy can "replace" the work of the lost ovaries is misleading. Our new data on the other hormones produced by the ovary shows that it can't. Women who have their ovaries removed often don't feel normal when only estrogen is "replaced." This may relate to libido, orgasm, and just general well-being. Because of this complaint, the new fad is to add testosterone to the mix (see Chapter 15).

The earlier menopause caused by ordinary hysterectomy (removing only the uterus) suggests that there may be a connection we haven't yet discovered between the uterus and the ovaries—something akin to, or part of, the feedback loop of the brain, hypothalamus, pituitary, and ovary. The uterus may produce a hormone that responds to the ovary. Then, when the uterus is gone and the feedback ends, the ovary realizes it doesn't have any place to drop its eggs, so it stops trying.

The ovaries are highly sensitive to any change in the reproductive environment. One study reported that four out of seven women who had had tubal ligations produced less estrogen afterwards. This could be because the operation disrupted the blood supply or because there's a hormonal connection we currently don't know about. This shouldn't be too surprising; as an environment, the body isn't all that different from the planet. If you cut down a rain forest, you affect more than just those trees; the whole ecology changes, causing the death of animals who would normally hide in the trees, the extinction of plants that flourish in the shade, and even damage to the ozone layer that will affect people on the other side of the earth. All environments consist of interwoven elements, and interfering with one affects the others.

As with all operations, complications can result from any form of hysterectomy. The most common is urinary tract infection. Bleeding is also common, and it can necessitate a return to the operating room for further surgery. You may have problems getting your digestive system working again. The wound can get infected. Because the organs are so close together, you may have damage to the bladder, rectum, or ureters (tubes that carry urine from the kidneys to the bladder).

There are also long-term effects. Thirty to 50 percent of women who have hysterectomies suffer from depression, although this is usually minor and short-lived, like postpartum depression. Other women complain of hot flashes, weight gain, and lack of interest in sex. Many women say that their orgasms change. This probably happens because the uterus produces prostacyclin, a hormone that may be involved in orgasm, and, often, because the cervix has been amputated. The cervix has many nerves and pelvic thrusts, literally, have an impact on it. Finally, many women miss the rhythmic contractions of the uterus that often accompany orgasm.

Most women say it takes almost a year to recover, and some spend many more years tinkering with their hormones in an attempt to feel normal again.

So these operations aren't as benign as they may seem. You can't just pluck out an organ or disturb the body's balance without paying a price.

This isn't to say that no one should ever have a hysterectomy. It may be the only way to stop perimenopausal heavy bleeding or to deal with huge fibroids, after you've tried all the other options. But it's crucial that you know what you're getting into. Since at least one third of the hysterectomies done in this country are unnecessary, it's important that you get a second and even a third opinion before you proceed. There are very few conditions that require an emergency hysterectomy. Bleeding can be temporarily stopped with Lupron long enough for you to consider your options.

VAGINAL DRYNESS

Loss of vaginal lubrication is often described as an automatic result of menopause. As I've said, however, it certainly isn't universal; and it can be transient. Nonetheless, if you're suffering from vaginal dryness, it can have a major impact on your quality of life. Most often, this dryness sneaks up on you. Then on a particularly romantic night you attempt to have intercourse, and it hurts. This tends to make you less eager to try again. And so a cycle begins: less and less sex and more and more dryness. This leads to a significant change in your life; but don't despair—there are a variety of approaches you can use to get things back to normal.

Approaches for Vaginal Dryness

Lifestyle: *sexual exercise (masturbation and sexual activity with a partner as often as you like)*
Supplements: *homeopathic remedies such as bryonia, lycopodium, and belladonna*
Lubricants: *Astroglide or others (be sure they're compatible with latex condoms if safe sex is a consideration)*
Treatments: *Replens, vitamin E, Chinese herbs, acupuncture*
Drugs: *vaginal estrogen*

Lifestyle Changes for Vaginal Dryness

The vagina is one organ where use makes a difference. Sexual exercise—either masturbating or with a partner—will increase your natural lubrication.

Drinking lots of water—eight 8-ounce glasses a day—can help your whole body, including your vagina, stay hydrated. You can drink your water in the form of fruit or vegetable juices or herbal teas. Coffee and alcohol, on the other hand, will dehydrate you. There are some reports that women with vaginal dryness have more urinary tract infections. Of course, infections can occur for other reasons too. But in any case drinking lots of water can help both problems at once.

There's one study on the use of phytoestrogens for vaginal dryness.[39] Women supplemented their usual diet with 45 grams of soy flour (about six tablespoons) and 25 grams of flaxseed (about two tablespoons) daily. Researchers monitored the estrogenic effects on vaginal mucus. After six weeks the women had quantifiable estrogenic changes. Their vaginal moisture remained elevated for two weeks after they stopped their diet, but after eight weeks, the women were completely back to their pre-diet state.

There are lubricants that you can use at the time of intercourse that will make you more slippery. These include K-Y Jelly and Astroglide. One of my friends said that even though she didn't have vaginal dryness, she liked to keep a tube of Astroglide next to her bed because it made her feel so sexy. (Be careful of petroleum jelly, though, because it can break down the latex in a condom, increasing your vulnerability to HIV—the virus that causes AIDS—and other sexually transmitted diseases. Always check with your pharmacist to see whether a lubricant is compatible with latex.)

There are also products you use not specifically at the time of intercourse, but on a regular basis to eliminate vaginal dryness. These include Replens, which, applied vaginally, will cause your vagina to absorb water and become more supple. A randomized controlled study comparing Replens with vaginal estrogen found that they were equal in treating vaginal dryness.[40] You can also open vitamin E capsules and apply the oil daily inside your vagina, for a week or two at first and then once or twice a week.

Alternative Approaches for Vaginal Dryness

Herbalists suggest that taking motherwort tincture or dong quai in any form by mouth for three to seven days generally improves vaginal lubrication. Ginseng, which we'll discuss at length later, can also help.[41] Homeopathic remedies suggested include bryonia, lycopodium, and belladonna, but I could find no good studies in support of these recommendations.

Drugs for Vaginal Dryness: Vaginal Estrogen

Vaginal estrogens can be very effective in treating dryness. There are a number of methods for taking estrogen vaginally, but only one of them—vaginal cream—is currently available in the United States. We have two forms of this, Premarin cream and Estrace (micronized estradiol). Both are very well absorbed and raise your blood levels of estrogen much the same as estrogen pills.

Estriol vaginal cream is available in other countries, but not here. It's very well absorbed, producing blood levels that are about a quarter of those produced by the pill of the same dose.

Some women think that because you apply the cream only inside your vagina, none of it will get into the rest of your body. That isn't the case. Some of the estrogen will always be absorbed in your blood. How much is absorbed depends on which form of estrogen dominates the preparation and how much you use. Estradiol is absorbed very well and raises blood levels. Premarin, which is mostly estrone, isn't as well absorbed.

An example of how well vaginal estrogen can be absorbed was reported in a letter to the *New England Journal of Medicine.* A seventy-year-old man came to his doctor complaining of a lump in his left breast. The lump was removed and found to be benign. But two months later he was back with a lump on the other side. This time the doctors checked his history before operating. It turned out that his wife had been using vaginal estrogen for eight years. She applied the cream twice a week for vaginal dryness and then two to three times a week as a lubricant right before intercourse—something, as we'll discuss shortly, that she shouldn't have been doing. The poor man had been absorbing this estrogen during intercourse. As soon as his wife stopped using it for lubrication, his breast lump disappeared.[42]

Depending on the dose, you can use vaginal estrogen for all your symptoms, or to help prevent osteoporosis and perhaps heart disease, just as you do oral estrogen. But if the dose is large enough to affect your bones or your heart, it will also be large enough to increase your risk of breast cancer and the other cancers that oral estrogens can cause.

Most women who use vaginal cream aren't thinking about preventing disease—they just want to get rid of vaginal dryness. This requires only a very low dose, which doesn't appear to have dangerous side effects. One study found that you can get effective relief from vaginal dryness with only 0.1 milligram of estrogen per use. For some reason (could it be that they want you to buy more?) the manufacturer's recommended dose is ten to thirty times that: 1.25 to 2.95 milligrams. But you're under no obligation to follow the manufacturer's recommendation. Remember what they used to say in the old Brylcream commercial—"A little dab'll do ya." This is particularly important for women who have had breast cancer and don't want to risk a recurrence by using large amounts of estrogen. But it's also relevant to anyone who fears the increased risk of breast and endometrial cancer, whether or not she is at particularly high risk for these diseases.

When you start using vaginal cream, you apply a small dab just inside your vagina daily for three to four weeks. Then you can reduce it to once or twice a week. If you apply it daily for more than four to six weeks, it becomes less effective. It's important to remember that this is not a lubricant—use something else to lubricate your vagina right before intercourse (or you could end up with a partner with breast lumps).

In Europe, there's a low-dose estrogen ring that's placed in the vagina much like a diaphragm. It releases small amounts of estradiol over time. As you might imagine, it's less messy than the cream. It's not yet available in the United States, but it's coming soon.

Estrogen pills or a patch will often help vaginal dryness. They don't always do so, however. At a recent medical meeting, one woman doctor said that I should tell my readers that in her case, Premarin alone was not enough to treat vaginal dryness—she needed the vaginal cream too. If you're taking Premarin for hot flashes or for one of the long-term reasons we discuss elsewhere, it may help your dryness, but as my friend says, it may not, and you'll need to add one of the remedies we've discussed. But if you're using the pill or the patch just to address dryness, it's overkill. Most of it goes into your bloodstream and from there into other parts of your body. You're better off with estrogen cream alone.

INSOMNIA

Approaches for Insomnia

Lifestyle: *exercise, good sleep habits*
Supplements: *motherwort, valerian, chamomile, passion flower, melatonin*
Treatments: *Chinese herbs, acupuncture*
Drugs: *natural progesterone, estrogen therapy, hormone therapy*

Lifestyle Changes to Help You Sleep

Insomnia can really mess up your life. As we mentioned in Chapter 3, some insomnia can be caused by night sweats; and when that's the case, you treat the insomnia by treating the night sweats. However, there is probably another component, unrelated to flashing.

Again, some of the lifestyle approaches are obvious. Cut down on caffeine and alcohol. It's ironic that people often use liquor to help them sleep, when it's far more likely to keep them awake or disturb the quality of their sleep. Don't eat a big meal right before bed. Keep your bedroom cool and dark, unless you're among the people who feel insecure in total darkness, in which case you might want to use a small nightlight. Use cotton sheets, which will make you sweat less.

Exercise is good for insomnia, for two reasons. First and most obvious, it makes you more tired. When you exercise, your natural blood levels of melatonin, a hormone that promotes sleep, decrease initially for a few hours. Perhaps this is the reason that exercise is invigorating. Later, your melatonin levels rebound and go up at night. This, in addition to the physical exhaustion, helps you fall asleep.

The relaxation response (see page 218) and meditation practiced regularly during the day have also been found to fight insomnia. And it wouldn't hurt to try visualization and affirmations. Visualize yourself sleeping soundly on your bed—you can even hear yourself snoring if that makes it more vivid. Say to yourself, "I choose to sleep soundly tonight."

Alternative Approaches for Insomnia

Herbalists recommend motherwort to help fight insomnia. Chamomile tea has become a popular treatment for sleeplessness—there's even a specific tea called Sleepytime, which combines chamomile with spearmint and other herbs. Oatstraw, nettle, and black cohosh are also used. Valerian (*Valeriana officinalis*) has a reputation as a powerful plant sedative—practitioners recommend that you take twenty to thirty drops just before bedtime to help you sleep. Be careful, though, since valerian can be habit-forming, as can any sleeping aid. I could find no studies on its use, but I know of many women who swear by it.

Drugs for Insomnia

Melatonin, a hormone available as a supplement, has received a lot of attention lately as a "natural" way to combat insomnia. In fact, there are several good randomized studies of the use of melatonin in both men and women. It helped them sleep, it could be differentiated from a placebo, and it didn't cause a hangover.[43, 44]

There are, of course, many soporific drugs and over-the-counter sleeping pills. Most of these are benzodiazepines, such as Valium, Xanax, Dalmane, Halcion, Restoril, and Ambien. They can be lifesavers at certain critical times in your life, but you should never use them for more than two to three weeks. They all have side effects, including loss of memory the next day, confusion, anxiety, and excitability. Use them only under a doctor's supervision.

Surprisingly, estrogen will improve insomnia almost immediately, not only by decreasing hot flashes but also by improving the quality of sleep itself. Micronized progesterone can also help—in fact, sleepiness is one of its side effects. Because of this, doctors recommend that you take it before bedtime.

MOOD SWINGS AND DECREASED LIBIDO

Approaches for Mood Swings and Decreased Libido

Lifestyle: *exercise, diet, stress reduction, support group*
Supplements: *motherwort, black cohosh (Remifemin), dong quai, Bach flower remedies*
Treatments: *Chinese herbs, acupuncture*
Drugs: *estrogen therapy, hormone therapy, testosterone*

Lifestyle Approaches for Mood Swings

The lifestyle approach to mood swings really comes from reassessing your life. This is the time to look at how much alcohol and caffeine you consume, along with the rest of your diet. Eating a diet high in fruits and vegetables, incorporating exercise in your life, and reducing your stress can do wonders for smoothing out your moods.

Many women find a support group of perimenopausal women like themselves to be of enormous help. It's a place where you can share your feelings as well as remedies that have been helpful to you.

Meditation and the relaxation response have been shown to help enormously in evening out your moods. Randomized controlled studies have demonstrated the effectiveness of meditation on anxiety and premenstrual syndrome, even if it hasn't been specifically studied for perimenopausal mood swings. Try visualization and affirmations. You can imagine yourself smiling and calm, and you can develop affirmations like "I am serene and comfortable with myself and my surroundings." As Rodgers and Hammerstein said, "Whistle a happy tune."

Yoga is especially good for women with mood swings.

Alternative Approaches for Mood Swings

Many herbalists recommend oatstraw as a safe herb that helps "nourish the nerves" (see Chapter 13). Garden sage, ginseng, black cohosh, and dong quai can all help with stress. Five to ten drops of motherwort is said to help when you feel your nerves starting to go. Dong quai is used for palpitations. Ginseng has a reputation for helping with libido. Regular use of vitex (chaste tree) for six to thirteen months is said to relieve all symptoms of PMS. These symptoms have not been very well studied, however, and I could find no scientific literature to support these recommendations.

One variant on Western herbs is specifically useful here. The Bach flower remedies are all compounded to soothe various emotional states. Their creator was a Harley Street physician in the 1930s who believed that the only way to really deal with illness was to treat underlying emotional causes. There are nearly forty of these remedies,[45] each one designed for particular symptoms of depression. To my knowledge there have been no studies on the remedies, but there is anecdotal evidence. Both my coauthor and my assistant have found Rescue Remedy, the most powerful of the flower remedies, extremely helpful. The remedies come in small bottles; you either put a drop directly on your tongue, or put four drops in a glass of water and sip it throughout the day. Aside from Rescue Remedy, the following are a few that practitioners suggest may help. The descriptions are quite evocative.

- Wild rose, larch, mustard, gorse, and gentian are said to help relieve apathy, resignation, despondency, self-doubt, and gloom.
- Cherry plum is used to help women who are filled with rage and feel that they are about to do something desperate. The usual dose is one to four drops taken frequently under the tongue.
- Mustard is for deep gloom.
- Aspen mimulus and red chestnut are for fear.
- Rock rose is for easing terror and panic.
- Walnut helps those who are too sensitive.
- Impatiens is good for impatience.

Because the essences are preserved in brandy, you'll get a minuscule amount of alcohol when you take them.

Homeopathic remedies are also used for specific mood problems. As I said earlier, it's much wiser to go to a practitioner and have a specific formula prescribed for you. Here are some common homeopathic remedies that have been suggested for mood problems.

- Lachesis is used to even out moods.
- Sepia is for when you want to be alone, have no libido, and are irritable with friends.
- Arum metallicum is for when you're feeling unloved and joyless.
- "Calms forte" is for depression with crying.
- Mulimen and belladonna are also used for mood problems.

Drugs for Mood Swings and Libido

Antidepressants are often used for mood swings. They're strong drugs, however, and should be used only under a doctor's care. Tranquilizers such as Valium and Xanax are also helpful. They're habit-forming, so you should use them only for short times, and only under medical supervision.

Studies have shown that estrogen therapy is not helpful for depression. In fact, estrogen therapy and hormone therapy with estrogen and progestin can actually *cause* depression. Provera especially has been found to cause depression in some women. If this is the case for you, the best thing to do is to stop taking these drugs.

Testosterone has been suggested to treat women with decreased libido. There are no good studies on its efficacy or safety. In some women it will improve libido, and they will feel wonderful; in others, it can cause serious side effects (see Chapter 15).

FUZZY THINKING

Fuzzy thinking is probably the most disturbing symptom of perimenopause. It's known to be transient, but most women can't just stay home from work for a few months or years until their thinking clears up.

Lifestyle Changes to Help Your Thinking

As with the other symptoms, decreasing your use of alcohol and caffeine will help your thinking. So will a good diet high in vegetables and fruits. Increased physical activity seems to decrease the symptoms of aging; by increasing reaction time and blood flow to the brain, exercise may increase cognitive ability as well.

Exercising your brain will also help. My eighty-six-year-old Swiss grandmother decided that she'd memorize the capitals of all of the states as an exercise for her brain and a way to wow her grandchildren. Join a book club, go online, play bridge, or go back to school. As with your vagina, use it or lose it.

Alternative Approaches to Help Thinking: Herbs

According to Susun Weed, sage will help you "gain mental clarity, a strong memory and a calm 'craziness.' "[46] (This sounds like my usual state.)

Ginseng is also said to help memory. It comes in a number of forms: oriental ginseng (*Panax schinseng*), American ginseng (*Panax quinquefolius*), tienchi ginseng (*Panax pseudoginseng*), and Siberian ginseng (*Eleutherococcus sentico-*

sus). Many of the beneficial effects of ginseng are notable during stress. It will not only help you cope but will also sharpen your mental abilities.

There are more studies in the scientific literature on ginseng than on any other herb I've researched. It's considered by the Chinese to be the king of herbs. It's been found, in good studies, to decrease anxiety in people and to improve a rat's performance under stress.[47]

Quality control can be a problem with ginseng, however. The majority of products in the marketplace contain only a trace of ginsenoside (its active ingredient), and some contain none at all.[48] Look for products that are standardized in terms of their ginsenoside content. According to Michael Murray, author of *The Healing Power of Herbs*,[49] if you get a high-quality ginseng root extract containing 5 percent ginsenosides, your dose should be 200 milligrams. It's best to start at a low dose and gradually increase it. Susun Weed prefers American ginseng, but you can experiment with different varieties. Weed finds that wild panax roots are the most effective. The kind of ginseng that's powdered in capsules or in foil wrappers is considered by most herbalists to be less effective.

Ginseng should not be taken with vitamin C, as it isn't as well absorbed with acid. But ginseng can be enhanced by taking it with vitamin E or flaxseed oil.

The dosage is five to forty drops of fresh root tincture thirteen times daily, or four to eight ounces of dried root infusion or tea daily. Usually, you'll notice an effect within two to three weeks. If you don't mind the taste, you can "chew a root as big as your little finger" daily for six to eight weeks.

One side effect of ginseng is a jittery, overstimulated feeling. It can also cause postmenopausal bleeding; if this happens you should stop using it. Other side effects include high blood pressure, nervousness, insomnia, skin eruptions, and diarrhea. It can also exacerbate fever and cause euphoria (but that might not be so bad). Women taking panax ginseng may experience breast tenderness.

The Chinese herb ginkgo biloba is supposed to help memory. Although there has been much publicity surrounding this herb, I could find only one study. It was a randomized controlled study of forty-eight patients and did find some effect on age-associated memory impairment.[50] Some herbalists also recommend clematis, one of the Bach "flower remedies" discussed above.

Drugs to Help Thinking

As we reviewed in Chapter 3, estrogen therapy may well help sharpen your thinking. But you don't have to take it forever. I suggest that you take it for two to four years and then taper off and see how your thinking is doing. It may be that your hormones have largely balanced out by that time.

URINARY INCONTINENCE

Lifestyle Changes to Deal with Incontinence

Treatment of urinary incontinence depends in part on the problem. If the problem is urgency (always feeling as if you have to go, but then producing only a little urine), there are behavioral modifications you can make, such as slowly training yourself to wait longer before emptying your bladder—one hour, then two hours, and then three.

If the problem is stress incontinence (losing urine when you laugh or sneeze), you should first try Kegel exercises to strengthen your bladder. This involves exercising your pubococcygeal (PC—no, that does not mean it's politically correct) muscle. (I told you exercise was good for everything.) To find the muscle, simply stop your flow while urinating: it's the PC muscle that contracts to do this. Practice a few times to get used to the feeling of the muscle. Stop and start your flow at will. Try some stronger and weaker contractions until you can contract the muscle when you're not urinating. You can do your Kegel exercises anytime you wish, while waiting for the bus or walking down the street, sitting at your computer or sitting in traffic. There are several different exercises. One is to contract your PC muscle for three seconds and then release it for three seconds; repeat this six times three times a day; then go to twelve times a day. Second, you can contract your PC muscle strongly for one second and then release it for one second; repeat this twenty times, three times a day. Speed up the contractions until you have a fluttery feeling. Another exercise is to contract the PC muscle for ten full seconds, working at holding the contraction. Repeat this five times three times a day. Once you have your PC toned and can do all of these exercises well, you can do them just once a day. As with most exercises, it helps to have a routine. Lest you think I am making this up, there are actually randomized controlled studies showing that these exercises can help incontinence.

Studies have shown that drinking one or two 8-ounce glasses of cranberry juice a day can help stave off urinary tract problems.

Alternative Approaches for Incontinence

If you're having trouble actually finding and feeling the PC muscle, you can use biofeedback to help you. (You'll need to go to a specialist for this.)

Biofeedback is really the first step for any problems of urinary incontinence, in my opinion.

A pessary is a plastic ring you insert just inside your vagina, above the bone, to help keep the organs in proper alignment and decrease leakage. It's especially helpful if the problem is weak pelvic muscles, which can result after many pregnancies.

There's actually an even simpler tool you can use—one that you probably already have in your medicine chest. One study looked at three groups of women with stress incontinence.[51] One group used pessaries, the second used normal menstrual tampons, and the third used nothing. The women drank three glasses of water and then did aerobics. In this situation, the tampon worked best. You might consider using a tampon to help prevent stress incontinence. (If you do use a tampon, remember to change it often to prevent toxic shock syndrome.)

Black cohosh is used for incontinence. The dose recommended by herbalists is one teacupful a day or ten to sixty drops a day of tincture. Cohosh shouldn't be used if you are having menstrual flooding or might be pregnant. The side effects—headache, dizziness, nausea, and visual disturbances—appear to be worse with the dry powdered roots in capsules. So if you try the capsules and are having any difficulty, switch to the tinctures.

Drugs and Surgery for Incontinence

Estrogen, especially vaginal estrogen, can be helpful if incontinence is related to vaginal dryness. Estrogen won't help stress incontinence, however. If you're going to try vaginal estrogen, you need only a little, as we described when discussing vaginal dryness.

Finally, surgery is sometimes done for incontinence. In certain specific situations it may be helpful, but I'd use it as a last resort.

OTHER SYMPTOMS

Obviously, we have touched on only the most common symptoms. If you have symptoms I haven't discussed, you should research them in a similar manner. What are the lifestyle approaches to this symptom? What are the alternative approaches? See an herbalist, homeopath, naturopath, or traditional Chinese doctor and get a recommendation. And consider drugs or surgery as well. Be aware of all of the options open to you. Sometimes one practitioner may have a solution that another is not aware of.

Ellen Brown and Lynn Walker, in their book *Breezing Through the Change,*[52] tell the story of a woman who said that her tongue was burning hot. Her doctor said that she'd just have to live with it. She saw an herbalist who suggested a Chinese herbal remedy, and her symptoms went away. On the other hand, Marcie Richardson, the gynecologist I mentioned earlier, told me about a neighbor of hers who had heavy perimenopausal bleeding and thought it was from a fibroid. She wanted to avoid surgery and went to an acupuncturist. He examined her, then told her that her bleeding was coming not from fibroids but from endometriosis, and recommended that she see a surgeon. His diagnosis was correct. She had a hysterectomy and now feels much better. No competent practitioner will try to steer you wrong. Explore all of your options—the menu is vast.

CHAPTER 12

For Prevention:
First Look to Your Lifestyle!

Menopausal symptoms, disrupting though they can be to your life, aren't dangerous. The diseases that you become more vulnerable to as you grow older *are* dangerous. Further, the methods you use to avoid these diseases often have their own dangers. And since prevention is a lifetime commitment rather than a short-term remedy, the implications of a preventive treatment are far different from those of a treatment for controlling symptoms.

In chapters 12 through 15, we're going to look at various ways you can try to prevent heart disease, osteoporosis, and other diseases of aging. I'm not going to give you "the" answers, because there aren't any definitive answers. Each of you reading this has her own set of needs, her own concerns, her own symptoms, her own history, her own lifestyle. Each of you will come up with your own approach.

As with our discussion in chapters 10 and 11 about the treatment of symptoms, I've divided the discussion of prevention into three categories: (1) lifestyle changes, (2) alternative treatments, and (3) drugs and hormones. And as with the treatment of symptoms, what you choose to do for one problem may well have implications for others. The estrogen you take for your hot flashes will also help protect your bones, as long as you keep taking it. The stress-reduction techniques you use to control mood swings will also help your heart.

Remember, none of this is either/or. You may decide to start an exercise program *and* take estrogen. You make your own rules, and you reexamine them as you get more information and your needs change. And you can always choose to "manage" your menopause simply by living with it. Consider chapters 12 to 15 as a survey of all the possible approaches to prevention. Then, the last chapter—Chapter 16—will offer suggestions for incorporating all the information in the book into a personalized formula that you can use to help you determine what, if anything, you want to do.

TAKING STOCK

The least risky and most natural approaches to preventing disease are the same as those for symptoms—lifestyle changes. These changes can have great psychological, as well as physical, benefits. Menopause is, after all, a rite of passage. Your reproductive life is over; you've moved from one stage of your life into another, and you're a bit closer to mortality. This is a good time to take stock of your life—and, pragmatically, to begin to take better care of your body, so that it will continue to serve you well as you grow into old age. The great thing about the kinds of lifestyle changes we're talking about is that while they're helping to avert heart disease and osteoporosis, they're also helping your overall health and sense of well-being—so that something that starts off as an attack on high cholesterol levels can end up giving you an energy and zest for life that you've been missing for years.

If you're going to make lifestyle changes, however, you need to set reasonable goals for yourself and develop a reasonable system for meeting them. Changing a habit or habits isn't as easy as popping a pill every morning. If you smoke two packs of cigarettes a day, eat steak every night and wash it down with a vodka martini, never exercise, and find the idea of meditating faintly embarrassing, you're not going to turn into a salad-chomping, teetotaling, nonsmoking, transcendentally meditating jock in the next two weeks. Some people need to change slowly. They should focus on just one facet and work on it for a month or two. Make an inventory of your habits, decide which habits you want to change, and then focus on the most important one. Start working on that one first: "For the next two months, I'll work on adding more fruits and vegetables to my diet." Others, like me, prefer to make big changes all at once. (I drive my family crazy when I suddenly make a major dietary change while the refrigerator is still stocked with last week's fad.) Either way, with a strong balance of self-discipline, self-awareness, and patience, you can make as much change as you want.

I recommend that you get a complete physical exam and blood cholesterol check before you begin any new diet or exercise program. It's good to know what your general health is, and a checkup can help you decide where you want to focus your efforts, and perhaps give you a sense of what limits you may need to impose on yourself. If you've been out of shape for years and have a sudden conversion experience, you'll need to know that you can't start running ten miles a day and lifting twenty-pound weights all at once.

DIET

"You are what you eat." We all know what good eating habits are—lots of green leafies and go light on the cheesecake. (No, cheesecake is not a good way to get calcium.) Most of us, however, are more likely to eat lots of cheesecake and go light on the green leafies.

With menopause, your metabolism begins to change, and some eating habits that haven't visibly affected you before may start to show up in your waistline and your digestive system. Sometimes, you may even find that your tastes are changing. So maybe it's a good time to look at your eating habits and change some of them. They all have an impact on both menopausal symptoms and the diseases of age that you're most likely to be worried about.

Watch Your Fats and Cholesterol

A diet low in fat, especially saturated fat, and high in fiber is important for prevention of breast and colon cancer and heart disease. To help prevent heart disease, you also want to maintain your cholesterol at a safe level.

What's a safe level? According to the American Heart Association, blood cholesterol of over 240 milligrams per deciliter (mg/dl) puts you at high risk of heart disease; 200 to 240 mg/dl is borderline. Thus less than 200 mg/dl is what you should aim for (see Chapter 6). Getting your cholesterol down isn't as easy as it may sound. It's not just a matter of avoiding foods with high cholesterol (although you should try to consume less than 300 milligrams a day). We've discovered that the cholesterol you eat probably isn't as dangerous as the cholesterol your own body makes.

Fat affects your cholesterol. Fats in foods come in three main varieties: polyunsaturated, monounsaturated, and saturated. *Saturated* fats are especially dangerous. Any fats that stay solid at room temperature are highly saturated. Some vegetable fats that don't have any cholesterol are high in saturated fats—such as chocolate and hydrogenated vegetable shortenings (corn oil). Although they don't have to have cholesterol, they create it—which is actually worse for you. So a diet low in saturated fats is probably more important than a diet low in cholesterol. Among foods high in saturated fat are meats, milk, eggs, cheese—foods high in animal fat. However, the problem isn't in the fact that something is an animal product; some animal products—skim (nonfat) milk and other nonfat or low-fat dairy products, lean meat, and egg whites—are fine.

Polyunsaturated fats and *monounsaturated* fats are usually oils. Greeks and Italians are only half as susceptible to heart attacks as Americans, because the traditional Mediterranean diet is low in saturated fats and the fat most commonly used is monounsaturated olive oil. This kind of diet helps lower LDL ("bad") cholesterol and also helps protect against oxygen-free radicals, which help to oxidize the LDL when it's trapped in the artery wall. (Remember that rotting garbage next to the freeway in Chapter 6?)

When you use monounsaturated fats in place of saturated fats, you get a bonus: a lower risk of breast cancer. But don't go overboard. Monounsaturated fats don't lower cholesterol unless they're taking the place of a saturated fat in your diet. Too much fat of any kind is not good for you. Some people have interpreted the data on monosaturated fats to mean that they should douse everything with olive oil. It doesn't work that way. What you should do is eat a diet low in fat (I'd aim for no more than 20 percent of your total daily calories from fat, only 7 to 10 percent of it saturated) and when you need to use fat in cooking and salad dressings, use olive oil, canola, or peanut oil. And use it sparingly.

You should also avoid oils high in polyunsaturated fats such as corn, safflower, and soybean oils. The structure of the fat helps determine its function. They are omega 6 fatty acids, and there's some evidence that they weaken the immune system and increase the chance of getting cancer. (The fact that soybean oil falls into this category is ironic because, as you'll see shortly, soy itself is one of the best things you can possibly eat.) On the other hand, omega 3 fatty acids—such as those found in salmon, mackerel, tuna, bluefish, Atlantic sardines, herring, whole grains, flaxseed, beans, seaweed products, soy, shellfish, and fish oil—may prevent cancer as well as heart disease.[1] (Omega 3 fatty acids in fish are better absorbed, but those in soy and flaxseed have phytoestrogens as well; see page 161.)

In his book *Dr. Dean Ornish's Program for Reversing Heart Disease,*[2] Ornish points out that a very low fat (10 percent) vegetarian diet combined with exercise and stress reduction not only prevents hardening of the arteries but can even reverse it. The Women's Health Initiative (the randomized controlled study of menopausal women's health) is specifically looking at the effects of a very low fat diet on heart disease, osteoporosis, colon cancer, and breast cancer.

Eat More Fiber

Fiber is found in whole grains, beans, fruits, and vegetables. Increasing the fiber in your diet helps you to decrease cholesterol and lower the risk of colon cancer. There are two kinds of fiber—insoluble and soluble. Insoluble fiber increases the bulk of stool your body produces. It helps to move things through at a faster clip, removing toxins in the process. Wheat bran is a major source of insoluble fiber. Notice that I said wheat *bran*—not refined wheat. The refining process strips away most of the fiber. Look for products that say "100 percent whole wheat."

Soluble fiber helps prevent the absorption of cholesterol by forming a gel in your intestine that traps some of the fat. Oat bran, rice bran, rolled oats, carrots, and guar gum (found in beans) are all soluble forms of fiber. They have been shown to decrease cholesterol and balance your blood sugar.

Aim for 30 to 35 grams of total fiber a day. Fiber is best found when a food is in its most natural state. Plenty of whole grains, fruits, and vegetables should do the trick. You get more fiber from eating a grapefruit than from drinking grapefruit juice. But I must caution you: if you start on your fiber kick all at once and load up the first day, expect to have a gaseous time of it. It's better to introduce fiber into your diet gradually so that your intestine has time to become accustomed to the change.

Don't Overdo Animal Protein

If you're like me, you were raised on a serving of meat every night (except for fish sticks on Friday). We were told that it was important to eat enough protein, and that the best way to do this was to eat meat. Red meat, and lots of it, made us strong, healthy, and somehow more American. There was no such concept as too much protein.

In recent years, I've instinctively backed away from that. At this point in my life I find myself an "almost vegetarian" (I still eat an occasional hamburger). This shift to a lower protein diet has happened gradually, as I lost much of my taste for meat. It turns out that for once I may have developed a good habit on my own.

There *is* such a thing as too much protein—in fact, there is too much protein in the diet of almost all Americans. A diet high in animal protein can interfere with the absorption of calcium. The body uses calcium to buffer acids produced when we digest animal protein; the calcium then gets excreted in urine. Thus foods rich in protein but low in calcium (such as red meat) can cause us to lose calcium. A 50 percent increase in protein above the recommended 15 percent of total daily calories can cause you to lose 32 milligrams of calcium a day. In the United States and Western Europe, we eat a lot of meat. This may be why osteoporosis is most common in high socioeconomic countries.

If you consume 1,500 calories a day, aim for about 56 grams of protein. Not all protein is equal, however. Although doctors have tended to tell postmenopausal women simply to limit their protein intake, I don't think that is necessarily correct. The real problem may be with *animal protein*. While I was writing this book, a study came out that confirmed what I had suspected.[3] In the study, women who ate a high-protein diet had more wrist fractures, but this appeared to be a risk only for the meat eaters: women who ate five or more servings of meat a day. (A serving was defined as 3 ounces—about the size of a pack of cards.) Women who ate plant protein did not have more fractures. Thus it's probably not protein itself that's the culprit, but animal protein. Shifting to a largely plant-based diet, with only occasional meat or fish, appears to be much better for your bones. This was confirmed in one observational study: women who ate meat regularly lost 35 percent of their bone mass between the ages of fifty and eighty-nine, while vegetarians who ate eggs and dairy products lost only 18 percent, even though both groups had the same amount of calcium in their diets.[4] Another study found that vegetarians had higher bone density at age seventy than meat eaters at age fifty.[5]

So don't eliminate all protein from your diet. Substitute beans for steak and tofu for hamburger, and you'll have less fat and more fiber—and end up with stronger bones. A great way to get plant-based protein is in soy (discussed in detail below). Don't be misled by the cheese and eggs in that one study: eggs are full of cholesterol and high in calories, and most cheeses are high in fat. Use them sparingly.

Soy: The Wonder Food

We spoke earlier (see Chapter 11) about phytoestrogens. From all the evidence we have, these appear to be close to a natural wonder drug—able to treat menopausal symptoms while helping to prevent heart disease, osteoporosis, and breast cancer. Remember those Japanese women who had lower rates of breast cancer, heart disease, and osteoporosis? They also had little trouble with hot flashes. There's some evidence that all of this is connected with their high consumption of soy protein, which contains phytoestrogens called isoflavones. As we saw in Chapter 11, at least one study has found that soy flour can prevent hot flashes; and two further randomized controlled studies are being conducted at Tufts and Bowman Gray.

The discovery of the estrogenic effect of these plants is fascinating. It began in Western Australia in 1946, when sheep grazing on red clover became infertile.[6] Much to everyone's surprise, studies showed that the clover the sheep had been eating was high in plant estrogens. The estrogenic clover decreased sperm transport in rams and blocked ovulation in ewes.[7] Since then, animals as diverse as cattle, mice, and quail have been found to become infertile from dietary phytoestrogens. In fact, one researcher, Claude Hughes,[8] has gone so far as to suggest that plant estrogens (phytoestrogens) are defense substances produced by many plants to decrease the fertility and therefore the population of plant-eating animals. Nature is pretty clever. (But don't be alarmed by these animal studies—soy doesn't cause infertility in humans, so your kids can eat it safely.)

Nature comes to *our* assistance, as well. These forms of plant estrogen are turning out to be one of the best dietary alternatives to estrogen drugs for postmenopausal women. One of the best sources of isoflavones is soy (they're also found in chickpeas, but at much lower levels). Soybeans are loaded with the two main isoflavones, genestein and diadzein (see Table 12.1). Another is flaxseed (see page 199).

The soybean has a lot going for it. It's a high-quality protein supplying most of the essential amino acids needed by an adult or child. It has more protein and less fat than other beans. It's also a lactose-free, cholesterol-free source of omega 3 fatty acids and calcium (equal to one third the calcium content of milk). These characteristics alone would make it good to eat. But this wonderful bean appears to have other important effects as well.

Soy and Your Heart

One of soy's more exciting benefits is in battling heart disease. As little as 25 grams of soy protein a day can lower cholesterol in people with high cholesterol. A recent article in the *New England Journal of Medicine* reported that an average intake of 47 grams of soy decreased total cholesterol by 9.3 percent, LDL by 12.9 percent, and triglycerides by 10.5 percent. HDL, "good cholesterol," went up a little (2.4 percent) though not a significant amount.[9] In a study of monkeys whose ovaries had been removed, the equivalent of a half cup of tofu a day was enough to produce a dilation of coronary blood vessels similar to that seen with estrogen.[10] This would suggest that soy works like estrogen on preventing heart disease (see Chapter 6).

Soy and Your Bones

What about osteoporosis? The isoflavones in soybeans may directly inhibit bone resorption. More important, they seem to help the body hold on to calcium. Normally, as I've mentioned, animal proteins increase the amount of calcium lost in urine. Soy protein doesn't seem to work that way, however.[11] In a study on rats whose ovaries had been removed, there was also evidence that soy helped increase the intestinal absorption of calcium, much as estrogen does. The rats had higher bone density as a result.[12] A soy-based drug called Ipriflavone is being used in Japan and Italy to treat osteoporosis (see Chapter 14).

Soy and Cancer

If soy helps the heart and bones, it must hurt the breast, right? Wrong! Here's where soy has the edge on estrogen.

First of all, soy has been shown to help breast cells mature and therefore become more resistant to carcinogens. Unfortunately, this effect is probably too late for you, since it takes place around the time of puberty, but at least you can tell your daughters and young friends about it.

Soy also tends to lengthen the menstrual cycle by increasing the length of the first part of the cycle (the follicular phase) by three to four days, and decreasing the surge of luteinizing hormone (LH) and follicle-stimulating hormone (FSH) at midcycle. These effects are similar to those seen with tamoxifen, a drug used to treat breast cancer that acts like both estrogen and an estrogen blocker.[13]

Epidemiological data also indicate that as little as one serving of soy food per day (one cup of soymilk or half a cup of tofu) can lower your risk of a wide range of cancers.[14] Soy appears to suppress mammary tumors in rats. It blocks tyrosine kinase, an enzyme important for the growth of cancer cells. It also blocks new blood vessels from growing in breast cancer tumors. A study in Singapore compared the amount of soy in the daily diets of 200 women with breast cancer and 420 women without breast cancer. The healthy women with the lowest risk of breast cancer ate about 55 grams of soy a day and had less than half the risk of breast cancer.[15] Several studies have now been started to look at whether a diet high in soy protein (50 grams a day) can prevent recurrence of cancer.

By now, though, you know that nothing is ever entirely clear. The epidemiological data would suggest that dietary soy helps prevent breast cancer through several different mechanisms, but studies of isoflavones (genestein and daidzein), the "active ingredients," alone with cancer cells in a petri dish show that low levels actually stimulate estrogen-sensitive cells to grow, although high levels block both estrogen-sensitive and estrogen-resistant cancer cells.[16]

Should women with estrogen-sensitive (receptor-positive) breast cancer worry about soy? I really don't know. As I said in Chapter 11, the epidemiological data are strong, but the answers aren't all in. A recent study of dietary soy did not show the decrease in breast cell activity that scientists had expected.[17] The active ingredients alone may not have the same effects as those in whole foods, and breast cancer cells in a petri dish are not the same as those in a woman.

Although not all of the claims for soy have been proven in a rigorously scientific way, the evidence we have so far is fairly convincing, and there's no risk involved in increasing the amount of soy in your diet. (It's impressed me enough personally that I now eat soy in one form or another every day.)

The average American eats 1 to 3 milligrams of isoflavones a day, while the average Asian eats 100 milligrams a day. Can too much soy be harmful? A study of cheetahs in a zoo who were eating a very high soy diet found that the animals were dying of liver failure.[18] Prolonged feeding of raw soy flour to rats resulted in the development of cancerous and noncancerous nodules of the pancreas.[19] But the amount of soy that we are talking about here doesn't come near the amount used with these animals. The worst you're likely to get if you pig out on soybeans is an increase in gas.

Varieties of Soy Products

Now that I've convinced you of the benefits of eating soy, how do you actually do it? Fortunately, there are a number of possibilities.

You can buy *fresh soybeans,* especially in Asian grocery stores in the summer. Boil the pods for fifteen minutes in salted water and eat them by putting a whole pod in your mouth and drawing it through your teeth to free the beans. In Japanese restaurants this is called *edamame.*

You can find *canned* or *frozen soybeans* in Asian markets and *dried raw soybeans* in health food stores and in some supermarkets. Like some other beans, dried soybeans need to be soaked in water overnight and then cooked for three hours. They can be used in soups, casseroles, and salads. Soy sprouts are similar to mung bean sprouts.

Soynuts are made from soybeans. You can buy them in health food stores or make them yourself by soaking the beans for three hours and then roasting them in the oven for about fifteen minutes.

Soymilk is the liquid expressed from soybeans that have been soaked and pureed. You can get it in different flavors, as well as low-fat and nonfat.

Tofu, produced from curdled soymilk, is the most common form of soy. It's available in soft, medium, or firm, and it also comes in a low-fat form You can use it in soups, stews, and casseroles. You can also puree it to use as a substitute for sour cream, to make mock mayonnaise, and to replace an egg in baking. You can slice and bake it, to use on sandwiches.

One of my favorite forms of tofu is *tempeh,* a combination of fermented soybeans and grains. It has a distinctive taste and is a good substitute for meat in soups, chili, or stir-fry dishes. After marinating in soy sauce, it can be grilled like a burger. It comes in sandwich-sized squares and makes a good, easy lunch food.

Miso is fermented soybean paste, most familiar as a salty soup.

You can use *soy flour* in some baking. Soy flour is made from soybeans that have been hulled, cracked, and heat-treated. It can be mixed with other flours, but it contains no gluten and inhibits rising, so it isn't good for baking on its own.

You can buy *soy protein powders* through the mail (as you can a number of soy products; see Appendix 2) and in health food stores. These powders come in several flavors and can be mixed with water or juice. Two scoops give you 35 grams of isoflavone. Although these powders are convenient, it is not clear that the isolated isoflavone will have the same beneficial effects as dietary soy.

Other products include *roasted-soy butter* and Nutlettes, a breakfast cereal. *Textured vegetable protein* (TVP) is made from defatted soy flour compressed until the protein fibers change structure. It can be rehydrated and used in place of ground meat. This is my coauthor's favorite. It makes a decent burger and great sloppy joes. It's also popular with campers, who use it with canned soup to make a dish popularly known as glop. A caution: one study showed that TVP used in a diet high in wheat flour wasn't well absorbed.[20] This study, however, isn't conclusive. Ongoing research will give us more information about this in the near future.

Unfortunately, soy sauce doesn't have an estrogenic effect, because the genistein is leached out in the processing. Other products that appear not to have much in the way of isoflavones are soybean oil, canned meal-replacement drinks, soy cheese, soy hot dogs, soy bacon, and tofu yogurt. Soy foods made from soy protein concentrate, such as veggie burgers, vary considerably in the amount of isoflavones they have, depending on the processing. Just because a product says "soy," then, doesn't mean that there are isoflavones in it. As with TVP, studies now taking place should tell us in a few years how valuable some of the processed soy products actually are.

Flaxseed

While soy's claim to fame is genistein, flaxseed has lignans—between 75 and 800 times more lignans than any other food. And there is growing evidence that this strange-sounding substance may have anticarcinogenic properties[21] as well as the symptom-reducing properties of plant estrogens. It also can lower LDL[22] significantly and may prevent bone loss. Flaxseed also contains five times as much omega 3 essential fatty acids (see page 193) as any other commonly available plant food.[23] One tablespoon of flaxseed is roughly equivalent to one serving of soy. As we mentioned in Chapter 11, you can grind it up in a coffee grinder and sprinkle it on your cereal, or soak it overnight and drink the liquid and seeds for breakfast.

How much flaxseed and soy should you eat? Mark Messina and Stephen Barnes[24] estimate that 200 milligrams of soy equals 0.3 milligram of pharmaceutical estrogen. Another estimate is that half a cup of soybeans

TABLE 12.1   Isoflavones

Food	Serving	Isoflavone (mg)	Calories	Fat (g)
Nutlettes breakfast cereal*	½ cup	122	140	1.5
Beef(Not) textured soy protein granules*	¼ cup dry	62	70	1
Roasted soynuts	¼ cup	60	195	9.5
Tempeh	½ cup	35	165	6
Low-fat tofu	½ cup	35	45–75	1.5–2.5
Regular tofu	½ cup	35	105–120	5.5–6.5
Take Care high-protein beverage powder*	2 scoops	35	100–130	1–1.5
Regular soymilk	1 cup	30	130–150	4
Low-fat soymilk	1 cup	20	90–120	2
Roasted-soy butter	2 tbsp.	17	170	11

Note: Isoflavone values are approximate, except for Take Care high-protein beverage powder.
*Ordering information: Nutlettes and Beef(Not): Dixie USA, 1-800-347-3494.
Take Care high-protein beverage powder: Nutritious Foods, 1-800-445-3350.
Source: Adapted from "Menopause Naturally," *Prevention Magazine*, August 1996, p. 67.

and two snacks equal about 200 milligrams of plant estrogen. According to Nina Shandler's cookbook *Estrogen: The Natural Way—Over 250 Easy and Delicious Recipes for Menopause*, one tablespoon of flaxseed or between one and two servings of soy a day should reduce the risk of breast cancer; two tablespoons of flaxseed or one serving of soy (50 milligrams) will decrease the symptoms of menopause; and three to five teaspoons of flaxseed or two to three servings a day of soy will decrease cholesterol. To reduce the risk of osteoporosis, you may need as much as six to eight teaspoons of flaxseed or six to eight servings of soy a day. All this can seem quite daunting until you start considering flaxseed and soy as ingredients rather than as endpoints in themselves. As Shandler says, you have to think of tofu the way you think of flour. "It is not how tofu tastes straight out of the package that matters," she writes. "It's what I can do with the stuff."[25] Soy cookbooks are cropping up all over. Shandler's showed me how I could get all of my estrogen needs for the day satisfied by one serving of homemade flaxseed and soynut granola. I've become a convert.

If your family objects to this new cuisine, remind them that soy and flaxseed can help all of them. It helps to prevent prostate cancer and to lower cholesterol in men. Remember too that the immature breast tissue in girls is more sensitive to the carcinogens leading to breast cancer. Soy will help mature that tissue better than anything besides teenage pregnancy— with none of the drastic consequences of that condition.

Bringing your family around may not be easy, of course. My eight-year-old keeps making nasty faces at the tofu chocolate pudding I make her. (I'm not giving up, though—I've only gotten up to recipe number 52 in Shandler's cookbook.)

Get Enough Fluid

As you get older, you need more fluid. Drinking enough water helps ensure that your kidneys will work well and thus that you'll be able to rid yourself of toxins. During perimenopause, water is even more important. You lose a lot of fluid when you bleed heavily, or when you sweat profusely with hot flashes. Make sure to drink at least eight 8-ounce glasses of water or fruit juice a day. I often drink my water as mineral water, which contains calcium, thus killing two birds with one stone.

Caffeine, like protein, causes you to lose more calcium in your urine, so you lose much of the effect of water when you drink coffee or caffeinated tea. However, once again life is never simple. A new study, which came out as I was writing this book, found that among women who drank two or more cups of regular, caffeinated tea a day, the rate of cancer of the digestive tract and urinary tract was only 40 to 70 percent of the rate for women who drank tea infrequently.[26] Green tea (which also contains caffeine) and black tea are being studied to determine how they act to prevent cancer. But while the scientists are looking for the active ingredient, you can decide— again—whether you're more worried about your bones or about cancer.

Alcohol, in addition to its other dangers, can dry you out. Sugared drinks provide fluid but create other problems, so use them very sparingly. Low-fat and nonfat milk and soymilk are also excellent ways to get your daily fluid.

Get Enough Calcium

Calcium is very important for women, and it becomes even more important as you grow older. You need it for your heart, bones, and nerves. If you don't consume enough calcium, your body will steal it from your bones. Calcium absorption decreases naturally with age, and even more postmenopausally, so it's important to increase your intake to compensate. Getting enough calcium—along with exercising—will increase your bone density.[27, 28]

Premenopausal women should get at least 1,000 milligrams of calcium a day (more if they're pregnant or nursing). Perimenopausal women should get 1,200 milligrams. Postmenopausal women should get 1,500 milligrams. According to government studies, however, the average woman consumes only 450 milligrams of calcium a day—a third of what she needs if she's perimenopausal, and only a bit more than a fourth of what she needs if she's postmenopausal. This alone could account for the 15 percent decrease in bone mass most women experience between ages fifty and sixty.

The best way to get calcium is in your food. Calcium is found in many foods, especially cheese, yogurt, and milk products. (Remember to use low-fat or nonfat dairy products whenever possible.) You can actually get 25 percent (350 to 400 milligrams) of your daily calcium needs from one cup of yogurt or milk, an ounce of hard cheese, or half a cup of ricotta cheese. Calcium is also found in many green leafy vegetables. One cup of cooked broccoli, kale, turnip greens, or mustard greens contains 200 milligrams of calcium. (Sadly, you won't get much calcium from some otherwise excellent green leafies: spinach, chard, beet greens, parsley, and rhubarb. They contain oxalate, which binds to calcium and makes it harder to absorb.)

Other sources of dietary calcium include shellfish, almonds (one cup equals 304 milligrams), Brazil nuts (eight nuts equal 50 milligrams), tofu made with calcium sulfate (check the label—one ounce equals 36 milligrams), and canned salmon or sardines with the bones (587 milligrams in 8 ounces).

Further, calcium has been added to some foods that don't naturally contain it. Minute Maid orange juice is one of these (one cup of Minute Maid contains 320 milligrams).

One of my more delightful discoveries while doing this book is the fact that calcium can be found in some of the ubiquitous mineral waters so many of us drink these days. (Lest we forget, calcium is a mineral.) Check the labels. My local supermarket stocks Pellegrino, a naturally sparkling mineral water with 5 percent of your daily requirement of calcium in each 8-ounce glass. (A German brand called Gerolsteiner Sprudel has 8 percent of the daily requirement.) Mineral water is surely not the main way to get your calcium, but if you're choosing between brands you may want to drink the one with calcium in it.

Herbs such as valerian, nettles, peppermint, oatstraw, sage, raspberry leaf, and many others also contain calcium.

Caffeine, alcohol, and soft drinks (which are high in phosphorus) all *decrease* your absorption of calcium. A high-salt diet causes you to excrete more calcium.

Watch Your Weight

With middle age, your metabolism starts to slow down. You also tend to decrease your activity. Together, these two tendencies lead to the gradual increase in weight you see in most middle-aged people.

In this country, obesity—defined as being at least 20 percent over your healthy weight, or target weight—is a serious health problem. In the Nurses' Health Study,[29] weight gain between ages thirty and fifty was the biggest risk factor for later breast cancer. Certainly heart disease is higher in women who are overweight, as is diabetes. About the only advantage to being heavy is a decrease in hot flashes and osteoporosis. Thus it's important to stabilize your weight at a reasonable level for you.

Avoid Crash Diets

If you're 20 percent over your target weight, start trying to lose weight gradually and sensibly. You all know how to find your target weight: look at one of those horrible charts put out by the insurance companies, the ones where you always need to decide that yes, you *are* big-boned and deserve to be in the heaviest category. (It's amazing how many "big-boned" women I know!) Bit by bit, decrease the amount of food you eat. This doesn't mean eating like a rabbit. Perimenopause is not the time for a crash diet. One of the causes of decreased peak bone mass is the continual dieting too many of us engage in for too much of our lives. Also, extreme dieting can lead to anorexia, a serious disorder that is certainly more dangerous then a few extra pounds. On average, you'll need 400 *fewer* calories a day to maintain the same weight at age eighty than you do at age fifty. Make what you eat count nutritionally, cutting down on fat and increasing fiber, fruits, vegetables, and soy.

Avoid Late-Night Meals

It's also very important to look at *when* you eat. Many of you are probably like me: you tend to eat a small breakfast or none at all, grab a quick lunch on the run, and nibble throughout the workday. When you get home, you're starving. So you sit down to a big meal at seven o'clock, finish at eight, and then go to bed an hour or two later. This is the worst way to eat.

There's a fascinating study about this.[30] Some researchers wondered why Japanese sumo wrestlers are so obese, when the Japanese diet is so healthy—low in fat and high in soy. So they interviewed a group of the wrestlers about their eating habits. It turns out that basically a sumo wrestler's diet is no different from that of the average Japanese man, except for two factors. Sumo wrestlers consume more calories, and they make sure to eat a big meal just before going to bed. The latter appeared to be the most important factor in their weight gain. For a sumo wrestler, weight gain is useful—but if obesity isn't in your job description, you can help avoid it simply by shifting the timing of your meals.

A less colorful study showed why this happens.[31] Robert Superko at the University of California at Berkeley found that the triglyceride levels are highest four hours after a big meal. If you have that big meal during the day, you can burn up these triglycerides. If your triglycerides peak at two A.M., however, they are stored as fat.

So you should either eat your larger meals earlier in the day, or just eat a number of small meals instead. This advice is difficult to fit into your lifestyle if you're working and your only time with your family is when you all sit together at the dinner table at seven o'clock at night. Still, you can decrease the amount you eat at the family meal while maintaining the ritual.

Watch Both Fat and Calories

In the old days, the buzzword was "calories." You were told to avoid anything that was high in calories, and that was pretty much all that mattered. Then we did a turnaround: it wasn't calories that mattered, it was high fat content. So the current style in dietary circles has been a diet low in protein and fat and high in complex carbohydrates. But as is so often the case, the baby got thrown out with the bathwater. Calories *do* make a difference—especially if you're overweight. The huge bowls of pasta we're eating aren't making us thinner. Pasta is a good food, but a lot of it has a lot of calories.

Further, since "low-fat" and "fat-free" are our current magic words, it's easy to see them jumping out at you in large letters on the front of the package and ignore the rest of the label. Look very carefully at every label on the food you buy. Often the reason a low-fat product tastes so good is that it contains a lot of sugar. Sugar isn't fat, but it turns into fat in your body, so replacing fat with sugar isn't really improving anything. Also, beware our other magic word—"natural." Many products boast that they have "all-natural" ingredients. Remember that sugar is a natural ingredient, and it's in a lot of those "healthy" foods.

A combination of choosing nutrient-rich foods and eating smaller portions more often may be a better choice than all those big platefuls of pasta. Nutritionists disagree about that, as they do about some of the other finer points of diet. Everyone agrees, however, that we don't need a high-fat diet and that we all should eat at least five servings of fruits and vegetables a day.

What If You're Too Thin?

There are some women who are too thin. These are the ones who are at risk for osteoporosis and more hot flashes. For some, being underweight is a matter of metabolism alone. Others have dieted most of their lives to get to that weight, and for them the problems are worse. These women might actually consider gaining a few pounds to help them through the menopausal transition. I know this sounds like absolute heresy in our culture, which is obsessed with thinness and in which any weight gain is often accompanied by feelings of guilt and anxiety. We've been told our whole lives that gaining weight is the ultimate sin. But in reality, "middle-age spread" can have some good points. Susun Weed, in her book *Menopausal Years*,[32] actually recommends that premenopausal women who aren't overweight begin to gain slowly—a pound a year—to prepare themselves for perimenopause. She feels that ten "extra" pounds are the "best ally you can have on your menopausal journey." I find her argument persuasive. There may be a reason your body wants to gain weight for menopause: those extra pounds keep bones strong, reduce hot flashes, and cushion you against falls. Still, before you make a beeline for the cream puffs, remember that we're talking about a *few* pounds. And those extra pounds shouldn't be all fat—they should be a combination of fat, muscle, and bone.

The key here is that good old-fashioned virtue: moderation. It's important to avoid both obesity and fanatical weight loss. We spend much too much time on dieting and weight loss and not enough on good nutrition and a healthy lifestyle.

So how do you gain a little weight but not too much? If you're among the rare people who don't put on weight with middle age, add a bit more complex carbohydrate to your diet. You can have a bigger plateful of pasta than the rest of us or add an extra slice or two of bread.

Diet and Cancer Prevention

Eating foods high in antioxidants, beta-carotene, and retinoids will help you lower your risk of cancer. In addition to the leafy greens, go for the fruits and vegetables that are orange and yellow; they're highest in antioxidants. A low-fat diet high in soy protein, fresh fruits and vegetables, and antioxidants can help prevent breast cancer, colon cancer, and heart disease. This is important to all women, but it is especially important if you're on hormone therapy, which increases risk of breast cancer. A recent study in the *Journal of the National Cancer Institute* showed that women who eat a lot of fruits and vegetables (more than five servings a day) have less breast cancer then those who eat less than three servings a day.[33] (Interestingly, some studies have shown that supplements of beta-carotene, one of the antioxidants, don't have the same effect as the real thing.)[34] In other words, do what your mother told you—eat your vegetables, especially your broccoli and carrots.

Developing Good Eating Habits

Keep a Food Diary

It usually takes work to develop good eating habits—most of us are too used to a high-fat, low-fiber diet to switch smoothly into a healthier mode. The best way to start on a diet like this is to keep a "food diary." Every day for a week, write down everything you eat. This means *everything*—not just what you eat at meals. The snacks and the little "extras" are usually what do you in. I suggest a week because one week is usually long enough to include all of the circumstances you're usually up against—including a weekend dinner in a restaurant or fast food at a ball game.

This dietary diary is for your eyes only, so you can be brutally honest. This kind of honesty can be very revealing: one well-known nutrition researcher told me that once he started keeping a food diary, he stopped eating his beloved chocolate eclairs. When you look at your own diary after a week and see everything you've been consuming, you're likely to be surprised—and maybe even appalled.

Once you've written your food diary, use one of the many books or computer programs available to calculate exactly how many calories you're getting from fat, protein, and carbohydrates. (To calculate calories, for every gram of fat multiply by nine; for every gram of protein and carbohydrate, multiply by four.) Then calculate what percentage of your diet is fat, carbohydrate, and protein.

The average American diet is 30 to 40 percent fat, when it should be 15 to 20 percent. Once you see where you're starting from, it becomes easier to see how to get to this goal. We provide several good sources of recipes and menus in Appendix 3. Although these can be helpful, they often don't take your individual circumstances into consideration, so you'll probably want to spend a little time tailoring them to your needs.

Other Techniques for Limiting Fat

A food diary is not the only way to develop better eating habits. If counting fat calories seems too obsessive to you, you can reduce fat to a certain degree simply by watching, and controlling, what you eat. Decrease the amount of meat or poultry you eat to one serving a week. (It's important to remember that a "portion" or "serving" is 3 ounces, or a piece the size of a pack of cards. Most Americans think a serving is two or three times that large.) When you do eat red meat or poultry, trim the fat or skin off. Eat fish and shellfish once or twice a week—most seafood is high in polyunsaturated omega 3 fatty acids, which help prevent heart disease. If you're a vegetarian, or an observant Jew who doesn't eat shellfish, you can increase your soy. Choose low-fat or no-fat dairy products. When you have to use oils or fats in cooking, use monosaturated forms such as olive oil and peanut oil. Stay away from fast foods and processed meats.

As you decrease fat and animal protein, increase fresh fruits, vegetables, and plant protein—especially soy. A diet high in a variety of fresh fruits and vegetables will supply many of the vital vitamins and minerals women over forty need. (Sometimes you may want to take vitamin and mineral supplements; we'll discuss those in the next chapter.)

ALCOHOL IN MODERATION

Sometimes improving your health is a matter of subtraction rather than addition. Alcohol is a ritualistic part of many of our lives, but many of us overuse it.

Moderate use of alcohol has mixed effects. One drink a day—a 4-ounce glass of wine, a 12-ounce can of beer, or 1 ounce of hard liquor—may help to decrease heart disease and osteoporosis. Alcohol has bioflavinoids and phytoestrogens in it, so it presumably raises your estrogen levels. Not surprisingly, then, one drink a day will also increase your risk of breast and endometrial cancer—even four drinks a week increases the risk of breast cancer. And heavy drinking is always bad for your health, whether or not you're an alcoholic.

Unfortunately, alcohol is worse for women than for men. A woman's body doesn't metabolize alcohol as well as a man's, and so the damage to the liver per drink is higher for a woman. Problems from drinking include pancreatitis; cirrhosis of the liver; cancer of the esophagus, head, and neck; and cancer of the liver.

What constitutes "heavy drinking"? Less than you might think: you don't have to be falling-down drunk to be a heavy drinker. For a woman, more than two drinks a day is "heavy." If you find that you're drinking to that extent, you need to reevaluate the role alcohol is playing in your life. Are you using it to reduce stress? Then maybe you should try one of the techniques we describe below instead. Are you using it to help you sleep? Alcohol can actually inhibit restful sleep. Try daily exercise or another method for improving sleep. One simple aid is to make sure you do something relaxing to wind down at the end of the day—watching light TV or reading a light novel, for example. If you need some kind of drink at night, make it chamomile tea, or the old standby warm milk. You could even make that warm soymilk. Is alcohol helping you tolerate a bad relationship? Then maybe counseling would be more effective.

I must admit this is an area I have difficulty with. I come from a large Irish Catholic family, and alcohol has always been part of my life. For me it's the easiest way to reduce stress, and I have to be continually on guard against slipping into the habit of drinking a glass or two of wine every night.

Unless you have a drinking problem, you don't need to give up alcohol completely. But it's really wise to keep it at no more than three drinks a week. This won't increase your risk of breast cancer, and it can still help lower your risk of heart disease. Save your drinking for specific times, and then savor it. Have a glass of wine with a special dinner. Celebrate with champagne when the occasion calls for it. Have a beer at the baseball game. And leave alcohol alone the rest of the time. If you don't drink, don't feel you have to start.

QUIT SMOKING

Why You Should Stop Smoking

There's no question that smoking is the single most dangerous thing you can do in terms of your overall health. It causes premature menopause (and wrinkles)—and that's the least of it.

Smoking is an enormous risk factor for heart disease. Among the women in the Nurses' Health Study,[35] one of the most comprehensive studies ever done, it was the greatest risk factor. If you quit smoking, your risk of heart disease will be reduced by 14 percent within two years, and after ten to fourteen years your risk is scarcely higher than that of people who never smoked.

Smoking also dramatically increases your risk of osteoporosis. In addition, it causes emphysema, cervical cancer, lung cancer, bladder cancer, cancer of the nose and mouth and throat, and cancer of the esophagus.

In some ways smoking is even worse for women than it is for men. A woman who smokes the same amount as a man is more likely than he is to get lung cancer. If you're on estrogen replacement therapy, you increase this risk even more.

How to Stop Smoking

Studies have shown that the most common reason women give for not quitting smoking is their fear of gaining weight. Smoking also serves many women as a major way to reduce stress. If you want to quit, you need to take this into consideration. It's important that you develop other methods of losing weight and reducing stress—such as exercise—before you try to quit smoking. In addition, give yourself permission to gain an extra eight or ten pounds, at least temporarily. If you deprive yourself of too much all at once, you're much more likely to go back to smoking.

Giving up smoking is never easy. You're giving up both a physical and an emotional addiction. It's a loss, and, as with any loss, you need time to grieve. You may be able to do it on your own, but you may also need some help. Look into comprehensive smoking cessation programs to help you succeed. Seek out other methods. There are lots of them out there—nicotine gum and patches, support groups, hypnosis, acupuncture. And don't give up if it doesn't work the first time. Try another approach. It often takes several tries before you can really quit.

I firmly believe you have to start by deciding in your heart of hearts that you want to quit. Then, you need to set a date. Next, you need to mobilize your friends and family to help you.

It can be done. I started to smoke heavily when I was twenty, and I kept it up for ten years. I decided to quit at age thirty because I felt I was now an adult. Besides, as a doctor I'd seen some of the horrors caused by smoking. I didn't succeed when I tried to quit on my own, however. So I made an appointment to see a hypnotist. On the way up to his office I smoked three cigarettes. They were my last. The most important thing the hypnotist said to me was that I would no longer think of myself as a smoker. It was hard, but the hypnosis, and my own determination, got me through it. I haven't had a cigarette in nearly twenty years—and I no longer even crave cigarettes.

Of all the changes discussed in this chapter, quitting smoking will have the most profound effect on your health. If you're a smoker and you're concerned enough with preventing disease to read this book, you can quit. Your life is worth it.

EXERCISE

If there were a drug that had as many good effects as exercise has, we'd all be buying stock in it and getting rich. Yet most people don't take advantage of exercise. It's free, it's familiar, and it's not a chemical. So we don't trust this simple thing nature has made accessible to us.

Exercise and Your Heart

Exercise can affect almost all aspects of your life. Regular exercise will decrease your risk of heart disease by raising the level of good HDL and lowering bad LDL. Sedentary women are three times more likely to die of heart attacks than women who exercise regularly. If you're at risk for heart disease, you can reduce your chance of dying of a heart attack 50 percent by becoming physically fit. This is the same figure that's been touted for Premarin—but somehow the drug companies don't seem to be quite as anxious to push exercise.[36] Studies have also shown that regular moderate exercise is as good as medication for lowering high blood pressure.

Exercise and Cancer

Exercise can also lower your risk of breast cancer. Premenopausal women who exercise 3.8 hours a week will decrease their risk of breast cancer by 70 percent if they have had full-term pregnancies and by 30 percent if they haven't.[37] Exercise may offer this protection in part because it lengthens your menstrual cycle, thus decreasing the overall amount of estrogen and progesterone your body is exposed to. Over time, this can add up to an enormous decrease, so it behooves every premenopausal woman to get onto a regular exercise program.

We don't know if exercise lowers the risk of breast cancer in post-menopausal women, but it's certainly worth a try, given all the other benefits it offers older women.

In addition, physically active women have less ovarian, uterine, and colon cancer than sedentary women.

Exercise and Your Bones

Women who have done a lot of muscle strengthening have stronger bones. This may have to do with increased estrogen production, especially since, as we saw in Chapter 11, women who exercise also have fewer symptoms of menopause. Until recently, it seemed that the only way to increase your own estrogen production after menopause was to gain weight. I always thought this was unfair. It *is* unfair—and what's more, it's untrue. My research has shown me that there are other possibilities. Like fat, muscle contains an enzyme called aromatase, which converts testosterone and androstenedione into estrone (a form of estrogen).

Researchers in St. Louis found that in less than twenty-two months women who exercised at least three times a week increased their bone density 5.2 percent, while sedentary women actually lost 1.2 percent of their bone.[38] After twenty-two months, the exercisers in the study had increased their bone mass by 6.1 percent—which is comparable to the changes seen with a medication such as estrogen or Fosamax. A recently reported randomized controlled study from Canada found that subjects who exercised for sixty minutes three times a week for a year stabilized their bone mass, improved their cardiorespiratory endurance, and had a better overall sense of well-being than those in the control group.[39] However, as with estrogen supplements, as soon as the women stopped exercising for a week or more, their bone density began to decline. Bone will grow again when you start exercising again, so it's important to choose an exercise program you can stick with—as we discuss later in this chapter.

Combining exercise with enough vitamin D and calcium (see Chapter 13) can decrease your risk of fractures by 30 percent. In addition, by making you stronger and improving your balance, it will decrease your risk of the falls that lead to fractures.

To help your bones, you've got to do some exercise against gravity. Jogging, running, or walking are the best forms of exercise because they use large muscles and make you support your own weight. Bicycling and swimming are next best. Although it was once thought that swimming didn't benefit bones, it now appears that it does increase bone density in your back.

Steven Blair at the Institute for Aerobics Research in Dallas found that people who engaged in regular physical activity had lower death rates from all causes. Death rates declined from 39 per 10,000 people per year among the least fit to 8 per 10,000 people per year among the most fit.[40]

Getting Started with Exercise

Ah, yes, you sigh. I realize now that I should have been exercising all these years. But the damage is done; it's too late to start now. And you fall sadly but comfortably back into the depths of your overstuffed chair.

Well, you're wrong. Although it's true that exercise is most effective if you start young, it can help you at any age. Studies have found that ninety-year-old women in nursing homes can increase their fitness when they start exercise programs.

Before you assume that this means you're condemned to a daily visit to purgatory, stop and think about all the activities that involve exercise. Many women have an allergic reaction to the notion of exercise—they don't want to stand in front of the television set imitating the gyrations of some cheery health guru, and they see the health club with its fancy machines as a modern-day version of the Tower of London's torture chamber. But if you give it some creative thought, you may be able to identify some kind of exercise that you can enjoy—or at least tolerate. Exercise means getting your body moving and using your muscles. It can be tap dancing, ice skating, step aerobics, swimming, walking, bicycling, in-line skating, gardening, ballroom dancing, tennis, basketball, softball, soccer, ballet, hiking, cross-country skiing, jogging—any number of things.

If you have arthritis and find all of these movements difficult (or even if you don't), you may want to look into water aerobics. Water is less stressful on the joints, and the resistance of water is great for strengthening muscles.

Even if there's no sport you really like, you can build exercise into your regular activities. My determinedly sedentary coauthor doesn't mind walking, so she works that into her daily life. There's a bus stop around the corner from her house that goes to her subway station—but she ignores it and walks ten minutes to the station and back. Often she gets off at the stop ahead of hers, adding another fifteen minutes to her walk. Adding this kind of exercise doesn't require any more time than the activity itself—no changing into sweats or going back and forth to the gym.

Of course, as I keep reminding my coauthor, not everyone hates to exercise. If you enjoy exercise, as I do, you're ahead of the game. Now you just have to make sure you do it regularly, and get in the basic kinds of exercise you'll need to stay in your best shape.

Creating an Exercise Routine

How do you start creating an exercise program suitable to your own goals? First, you have to identify those goals. The major goals include flexibility, increased muscle strength, and aerobic conditioning.

Stretching for Flexibility

Flexibility is best achieved by stretching. When you were a kid, you were flexible (I look at my eight-year-old sitting on the floor and marvel). But I don't have to tell you those days are gone. If you want to maintain flexibility, you need to work on it. Five minutes of stretching a day can increase your flexibility considerably and make you feel better. There are several books available that give you the outlines of stretching for a variety of activities. My couch-potato coauthor has grudgingly admitted that daily stretching exercises actually do make her feel better—more energized to focus on the reading and writing she prefers to spend her time on.

Stretching is often best done when your muscles are "warm." This means that you've been using them to exercise or at least move around a bit. You can combine stretching with the rest of your program by tacking it onto the end or doing stretches after you've warmed up a bit. Don't neglect it—the aches and pains that come after exercise are due as much to lack of stretching as to the exertion itself.

Building Muscle

Muscles have a tendency to weaken with age, adding to overall frailty and the tendency to fall, so you'll probably want to do some muscle-building exercises. These can also help increase bone density; bone attached to a muscle being exercised will increase in density. For example, squats increase the bone mass in your hips. Although all exercise will strengthen some muscles, it's best if you strengthen all of them. Jogging, for instance, increases the muscles in your legs but doesn't do much for your arm muscles.

The best way to strengthen your muscles is with weight resistance training. You can do this with machines, like those in a gym or health club, or by using free weights (small dumbbells of different weights) at home. There are books and videos that can help you get started, or you can hire a trainer for a lesson or two. Once you're in a routine, it becomes easy. You should start with muscle strengthening three times a week, every other day. (Take Sunday off.) Daily weight training doesn't give your muscles enough time to recuperate between efforts.

Aerobics

Cardiovascular training is also important. You can think of it as exercising your heart. This means aerobic exercise, which will get your heart rate into the target range. Aerobic exercise can take the form of walking at a brisk pace, bicycling (either outdoors or on a stationary bike), swimming, or any other activity that will get your heart beating faster.

Your target heart rate (beats per minute) is calculated by subtracting your age from 220, and then multiplying the resulting figure by 0.6 to 0.8. So, for example, if you're 50, subtract that from 220 and you get 170 beats per minute. Multiply that by 0.6 and you get 102; multiply by 0.8 and you get 136.

You can check your heart rate by feeling for the pulse in your neck, counting the beats for ten seconds, and multiplying by 6. Your heart rate should be between 102 and 136. This formula is fairly accurate for premenopausal women, though according to Morris Notelovitz,[41] it underestimates the target range for women in their sixties by 6.9 percent and for women in their seventies by up to 16 percent.

A breath test is an easier way to determine whether you're exercising aerobically. You should be able to sing "God bless America, land that I love" before taking a breath. (If, like my coauthor, you loathe "God Bless America," pick a song line that takes the same amount of time. She's settled on "Come to me, my melancholy baby.") If you can go on to the next line without taking that breath, you're exercising too little; if you need to catch your breath between words, you're working too hard. You shouldn't be panting, but you should have some feeling of exertion.

How Much Exercise Should I Do?

To keep your heart in shape, you need to exercise twenty minutes a day, three to four times a week. If you're interested in weight control as well, increase that to forty-five minutes every day. To build bone mass, you need twenty to thirty minutes a day of antigravity exercise—such as walking, jogging, or bicycling—two to three times a week. Add upper-body weight training (fifteen minutes of lifting two to three times a week). For stress reduction, thirty to forty minutes of brisk walking every other day will work wonders.

Yoga is a wonderful way to incorporate many of these elements and stress reduction too. Many women find it is a perfect way to maintain their fitness.

More Thoughts on Exercise

If you've been sitting on your duff for the past twenty years, let me remind you that you should have a physical examination before starting an exercise program. This should include tests for cholesterol level and blood pressure, which you can then use as a baseline. After six months of exercise, you can recheck them to see if your new habits have had an effect.

There are lots of aids available for exercising. There are videos for aerobics, for muscle toning, for flexibility, and for all three combined (see Appendix 3). If you prefer to exercise in the privacy of your home, videos may be the perfect choice. There are also audiotapes: I use music tapes on which a beat is maintained at a set pace to keep me going when I walk briskly or jog. You can get everything from rock to big band music to country and western, and from three to ten miles per hour.

If you prefer to work out with others, you can join a health club. Or you can get a group together to walk early in the morning, during lunch breaks, or after work in the evening. Often working out with a group, or even just one friend, can motivate you on those days when you're tempted to stay home and watch TV. (If you prefer, you *can* stay at home and watch TV—on your treadmill or exercise bike. You can even build in bribes to yourself: "I can watch *General Hospital* only if I do it while I'm exercising.")

But how do you put all these things together into a cohesive program? A one-hour program might include a five-minute warm-up (walking slowly or stretching) followed by fifteen minutes of weight training on machines or free weights; then thirty minutes of aerobics (brisk walking, running, bicycling, dancing, climbing stairs) followed by a ten-minute cool-down (stretching). A thirty-minute routine could alternate muscle strengthening one day with aerobics the next. But again, make sure you pick something you know you can stick to. It may be easier for you to space your exercise out. Walk to and from work, for example, and do your weight training every other evening.

The more research I did for this book, the more I became convinced that regular exercise was the most important lifestyle change I could make.

Although I've been involved with athletics throughout my life, I've also had intermittent periods of being fairly sedentary. This book started me back on a regular program. Now when my daughter is in school, I get up at five A.M. and walk or jog (or both) for ten minutes on a treadmill. Then I do two to three strength-training (weight-lifting) repetitions while my heart rate is still up. I then get back on the treadmill for ten more minutes and back to weights. I do this circuit three times for a total of thirty minutes of aerobics, and alternate upper-body weight training one day with lower-body weight training the next. It takes forty-five minutes all together, and I watch the news while I do it. Once I'm done, I stretch and then get my daughter up at six for school. I feel much better, sleep better, and definitely feel a sense of moral superiority. On weekends and in the summer, the dog and I go for an hour-long "power walk" or a slow jog along the beach, followed by ten to fifteen minutes of weights and stretching. This works for me. Not only does it make me feel healthier, but it gives me a sense of control over my body when being in perimenopause makes me feel out of control in so many other ways.

I realize that my heavy-duty routine isn't right for everyone. Some of you might be closer to my end of the spectrum; some might be closer to my coauthor's. She wants to do as little as she can possibly do and still get some benefit from it. As we worked on this book, she finally broke down and got some three-pound weights and a video and has started to do weight training for fifteen minutes every other day. She's added that to her walking and stretching. She's been sticking with it, and she's even beginning to enjoy it, much to her chagrin.

And that's the key. If my coauthor tried my heavy routine, she'd quit in a week. If I used her mild routine, I'd be bored to death. You have to find what will work for you. Remember, you're not just trying to find an exercise pattern for the next six weeks to lose an extra five pounds—your goal is to get fit and stay fit for the rest of your life. It's better to do a little less and stick with it than to do a killer regime for a couple of weeks and then drop it in despair.

There are also a number of small things you can do—with or without a regular routine—that can incorporate exercise. Use the stairs instead of the elevator or escalator. While I was still at UCLA, I got into the habit of walking the five flights of stairs to the clinic. At first I'd arrive huffing and puffing and dripping with sweat, but soon I could do it while remaining cool and collected. Walk to the store instead of driving (harder to do in L.A.). At home, don't save yourself steps by waiting for things to stack up before taking them upstairs—make all of those extra trips; they'll work your muscles. Look for ways to be active. Even standing up four hours a day can increase your bone density. Every little bit counts.

I like to think of exercise as a medical treatment without side effects, but that's not always the case. You have to be careful not to overdo it, especially if you're just starting. And you need to be conscious of your body's messages to you. Jogging and squats can be hard on the joints. If you're feeling frequent pain in your joints, check with your doctor and modify your routine. One of my friends walked around for months with pain in her foot, which her doctor said was nothing. She finally found a podiatrist who discovered a tiny stress fracture in her ankle: she'd gone from no exercise to strenuous walking without giving her body time to build up to it. I suddenly switched from walking to jogging in the hills around my house. Running downhill turned out to be too hard for my legs, but as soon as I changed to the relatively flat beach, I was okay. This doesn't mean that the slightest muscle ache should be your excuse to give up forever, but it does mean you should be sensible. Moderation counts, even here.

REDUCING STRESS

One of the worst threats to health is chronic stress. It increases blood pressure, respiratory rate, heart rate, and oxygen consumption. Stress isn't a bad thing in itself: it's the body's way of alerting you to danger, so you can do whatever is required to escape. But when it becomes chronic, it interferes with the body's resistance to illness and its ability to repair itself. When you're stressed, your body has a "fight or flight" reaction, pouring out epinephrine and norepinephrine, causing your heart to race and mobilizing your body for action. This reaction, which is great if you have to run away from an attacker, isn't the best way to handle sitting in traffic on the freeway. The results of chronic stress are heart disease, high blood pressure, and cancer.

I hate it when well-meaning friends tell people to cut out the stress in their lives, as if it were something you could remove surgically. Stressful situations are part of everyone's life, and, as we discussed in Chapter 3, the years when you're approaching or beginning menopause are often the time when new stresses are added to your life: the loss of aging parents, the departure of kids for college or jobs. What you can do, though, is change the way you deal with stress.

Health Benefits of Stress Reduction

Reducing stress—or dealing with it better—sounds like motherhood and apple pie. Of course it's a good idea. Of course you feel better. But did you know that in randomized controlled studies it has been found to lower blood pressure? There is even some evidence, which I'll discuss in Chapter

13, that it might affect the progress of life-threatening diseases like cancer and heart attacks. And as we saw in Chapter 11, it can reduce hot flashes.

Reducing Stress by Taking Time for Yourself

I met Susun Weed, author of *Menopausal Years: The Wise Woman Way,*[42] when we both spoke on a panel on hormones in Philadelphia, and I was impressed with her view of menopause. She sees this stage of a woman's life as no less than a metamorphosis, a complete change from one state of life to another. She says that the first step of menopause is a need for isolation. She uses a wonderful metaphor: a caterpillar who's been munching leaves with all of the other caterpillars until one day it looks up and says, "I don't want to munch another leaf. In fact, I don't even want to hear leaves being munched anymore!" So it moves away and finds a place to weave its cocoon.

We need our own version of that cocoon, Weed says, and she uses another image for the time menopausal women need—a "crone's year away." For a particular woman, that "year" may be only a month, a day, or even a few minutes, but we all need some time to ourselves, especially around perimenopause. The enormous physical changes we go through may be our body's way of telling us to wake up and readjust. Maybe irritability and mood swings are the body's attempt to drive everyone away so that we can have the time we need alone.

While I was writing this book and wiping off the perspiration from my hot flashes, I suddenly realized that I needed a break from my medical practice. I'd been caring for patients for almost twenty years; I needed to take a break to focus on caring for myself. As a result, I retired from seeing patients. I have many activities I'm still involved in, from research, teaching, lecturing, and writing to going back to school to get my MBA. Maybe I'll go back to patient care at some point, maybe not. I hadn't really thought that this change had anything to do with approaching menopause until I heard Susun Weed on that panel. But doing this for myself has made an enormous difference in my level of stress.

Your own "crone's year" may not involve anything as drastic as quitting your job. But it could include some major change—moving to a new home, taking a long-dreamed-of trip. On the other hand, it could be something as simple as finding a way to create time for yourself and to bring peace and relaxation into your life. Billye Avery, the founder of the National Black Women's Health Project, suggested (in a speech I heard in Provincetown) that all women give themselves an hour a day when they don't have to answer to anyone but themselves. You can meditate, exercise, pray, or listen to music—but do it alone. Above all, don't use your hour as a chance to catch up on chores or other work. Have a family meeting and announce that this will be your hour, and no one is to interrupt you. I know I just told you to find time for exercise, and now I'm telling you to find yet another hour from a day that's already too busy. But adding exercise and "alone" time will recharge your batteries, so you'll do the other things in your life more efficiently and more wholeheartedly. Just as menopause is a wake-up call for nutrition and exercise, it should be a wake-up call for incorporating techniques for stress reduction into your life.

Mind-Body Techniques for Reducing Stress

It's not hard to convince people that the mind can have a powerful effect on the body. Any woman knows that all she has to do is worry that she might be pregnant, and her period will be late. We all know of people who stay alive against all odds until a special event has occurred and then, as soon as they're ready, die.

Effects of mind-body have been inadvertently demonstrated by scientists in an interesting way. Remember the cholesterol studies we discussed in Chapter 6, in which even the control group, who took a placebo, experienced a change in HDL levels? This change was less than that among the groups that took hormones, but it occurred. The only explanation is that some of the subjects believed they were getting a remedy. This was hardly an isolated event: many studies find a significant change in subjects who receive placebos. Norman Cousins called the public's attention to this in his 1979 book *Anatomy of an Illness*,[43] in which he advocated a conscious use of the placebo effect to heal illnesses—and reported that he himself had done so.

The most common self-administered mind-body methods of stress reduction are meditation, mental imagery, autosuggestion, progressive relaxation, breath therapy (discussed here), and mindfulness (discussed later in this chapter). These are all variations on a single theme: getting in touch with your inner core.

The most important of these techniques is *meditation*. Herbert Benson, a doctor who has studied many alternative forms of healing, calls his own version of meditation the "relaxation response."[44] This was the basis of his work as director of behavioral medicine at Deaconess Hospital in Boston. With his colleagues, he ran several groups for people with a variety of diseases. One of the doctors who worked for a time in the group for cancer was the oncologist Leo Stolbach, who reported positively on the results. "What the relaxation response can do," Stolbach said, "is to slow down or even stop the continuous chatter the mind is constantly putting us through. It gives the mind a rest from those thoughts and then a chance to deal with the issues they raise." He described a number of physiological responses to the relaxation response: a decrease in pulse, blood pressure, respiration rate, oxygen consumption, and overall metabolism—all of which helped reduce stress.[45]

Meditation is easy to describe, although it's harder to do. There are many different ways to meditate, coming out of many different traditions. All of them are said to induce the relaxation response.[46] One of the most popular begins with finding a quiet, comfortable place where you can spend fifteen to twenty minutes. The next steps include repetition of a word, sound, phrase, or prayer, and a passive return to the repetition whenever thoughts intrude. The famous *om* is one such word—it comes from Eastern traditions—but you can use any word that has meaning to you, like *peace*, or a phrase from your favorite prayer.

There's good evidence that meditation measurably reduces stressful reactions in the body. One study compared meditation and exercise to see which had the stronger effect on beta endorphins (chemicals that act like narcotics in the brain) and corticophin-releasing factor (a hormone from the brain that tells the adrenal gland to release cortisol). They found equal effects in elite runners and experienced meditators, showing that you don't have to sweat to get a "runner's high."[47]

In my favorite study, researchers quantified the effect of adding meditation to a "happiness enhancement program." Those who meditated scored highest on the "happiness" measure.[48] I can't think of a greater role for any lifestyle change, any alternative, or any drug than "happiness enhancement." Excuse me while I go meditate.

Mental imagery—also known as *visualization*—can be used with meditation or on its own. We've already discussed the use of mental imagery for symptoms such as hot flashes. It can also work for generally calming yourself, and to bolster your system against future disease. This ancient technique, rediscovered in recent years by "new age" devotees, has as its basis the belief that if you create strong mental pictures of what you want, while affirming to yourself that you can and will get it, you can make virtually anything happen. It involves imagining that the changes you want to happen in your body (or in your life) are actually happening. For example, you might imagine that your bones are sturdy, rocklike structures impervious to decay. Or you might visualize one of your concerns metaphorically— LDL as an army advancing through your arteries toward your heart, and HDL as a defending army, defeating the LDL. There are many, many ways you can envision a problem and its solution. This technique has actually been found to increase immune function, and to achieve some remarkable cures. (You can also use it to help you achieve other goals, from getting a job to finding a parking space. Maybe you've always wanted to go to Paris: take part of your "alone" hour and visualize yourself walking along the

Seine. This may sound like hocus-pocus, but if you tell your mind something will happen, you open yourself to the possibilities that may have been there all along without your seeing them.)

Autosuggestion (also called *affirmation*) is similar to visualization, but it is a verbal rather than a visual approach. You use phrases rather than images to describe the changes you want. When the changes are health-related, you focus on the area of the body involved as you form words (in your mind, or out loud, depending on which you're more comfortable with and where you are). The phrase can be very simple—"I am calm and serene," or "My heart is strong and healthy." Whenever your mind wanders, bring your attention gently back to the phrase.

For autosuggestion to be effective, two things are very important. One is to use the present tense rather than the future: "I am healthy," *not* "I will be healthy." If that feels too discordant—as it sometimes does when you're feeling very uncomfortable and can't persuade your mind that you feel great—you can phrase it in terms of a choice: "I choose to be healthy." Formulating your wish in the future pushes it away from the present. As the song says, tomorrow is always a day away.

The second essential thing is to use positive, not negative, phrasing: "My bones are strong" rather than "I won't get osteoporosis." You don't want to insinuate into your mind the very idea you're trying to program it against.

If you want to try working with mind-body techniques on your own, there are a number of audiotapes and videotapes on relaxation and imagery that you might want to try out. If none of these tapes is exactly right for you, you can try creating your own. In *The Road Back to Health*, the psychologist Neil Fiore suggests a model for creating your own visualization tape.[49]

Progressive relaxation involves tensing each muscle for a count of ten and then releasing for a count of ten before moving on to the next muscle.

Breath therapy induces the relaxation response by concentrating on slow, deep diaphragmatic breathing.

Laughter and Stress Reduction

When Norman Cousins set about to cure himself of a degenerative illness, he came up with a creative form of therapy. This rather formidable intellectual decided to laugh his way back to health. "I discovered that ten minutes of genuine belly laughter had an anesthetic effect and would give me at least two hours of pain-free sleep," he wrote.[50] He researched and found the medical basis for this: laughter can stimulate endorphins.

Several of my patients have used laughter as an important part of their healing process. One woman had breast cancer twice, and laughter was an integral part of her treatment. "I told people I wanted to laugh. Friends sent me funny books, cut out cartoons, called me and said funny things," she reported. Eventually she died of her cancer, but her multilevel approach to fighting her disease had given her the strength she needed to live her life fully to the end—and to help launch the breast cancer political movement. Laughter can help heal, as it did with Cousins; and it can help improve the quality of your life, as it did with my patient. I have no doubt that, together with other approaches, it can help prevent disease as well.

Integrating Stress Reduction into Your Everyday Activities

Some techniques for reducing stress can be used during your normal life, apart from your special "hour apart." You can use deep breathing at any time, for instance, to work on a specific symptom as it's occurring (this is what makes it so good for hot flashes), or simply to program your mind to relax. Similarly, you can say "affirmations" at any time, and for any length of time.

One technique—*mindfulness*—is actually designed to work as part of everyday activities, rather than in a particular, set-aside time. Mindfulness is really a form of meditation. You become mindful of whatever is happening now and focus on it—whether it's washing the car, sharpening a pencil, or reading a bedtime story to your children. Whenever thoughts intrude, you bring your mind back to its focus.

Making meditation or the relaxation response or some other stress-reduction technique a habit can be one of the most important steps you take to improve the quality of your life and prevent disease. On the other hand, not every technique is good for everybody. Lawrence LeShan, in *How to Meditate*,[51] emphasizes that meditation is something you have to work at, and that it needs to feel right for you. Meditation, he says, should "make you feel better when you do it than when you don't do it." If it doesn't, you should stop doing it.

I would go a bit farther. There are times in your life when you have enough you need to work at, and the thought of one more pressure, one more obligation, is too much to deal with. If that's how you feel, even meditation or visualization, for instance, may be the worse possible use of your "crone time." Sometimes the most healing things can be the most apparently trivial ones. Your "alone" hour might be best used listening to music, reading a romance novel, or watching a sitcom and laughing. Or maybe you just need to sit and stare out the window, letting thoughts flit through your mind without paying much attention to them. The worst thing you can do is get all stressed out about the need to fight stress. Find what works for you—and if it stops working, find something else. "Cronehood" is a very creative state.

SOCIAL SUPPORTS

There is growing evidence that supportive interpersonal relationships are strongly related to better health. We're social beings; we need contact with others to survive. It's unrealistic, particularly during a time of transition such as menopause, to expect your spouse, partner, lover, or best friend to be all things to you. You may want to find a support group where you can discuss the changes going on in your body and mind. A night out with your friends, a religious club, a reading group, or an exercise class may also help serve your need for like-minded companions. In one randomized study of women with metastatic breast cancer, the women who were assigned to a support group lived on average eighteen months longer than those who weren't.[52]

CREATIVITY

Another important aspect of lifestyle is creative activity. The end of biological fertility can be a good, symbolic time to stress other forms of creativity. You may want to take up painting, music, or writing. Or you might want to run for political office, or do volunteer work for a cause you believe in. Involve yourself in something you're passionate about. Your soul, like your body, needs exercise.

Although I'm suggesting a lot of changes that, in most cases, take a lot of self-discipline, I think it's equally important to be a bit self-indulgent. Life needs to be enjoyed. You need generally healthy habits, but you also need a room for the occasional exception. I generally eat a low-fat diet based on fish and vegetables—but I've decided that chocolate is a vegetable. I try to exercise six days a week—and sleep late on one. Having fun is vital to your emotional health. The goal isn't to prolong life at all costs—it's to live a joyful, vigorous, healthy life for as many years as you're given.

CHAPTER 13

Alternatives:
Acupuncture to Herbs

Ideally, we'd all exercise regularly, eat a perfect diet, develop terrific stress-management techniques, never touch tobacco or booze, and sail through life in vigorous health, meeting a peaceful and painless death at the age of a hundred. But life isn't always ideal. Some people would find the elements of creating a completely physically healthy lifestyle so difficult they wouldn't want to live to a hundred. And for others, even the most rigorously healthy regimen doesn't always provide enough of a sense that they're doing all they can to prevent osteoporosis and heart disease.

Though the pharmaceutical companies would have you believe that for such women, drugs are the only solution, that simply isn't the case. Before you make a choice about taking hormones, you might want to consider some alternative approaches.

In this chapter we're going to look at some of the supplements, herbs, and alternative treatments used for prevention of disease. I'll talk about traditional Chinese medicine (which includes herbs, acupuncture, and other treatments), Western herbal traditions, and vitamin therapy, among other methods. All of these involve more risk than making lifestyle changes but less risk than taking drugs.

As we mentioned in Chapter 11, the medical establishment is becoming increasingly interested in these alternative approaches. At the 1996 meeting of the American Association for Cancer Research, there were several reports of studies on ginseng and dong quai, as well as on soy and green tea. All were being studied in a vigorously scientific way in animal models to see if they have a beneficial effect on cancer. Perhaps in the next edition of this book we'll be able to include more traditional scientific data.

My plan in this chapter will be to describe the different alternative approaches to health that I believe can be helpful in restoring balance at this challenging time of life. Part of this involves looking at how each approach views menopause to demonstrate alternative ways to frame the experience. I'll also review what I think are the most tried and true herbs and remedies and give you references in case you want to explore anything more thoroughly.

A FIRST STEP: FINDING A GOOD PRACTITIONER

My original intention in this chapter was to describe herbs and other treatments that could be used as alternatives to Western preventive drug therapy. As I became immersed in the research, however, I realized that picking bottles of herbs off the health food shelf and trying them without supervision or prescription could be as ridiculous as pulling drugs off the pharmacy shelf and trying them out. This is important even when you're considering such treatments for short-term control of symptoms, as discussed in Chapter 11. When you're thinking about them for long-term use in preventing disease, it's still more important, for the same reason that it's important with Western medicines. The longer you take a substance, the more vulnerable you're likely to be to its side effects.

The initial research is something you can do on your own by checking out the literature on these healing techniques or talking with friends who have used them. But before you decide to start using an "alternative" healing method, you should consult with a qualified practitioner. It's not as simple as saying, "This herb is good for this symptom, so I'll take it." Just as you need a Western medical doctor to get a prescription for estrogen, you should see the appropriate practitioner to obtain the correct prescription for a given alternative therapy. If anything, alternative practitioners tend to individualize their therapies more than Western providers; and for most of these treatments, you'll need to be evaluated personally if you're going to benefit.

In Western medicine, we treat everything as if one size fits all. (For example, most doctors who put you on estrogen will automatically give you 0.625 milligram of Premarin regardless of why you're taking hormones, or what your height and weight are.) But many of these other traditions treat the person rather than the symptoms, as they try to restore balance. This requires that you see a diagnostician who can individualize a regimen for you. In addition, although many of these approaches can be complementary to Western (allopathic) medicine, they often don't work together.

Chinese herbs may have one aim whereas Ayurvedic herbs may be trying to achieve something entirely different, for instance. Practitioners of each approach can help you decide which herbs will work together and which will counteract each other—as well as which will work with or counteract whichever Western medications you're using.

I also strongly recommend you keep all of your health care providers and practitioners informed about every drug or remedy you may be taking. You should be careful not to mix and match without help.

MINERAL AND VITAMIN SUPPLEMENTS

Not all alternatives are unfamiliar, exotic, or "new age." In fact, some are things you probably use already—such as mineral and vitamin supplements.

There's no question that the best way to get the vitamins and minerals you need is in food. That way they come packaged with all of the other factors that can help them work. For example, while beta-carotene may be the most "active" carotene, taking it alone in a pill does not replicate the benefits of consuming foods rich in all 800 carotenes and 1,000-plus carotenoids. This has been recently demonstrated in studies which found that adding a supplement of beta-carotene to the diet of smokers and asbestos workers did not prevent lung cancer, as had been hoped, but may have actually made it worse.[1] On the other hand, eating a diet high in fruits and vegetables *does* help prevent cancer. Maybe we haven't isolated the right active ingredients, or maybe the active ingredients need to be taken along with certain other substances (cofactors). Thus I think we need to be careful about equating supplements with what we can get from our diet.

Having said that, I must still acknowledge none of us is perfect. There may be certain vitamins or minerals that you chronically miss in your diet. Take another look at your food diary (see page 206) and make some calculations for a few typical days, to see what you're really getting in your diet. This will give you a better idea of whether you need a supplement and if so how much. The women who are most likely to be missing some vitamins or minerals are those who smoke, are dieting, are under stress, have heavy menstrual bleeding, are vegetarians, or have digestive problems. One study of both men and women found that girls and women were getting less than 80 percent of the "recommended daily allowance" (RDA) of calcium, magnesium, iron, zinc, copper, and manganese.[2] In another study—a two-year study of women—about 70 percent of the subjects consumed less than 70 percent of the RDA for calcium and iron, and about 40 percent of these women didn't get enough vitamin B6 or magnesium.[3] This may be even more serious than it appears, since the recommended daily allowances were set to prevent deficiencies, not to promote health. The metabolic changes of menopause can require different amounts of some vitamins and minerals than you needed when you were younger. For example, you'll need more calcium than the RDA to help prevent osteoporosis, colon cancer, and high blood pressure.

Minerals

Calcium Supplements

As we said in Chapter 12, calcium is important for our hearts and bones, and possibly to help prevent colon cancer. A meta-analysis of calcium and bone mass in adult women suggested that women could add 0.8 percent bone mass per year with calcium supplements. The author speculated that "up to half of the women who take calcium supplements might prevent the usual 2% loss in bone that occurs with aging, and . . . high calcium intake could benefit women in their early postmenopausal years."[4] Calcium (along with vitamin D) has been found to reduce the incidence of colon cancer in a study of men.[5] Though there haven't been studies of its effect on colon cancer in women, it's likely that such an effect exists. Calcium and vitamin D also lower blood pressure in women.[6]

Calcium supplements come in a variety of formulations. Calcium citrate (Citrical) is the easiest to absorb on an empty stomach. But calcium carbonate (Tums, Os-cal, and their generic equivalents) is the most commonly used. It's absorbed well when chewed and taken with meals. It's also the least expensive and has the highest concentration of calcium. (And it's very well advertised—with a catchy tune borrowed from *Dragnet* and an ad campaign that seems strongly focused on women.) Calcium gluconate and lactate are less concentrated, so you have to take more tablets to get the same amount of calcium. You want to *avoid* dolomite, bonemeal, and oyster shell, since they're generally contaminated with lead and other minerals.

Calcium, calcium carbonate, calcium citrate, calcium lactate, and calcium gluconate are all forms of calcium. But it isn't just overall calcium that matters—it's the amount of *elemental* calcium a supplement contains. Read the label carefully. For example, the label for one generic calcium says: "Each tablet contains 500 milligrams of calcium carbonate or 200 milligrams of elemental calcium, which is 20 percent of the USRDA for calcium." Since the RDA underestimates your real need, this means that you'd need to take seven to eight tablets to get your daily requirement if you have none in your diet. Since you probably eat some foods with calcium, taking two to three tablets in the morning and two to three before bed is probably about right (800 to 1,200 milligrams).

Up to 2,000 milligrams of calcium daily is probably safe for most women, but more than that can increase the risk of kidney stones, as well as potentially increase your intake of harmful trace metals (manganese, lead, cadmium, aluminum copper, and arsenic) commonly found in antacids and supplements.

Calcium supplements are best taken as divided doses, as only about 750 milligrams can be absorbed at once. According to Susun Weed, 500 milligrams taken morning and night provides more calcium than 1,000 milligrams taken at one time.[7] But if you take calcium only once a day, do it at night, when your body needs more calcium. I always feel that taking Tums at night is triply good, since it gives me calcium, prevents heartburn, and helps me sleep. (My more frugal coauthor prefers her drugstore's own brand, which is fine—but you need to read the label and make sure it's got all the same ingredients as Tums, not one of the other, aluminum-based antacids. Make sure it says "calcium carbonate" on the label.)

To absorb calcium, you also need vitamin D, magnesium, and boron (see below).

Magnesium

One study suggests that magnesium may even be more important than calcium for building bones.[8] Magnesium depletion causes bones to stop growing, decreases osteoblastic and osteoclastic activity, and results in low bone density and increased fragility. Not only is magnesium important for the absorption of calcium, but low magnesium can cause vitamin D resistance. One study found that women who combined calcium and magnesium were actually able to build bone, as opposed to simply stopping its loss.[9]

Luckily, most foods high in calcium are also high in magnesium. (You should aim to have calcium and magnesium in a ratio of 2 to 1.) If you're taking 1,500 milligrams of calcium, you should take 750 milligrams of magnesium (*not* the laxative magnesium citrate) along with it. If you're not getting enough of one in your food, you won't be getting enough of the other either. Foods high in magnesium include nuts, legumes, cereal grains, dark-green vegetables, and seafood.

Other Minerals

Calcium and magnesium aren't the only minerals important in the menopausal and postmenopausal years. If you have heavy bleeding, you may be losing a lot of *iron*, so you'll need to increase your iron intake, which may mean taking supplements. On the other hand, after menopause, when you're no longer bleeding, you need less iron and can decrease your consumption. Overly high levels of iron have been associated with heart and liver disease. One way you can keep iron levels in check postmenopausally is to donate blood. You help other people and yourself at the same time (unless, of course, you're anemic, but they'll check your blood count before you're allowed to give blood). Iron can be found in red meat, fortified cereals, fish, green leafy vegetables, poultry, and beans. Most nutritionists recommend 15 milligrams a day for women under forty and 9 milligrams a day for those over forty.

Zinc is a trace element that's needed for adequate immune function. You need about 30 milligrams of zinc a day. Larger doses can interfere with copper metabolism, and doses over 2 grams (2,000 milligrams) are toxic. Sources of zinc include pumpkin seeds, oysters, and spirulina. Herbs containing zinc include sage, wild yam, and nettles, to mention just a few.

Copper helps build bones, lower cholesterol, and strengthen muscles. The best sources of copper are seafood, organically grown grains, beans, nuts, leafy greens, seaweeds, and bittersweet chocolate. (I always knew that chocolate was good for me!) A supplement of 2 milligrams daily is enough. Herbs containing copper include skullcap and sage.

Boron also helps keep bones healthy. It's found in green leafy vegetables, grapes, raisins, apples, nuts, wine, and cider. If you don't eat enough of those, you can take a 3-milligram supplement. Boron is found in all organic garden weeds, such as chickweed, nettles, and dandelion.

Chromium helps reduce cholesterol and therefore is another useful trace mineral. You can get it in brewer's yeast, wheat germ, whole grains, brown rice, beans, cheese, beer, and meat. A supplement of 100 micrograms a day is reasonable. (A microgram is one-millionth of a gram, or one-thousandth of a milligram.) Chromium is found in such herbs as oatstraw, nettles, red clover, wild yam, and black cohosh.

Selenium in the diet has been linked to a lower risk of breast cancer and heart attacks. Although there are no definitive data, a few provocative studies have found that regions with low levels of selenium in the soil have higher rates of cancer and heart disease.[10] Selenium is found in seafood, liver, kidneys, grains, chicken, mushrooms, and garlic. A supplement of 50 micrograms is reasonable, although (as with beta-carotene supplements), it may not have the same effect as it does in foods.

Manganese is good for bones, hearing, and prevention of diabetes. Recent studies of women with osteoporosis showed that they had manganese levels 29 to 75 percent lower than other women.[11] This mineral is found in seeds and leaves grown in healthy soil, and in seaweeds. Herbal sources include raspberry leaf, chickweed, ginseng, wild yam, nettles, and dandelion. A supplement of 5 micrograms daily is sufficient.

Phosphorus is important in the formation of bones and teeth. But it can be harmful too. Some animal studies have shown that a low calcium-to-phosphorus ratio leads to bone resorption.[12] Women who consume little in the way of dairy products and green vegetables can have a calcium-to-phosphorus ratio as low as 1 to 4. Most junk foods and sodas are very high in phosphorus and should be avoided. The recommended daily allowance of phosphorus is 800 milligrams, but supplements aren't usually necessary, because virtually all of us consume adequate amounts in our diet.

To summarize, if you're over forty, you should be sure you're getting (daily) 1,500 milligrams of calcium, 100 micrograms of chromium, 3 milligrams of boron, 2 milligrams of copper, 5 milligrams of manganese, 750 milligrams of magnesium, and 30 milligrams of zinc—while keeping your iron intake down to 9 milligrams, unless you're losing a lot of blood. Should you get a blood test to see if you're getting enough? Not really. Most of these minerals are bound in the body, so that blood levels may not reflect the true amount you have or need. A minimal supplement that provides the amounts we have listed won't be toxic even if you're getting enough in your food. Megadoses of minerals (and vitamins) are a different matter and should only be taken under a practitioner's supervision. More isn't necessarily better and can even be harmful.

Vitamins

As with minerals, the advantage of obtaining vitamins from food is that they come automatically combined with the appropriate minerals and cofactors that make them easiest to absorb and most functional. Rather than take up a lot of space about which vitamins are in which foods, I'll just give an overview here. The detailed information is available in many other places. And there are few surprises. Except for vitamin D, you can get most of the vitamins you need by eating lots of fruits, vegetables, and whole grains. (I told you there were few surprises!)

Vitamin D

Preliminary studies have found that aside from helping absorb calcium, vitamin D may help protect against colon cancer and breast cancer. This vitamin is found in your skin, and it's activated by the sun. Fifteen minutes in the sun daily without a sunblock will supply it. Unfortunately, the same ultraviolet rays that give you the vitamin D also cause skin cancer. This means that you need a sunblock, but you'll get less vitamin D when you're wearing a sunblock and may need to be out in the sun longer. Morris

Notelovitz and Diana Tonnessen did a study showing that women living in Florida had twice as much vitamin D in their blood during the spring as did women living in Finland. They also cite another study, which found that half of a group of postmenopausal women living in Boston were deficient in vitamin D during the winter months. However, those who took supplement of 220 IU (International Units) of vitamin D a day blocked seasonal fluctuations in parathyroid levels.[13] In Chapter 5, we talked about how parathyroid hormone regulates the amount of calcium in the blood. If your calcium levels are low because an insufficiency of vitamin D is keeping your body from absorbing it, your parathyroid will go into action and leech calcium from the bone in an attempt to remedy the situation.[14]

If possible, therefore, walk or exercise outdoors (not at high noon, though, and not without an adequate sunblock). Try to make sure to get outdoors even in cold weather—you can still get vitamin D from winter sunshine, and you're less likely to get skin cancer. Vitamin D is hard to find in food, but some foods do have it—fatty fish (salmon, tuna, and mackerel), liver, and eggs. In addition, milk is supplemented with vitamin D, as are many cereals. Most multivitamins supply the 400 units of vitamin D you need each day. And those of you living in an area with cold, gloomy winters (I've gotten very smug about weather since I moved from Boston to L.A.!) should take a vitamin D supplement during that season if you don't spend much time outdoors. You can overdose, however, so you should avoid taking more than 1,000 units a day.

Antioxidants

Antioxidants are probably the most important vitamins for women who are aging. These include vitamins A, C, and E, and beta-carotene. As we noted in Chapter 6, it's the oxidation of LDL that is the first step in the hardening of the arteries. The oxygen-free radicals created in this oxidation process are now thought to be related to wrinkles, liver spots, rheumatoid arthritis, and cancer. Vitamin E is the best at neutralizing these free radicals before they can do too much damage. It reduces tissue damage after a heart attack, decreases damage caused by inflammation, and increases resistance to cancer cells. If you have cancer, however, you should be cautious about taking vitamin E as a supplement until more information is available (see page 163). An adequate dose of vitamin E is 400 IU.

Vitamin A and carotenoids (found in green and yellow vegetables) are also important sources of antioxidants. Beta-carotene decreased the incidence of heart attack and stroke by 50 percent in a group of male doctors (I know, I know) who took it every other day for six years. There has been some speculation that beta-carotene can prevent lung cancer in smokers, but as I mentioned, recent studies of supplements have been disappointing.

Vitamin A is also important for vision, and it can improve night vision, which often decreases as we age. You remember all those old jokes about how rabbits don't wear glasses because they eat all those carrots? Well, carrots are a great source of vitamin A. For a supplement, women need about 5,000 IU of vitamin A and 3 to 5 milligrams of beta-carotene daily. (Don't overdo it—15,000 milligrams a day may be toxic over time and can cause birth defects.)

Vitamin C also works with vitamins E and A to prevent oxidation of LDL, and it helps the immune system as well. As a million commercials have told you, there's a lot of vitamin C in orange juice—from which you might have guessed that there's also a lot in oranges. It can also be found in broccoli, hot peppers, green peppers, tomatoes, cabbage, green leafy vegetables, strawberries, and grapefruit. If you take a vitamin C supplement, divide it into three daily doses. You don't need a whole lot—between 500 and 1,500 milligrams a day.

B Vitamins

Vitamin B isn't a single vitamin but a whole collection—thiamine, riboflavin, niacin, pantothenic acid, pyridoxine (B_6), folic acid, cyanocobalamin (B_{12}), biotin, para-aminobenzoic acid, inositol, and choline. Vitamin B_6 is said to relieve PMS in premenopausal women, but there are no randomized controlled studies. A few clinical studies have shown that vitamin B deficiency may be the cause of some postmenopausal anxiety and irritability. B vitamins should usually be taken together as a B complex in order to achieve the best balance. If you're over forty, be sure you're getting at least 100 milligrams of niacin.

Multivitamins: Can One Pill Do It All?

A multivitamin supplement will often supply what you need. But how do you choose the right one from the multitude that are on the shelves? Sherry Sultenfuss offers advice in her book *A Woman's Guide to Vitamins and Minerals*.[15] First read the label. As with calcium supplements, you can get confused. It's important to see if an ingredient is listed plainly or in parentheses. If a label says "zinc picolinate 50 milligrams," this means that 50 milligrams is the combined weight of the zinc and the picolinate. If it says "zinc (picolinate) 50 milligrams," this means that there are 50 milligrams of zinc. Since you want to know how much actual zinc there is, you'd do better with the latter.

Taking a balanced supplement with vitamins and minerals is important. Inappropriate combinations can be a problem, as we saw with phosphorus.

Natural versus synthetic probably doesn't matter as much as you would think. Most natural vitamins contain other ingredients—such as rose hips, which include not only vitamin C but also flavinoids, fructose, malic acid, sucrose, tannins, zinc, and vitamins A, B, D, and E. You may be surprised to hear that a vitamin can (legally) be labeled "natural" if as little as 10 percent of its ingredients are natural.

Be sure to look at the expiration date on a bottle of vitamins before you buy it. Many vitamins and minerals can lose their potency quickly.

Finally, Sherry Sultenfuss says that it is better to take your supplement three times a day than all at once: the water-soluble vitamins have a greater chance of being absorbed. (Of course, you can't do that if you have one capsule a day, but taking timed-release formulations may help in this situation.)

So do your research. A vitamin ad may claim to have "everything a woman needs," but that doesn't mean it's true. Once you find a combination that truly provides you with the appropriate supplements, stick to it, while you keep trying to improve the variety and healthfulness of your diet. You can't lose.

HERBS

I discuss the use of herbs for symptoms at length in Chapter 11. In this chapter I'll focus on those herbs that are generally used for prevention. These herbs, as opposed to some of those we considered in Chapter 11, are not known to be estrogenic and therefore are considered safer for women with breast cancer. They are generally considered nourishing rather than medicinal herbs. I have not been able to locate any traditional scientific literature supporting their use. Therefore, you should consider these recommendations as unproved but probably not risky.

Horsetail (*Equisetum arvense*)

Horsetail picked in the spring is said to be especially good for preventing or reversing osteoporosis because it is rich in minerals, especially magnesium. It's also said to prevent clogged arteries by virtue of its silica, chromium, flavinoids, saponins, and astringent agents. It can be combined with stinging nettles for an even stronger effect. It also provides potassium and iron, which help increase energy and decrease fatigue.

Horsetail can be used in soup or dried for teas. The dosage is one cup (250 milliliters) of tea made from dried spring-gathered herb daily. (Ready-made teabags are less reliable in the amount and potency of the herb you will get. Nonetheless, they are probably safe.) Don't use horsetail if you experience sensations of nervous sensitivity or urinary irritability after drinking it.

Oatstraw (*Avena sativa*)

Oatstraw does indeed come from oats, just like oatmeal. It is rich in calcium and has a reputation for building tough, hardy bones. It also reduces cholesterol and therefore the risk of heart disease. The dosage is one cup or more of dried-leaf, stalk, and grain infusion daily. I bought some oatstraw tea, and I've found it very tasty.

Seaweeds

Seaweeds contain high levels of almost every mineral you need for good bones. They are also said to lower blood pressure and cholesterol. They have abundant antioxidants, which can help prevent heart disease as well as cancer. You can buy seaweeds in an Asian grocery store or a health food store. You can use them as a condiment daily and also as a vegetable. Try them with pasta, grains, eggs, salad, and popcorn. Because they're high in iodine, however, you should be careful if you're hyperthyroid.

Stinging Nettle (*Urtica dioica*)

Stinging nettle herb is a good source of calcium, magnesium, potassium, silicon, boron, and zinc, as well as vitamin D. It's therefore likely to be of some help in preventing osteoporosis. It can be eaten as greens all spring, when nettles are fresh; the dried plant can be drunk as a tea the rest of the year. The dosage is one cup or more of dried-leaf infusion daily.

CHINESE MEDICINE AND ACUPUNCTURE

Chinese medicine covers a variety of related systems of healing. It has been practiced for over 2,000 years in China and since the 1700s in the United States. It's based on a paradigm completely different from that of Western medicine.

One of the key principles involves *yin* and *yang*. These are generic concepts, representing any two opposite aspects within a single object that are interdependent and in constant flux. In the human body, health is a relative balance of yin and yang that's never static. Although they've been misinterpreted in the West as representing male and female, in nature yin and yang correspond to the natural principles of fire and water. The ultimate goal of Chinese medicine is to balance yin and yang. Marie Cargill describes this in *Acupuncture: A Viable Medical Alternative:*

> Yin and yang are dynamic states that continually create and regulate one another through many subtle transformations. . . . [They] define and constrain one another by striking a balance between excess and deficient energy levels. They are fluid states of beginning, acting, changing, resting—in short, the entire repertoire of balances that constitutes being.[16]

Another principle is *chi* (or *qi*), the "life force energy." *Chi* is thought to be responsible for the movement and transformation of the bodily fluids.

Finally, there is *jing*—the vital physical essence of the body. According to Honora Lee Wolfe, in *Menopause: A Second Spring,* menstrual blood is the outward physical manifestation of *jing* in women, as semen is in men.[17] In Chinese medicine, menopause, although it is a sign of aging, actually slows down the aging process by preventing unnecessary loss of blood and *jing.* Therefore it's a necessary, vital, stabilizing mechanism in a woman's body, slowing down the loss of *jing* and thus allowing the woman another twenty to thirty years of relative good health.

This view of menopause leads to a different approach. You're dealing not with a disease needing treatment, but with a stabilizing force that may need balancing. This balance relates to the individual's constitution and is affected by stress, overwork, emotional upset, and any illness. For this reason, there's no single treatment appropriate for all menopausal women. Each prescription is individualized.

Treatments in Chinese medicine include acupuncture, Chinese herbs (some of which are described in Chapter 11), massage (acupressure, shiatsu), and chi kung. Chi kung, one of the martial arts, is also a type of mind-body medicine that combines elements of meditation, relaxation training, visualization, movement, postures, and breathing exercises. It serves both for physical fitness and for self-healing.

Chinese Herbs

There are now several ongoing studies funded by the National Institutes of Health on the use of Chinese medicine in the United States. Some studies have already found that Chinese herbs can decrease symptoms resulting from chemotherapy and radiation treatment for cancer. Chinese herbs have also been found to reduce heart disease and cancer.

We've already discussed how Chinese medicine can be used to treat the symptoms of menopause. It's also used to help prevent future problems.

Some of the Chinese herbs are the same as the ones used by herbalists in the United States, while others are unique to China. Because the literature about them is mostly in Chinese, I've been unable to fully evaluate it. I suggest you consult a traditional Chinese doctor if you're interested in pursuing this course further. (There are, by the way, a large number of American practitioners of Chinese medicine, many of whom have studied in China. It isn't nationality or race that's important; it's the study of the discipline.) If you have had breast cancer, check Table 10.1 (page 154), on the estrogenic effects of herbs, for information about their safety.

Also, as we mentioned in Chapter 10, you need to be careful about the source of any herbal treatment or formula. There have been some reports of adverse reactions, usually involving herbs that contained other prescription medications or contaminants. These complications have included kidney failure, liver failure, coma, and death. Most of these drugs used in the United States come from Hong Kong, where there is no regulation. For example, in 1994 there was a report of two deaths following the use of an herbal formula containing aconitine, which is used for relief of minor muscle pain. When the herbal preparations were analyzed, it was found that the amount of aconitine was greatly in excess of the maximum recommended in the pharmacopeia of the People's Republic of China.[18] Analysis of another Chinese herbal medication that had led to complications found that the herbs had been adulterated with a nonsteroidal anti-inflammatory drug (mefanamic acid) and Valium.[19] I don't want to imply that all Chinese herbal formulas are dangerous. In fact, a study done in Hong Kong of 1,701 patients admitted to two general medical wards at Prince of Wales Hospital over eight years found that only three patients had been admitted for complications from Chinese herbal medicines.[20] I could find many more reports on serious complications of aspirin. Still, I do want to remind you that even though something is an herb, it may not be entirely safe. The best approach is to go to a reliable practitioner who will know the best and most reliable sources of these remedies, and the proper dosages. Also, keep your provider informed about all the medications and treatments you're taking.

Panax ginseng, as I mentioned in Chapter 11, is the Chinese herb that has been studied the most. It has been found to increase HDL and reduce total cholesterol and triglycerides in rats and humans. It was also able to decrease the stickiness of platelets (the component of blood that leads to blood clots), much as aspirin does.[21] It has also been found to inhibit the growth of cancer cells.

Salvia miltiorrhiza (a cousin of garden sage) has been found to dilate blood vessels, especially in the coronary arteries. It was studied in comparison to nitroglycerin and found to be better at improving cardiac function.[22]

Tochu bark extract was found—in a randomized controlled study of rats whose ovaries had been removed—to increase the absorption of calcium and increase bone density and muscle weight,[23] and so might help prevent osteoporosis as well.

Acupuncture

Acupuncture has been used for the prevention of heart disease, osteoporosis, stroke, cancers, and many other diseases of aging. I was not able to find any Western scientific literature supporting its efficacy, however.

AYURVEDA

The Ayurvedic system of preventive medicine and health care in India dates back more than 5,000 years. It has recently gained popularity in this country because of the work of Deepak Chopra. Chopra describes the purpose of Ayurveda in his book *Perfect Health:*

> The guiding principle of Ayurveda is that the mind exerts the deepest influence on the body, and freedom from sickness depends upon contracting your own awareness, bringing it into balance, and then extending that balance to the body. This state of balanced awareness, more than any kind of physical immunity, creates a higher state of health.[24]

Ayurveda accepts that the body is always changing but holds that some of this change can be controlled by a mind-body approach. Rather than seeing the body as simply a group of cells, tissues, and organs, this discipline views it as a "silent flow of intelligence, a constant bubbling up of impulses that create, control, and become your physical body. The secret of life at this level is that anything in your body can be changed with a flick of an intention."[25]

Ayurveda—like traditional Chinese medicine—has a concept of vital energy, which it calls *prana. Prana* can be absorbed through the breath; thus breathing and breathing exercises hold an important place in this tradition.

The goal of Ayurveda is to promote and enhance health. Diseases can also be treated within this tradition, but the approach generally is to work on a person's overall integration, balance, and harmony. Ayurvedic doctors try to increase your resistance rather than to treat your symptoms.

The core of Ayurvedic treatment is meditation. In the strict tradition of the Mahareshi Ayur-Ved, the development of consciousness through transcendental meditation is the basis of this science of mind-body. Other Ayurvedic practitioners also use meditation but feel that there are various ways it can be carried out. Both approaches, however, use a combination of meditation, diet, herbs, exercise, breathing exercises, aromatherapy, yoga, massage, and chronotherapy (paying attention to natural metabolic rhythms).

There is a body of scientific study on Ayurvedic medicine in India, and some initial studies are now being done in the United States. However, since this is a very individualistic approach, in which the treatment being proposed is specific to the individual rather than the disease, Western-style studies are difficult to perform. There is no readily identifiable endpoint to measure. Ayurveda does appear to be helpful in treating chronic diseases and preventing disease. It's less effective for acute or advanced diseases. Its emphasis on prevention and enhancement of health makes it an ideal approach to menopause. It can provide an individualized lifestyle approach that can help many women achieve the balance they need for the second half of their lives.

Ayurvedic practitioners in the United States aren't as well organized as practitioners of traditional Chinese medicine. In India, the training lasts five and a half years, and the degree is called bachelor of Ayurvedic medicine and surgery. A few Western (allopathic) schools offer specialization in Ayurveda. In the United States, there are no strict criteria for training, but there are several training centers, which are listed in Appendix 1. The best way to select practitioners is by asking about their training and experience, getting recommendations from friends, and interviewing them.

Ayurvedic herbs have been found to decrease cholesterol-induced atherosclerosis in rabbits.[26] Other drugs and herbs that have been studied and found effective include terminalia belerica,[27] maharishi ayur-veda herbal mixtures,[28] and modified anna pavala sindhooram.[29]

In addition to its herbs and medicines, the transcendental meditation used in Ayurveda has been found useful for patients with coronary disease in a randomized controlled study.[30] Another study compared transcendental meditation with muscle relaxation as a means of reducing stress in a group of older African-American men and women with high blood pressure. These researchers found that the group using transcendental meditation did much better at controlling their high blood pressure.[31]

NATUROPATHY

Naturopathy combines natural treatments from a variety of traditions, including those we've been discussing. In the 1980s the American Association of Naturopathic Physicians articulated the basic philosophy, taken from Hippocrates: "The body heals itself, and the task of the physician is to support this inherent healing potential."

There are six basic principles in naturopathy. First, respect the healing power of nature: the practitioner's job is to remove the blocks to healing and bolster the body's own ability to heal itself. Second, treat the whole person: health is a result of interactions of physical, mental, emotional, genetic, spiritual, environmental, social, and other factors. Third, do no harm. Fourth, use the least invasive treatment that will help the patient. Fifth, identify and treat the cause of the illness—by which naturopaths mean not bacteria or carcinogens but rather the patient's lifestyle, dietary habits, and emotional state. Sixth, prevention is the best cure. In all of this, the doctor is a teacher. The practitioner's role is to educate the patient and to encourage responsibility for oneself. Many of these principles have been absorbed by Western (allopathic) medicine, as "holistic" medicine becomes more and more popular. They make a lot of sense.

Naturopathic practitioners may use any of a number of methods, including clinical nutrition; physical medicine such as therapeutic manipulation, massage, and bodywork; homeopathy; botanical medicine; Chinese medicine; Ayurveda; and psychological counseling. There are no modalities that are the exclusive province of the naturopath; these practitioners hold that what distinguishes them is their adherence to the six principles.

There have been many studies of naturopathic treatments, though their connection with naturopathy isn't always noted. We've seen numerous studies of the results of diet and nutritional additives and their effect on the risk of cancer, heart disease, and other chronic diseases.

There is growing interest in natural approaches to prevention and treatment, not only because of their effectiveness but also because they're inexpensive. William Collinge, author of *The American Holistic Health Association Complete Guide to Alternative Medicine*,[32] reports that in Germany, naturopathic services have been found so cost-effective that the government now requires conventional doctors and pharmacists to receive education in naturopathic methods and botanical medicine.

According to naturopathic medicine, there are several main "gateways" in a woman's life. These include puberty, establishing a stable relationship, pregnancy and childbirth, and menopause. At any of these transitions, personality and health have an opportunity to undergo great change, for better or worse. Menopause can be a time of relief from troublesome periods, but it can also be a source of new problems if you're overextended. If you take care of your health during this transition, you can improve your constitution and enjoy the next phase.

Naturopathic medicine has much to offer the menopausal woman. It takes the best of many disciplines and treats the whole woman. And, like most of the other alternative philosophies, it views menopause as a time of transition, not a disease—a refreshing change from the attitude of Western medicine.

Naturopathic doctors are licensed in thirteen states in the United States and Canada. You can contact the American Association of Naturopathic Physicians to find out the situation in your state, and to help you find a naturopathic physician. Other resources are listed in Appendix 1.

MIND-BODY TECHNIQUES

In Chapter 12, I talked about several mind-body approaches you can use on your own—although for most of them, you're likely to do better if you have a few sessions, alone or in a class, with a practitioner. There are two mind-body techniques, however, for which a practitioner is essential: hypnosis and biofeedback.

Hypnosis puts you into a highly focused state that allows you to use imagery, relaxation, or autogenic phrases in a more powerful way. It's good for changing bad habits, such as smoking and overeating. We've had years of sitcom jokes about people being hypnotized and ending up quacking like ducks in the middle of business meetings; and a crime drama occasionally has a plot in which an innocent pawn is hypnotized into committing a murder. But hypnosis is unlikely to turn you into either a fool or a murderer—it can simply help you let your mind know you're serious about making a health-related change. I told you in Chapter 12 how I quit smoking through a hypnosis program. You do need a qualified practitioner, however. Amateurs playing around with stuff they don't know about can have a frightening effect on your mind.

As noted in Chapter 10, biofeedback is a method for learning to regulate certain bodily functions by using physical measurements. It can help control a number of symptoms, including headaches, chronic pain, asthma, and muscular problems.

MASSAGE THERAPY AND BODYWORK

Massage is one of the oldest forms of therapy, and it is a component of almost all healing traditions. There are over eighty different types of massage or bodywork, but they all have some principles in common. The first principle is that improving the circulation of the blood and lymph is good for health. A second principle is that release of tension and toxins promotes greater relaxation and well-being. A third principle is that mind and body are related: as the body is relaxed, the mind can also relax. This also leads to reduction of stress, and a fourth principle is that most modern chronic illnesses are related to stress. Many of the approaches to bodywork also use the concept that massage increases the flow of energy or opens up new channels for energy.

Although there is no direct correlation with or prevention of disease, massage plays an important role in treating various joint and muscular aches and pains, which is useful in helping you keep up an exercise program, since sore muscles can be discouraging. It can also help in stress reduction.

The best way to find a massage therapist is through the American Massage Therapy Association. Other types of bodywork are mentioned in Appendix 1.

There are many other alternative approaches, but in a book this length, I couldn't begin to cover them all—nor can I do full justice to those I've described. If you're considering treatment for menopausal symptoms or trying to prevent heart disease or osteoporosis, I would strongly recommend that you look into some of these before you try Western drugs. There are fewer dangers, and for the most part equally good effects. If you do decide to take hormones, some of these approaches can be of use in lessening the side effects of your drug.

CHAPTER 14

Drugs: Other Means of Prevention

We can talk all day about the benefits of a healthy lifestyle and the advantages of herbs, but there will always be women who need or want to go to the third and most risky level. Approaches at this level include drugs—hormones and others. Side effects are inevitable with drugs, but this doesn't mean that drugs are never appropriate for menopausal symptoms or for prevention of potential illnesses. For example, depending on your level of risk, Premarin may be a good part of your overall program to prevent a hip fracture. There are drugs that will lower your cholesterol when changing your diet doesn't work. New drugs are being developed to cure and even prevent osteoporosis.

We discussed surgery—which is also a third-level approach—in Chapter 11. In this chapter, I'll discuss the use of specific drugs for treating and preventing osteoporosis and heart disease. Because hormones are the drugs most commonly used to prevent these diseases in women, I'll devote Chapter 15 to the topic of hormones in all of their guises.

DRUGS FOR OSTEOPOROSIS

Calcitonin

Calcitonin, a hormone made by your thyroid gland, inhibits bone breakdown. There's now a version made from salmon that you can take to help block bone loss. It's been tested only in women who already have osteoporosis, and it's most effective in women with the highest bone turnover. In two-year studies, it's been found to increase bone density by 5 percent when taken with calcium; in comparison, women who were given calcium and a placebo had a 2 percent decrease in bone density.[1] It's not really clear whether the effect of calcitonin will persist beyond two or three years. There are data, however, indicating that women who took calcitonin had two-thirds fewer vertebral fractures in those first few years.[2] As of yet we don't know whether calcitonin can build bone or just prevent its loss.

One of the more dramatic effects of calcitonin is the decrease of pain caused by vertebral fractures from osteoporosis.[3] This alone may make it a good choice in certain situations.

Calcitonin is not absorbed very well orally, but there's a new nasal spray version, Miacalcin, that's been approved by the FDA. It appears to be especially good for women over sixty-five. The only reported side effect is nasal irritation. And it's rapidly metabolized, so you don't have to worry that it will stay in your body permanently—unlike the bisphosphonates, which we discuss next.

Bisphosphonates

Bisphosphonates are drugs that act by binding to the osteoclasts (the cells that resorb bone) and preventing them from functioning; this decreases bone loss in menopausal women. The fact that these drugs decrease bone loss, however, doesn't mean that they actually build bone. Also, although we know that they decrease fractures in the short term, we don't know what they do in the long term. Because they interfere with the balance between resorption and buildup, they may eventually affect the architecture of the skeleton.

Two bisphosphonates are already on the market: Didronel (etidronate) from Procter and Gamble and Fosamax (alendronate) from Merck. Soon to follow are Risederonate, which is being developed by Procter and Gamble and Pfizer; and Tiludronate, from Sterling-Winthrop. Two more compounds are being developed separately by the Japanese firm Yaminuchi and by Broehringer Mannheim in Germany.

The bisphosphonates—like estrogen—can give the illusion of creating bone growth, because bone growth already in progress doesn't stop: it completes its particular growing project. In Chapter 5, we drew an analogy with building a house. In terms of that image, it's like looking at one room that has been partially redone. The work on that room continues till it's finished, and it looks as if the house is getting nicely rebuilt. In fact, though, no more rooms are being added; it's just that a room that was already started is getting completed. This leads to an increase of bone of about 5 to 10 percent—the figure you see in most reports. But the growth continues only for a couple of years, after which bone activity levels off; and then it all stops—both growth and resorption.

That's why we're leery of long-term use of bisphosphonates. Your bones continue remodeling throughout your whole life. If you gain weight in the hips, they need to shore up the bone density in your pelvis and legs to be able to carry the extra weight. If you have arthritis and start walking differently (leaning to one side, say) to avoid pain in the hip, your bones need to shore up that hip and leg. What if you break a bone? You need to be able to repair it. So you don't want to block all bone turnover.

This concern led doctors to give the original bisphosphonates, such as Didronel, intermittently. You'd take them for three months and then stop for three months. There have been some reports of osteomalacia (soft bones) in women who took this etidronate for four years. Newer bisphosphonates such as Fosamax are less tightly bound by bone, and so it's thought—though not confirmed—that they can be given continuously.

A study done in the Netherlands[4] examined some aspects of bone turnover in women who took an early form of bisphosphonate for five to nine years and then stopped. The researchers found that the suppression of bone turnover was reversible once the drug was stopped, but that the beneficial effect on bone density and rate of fractures persisted for at least two years. As of yet we don't know what the correct duration of use should be, but this study suggests that it does not have to be indefinite.

Fosamax has been marketed very strongly as an alternative to estrogen. Although it has been tested only in women who already have osteoporosis, the implication is that it can be used to prevent the disease. I think this is a little premature. Two identical randomized placebo-controlled studies have been done on 900 women who had been postmenopausal for at least five years and had low bone density (2 standard deviations below the bone density of a premenopausal woman).[5] They took Fosamax for three years and showed an increase in bone density of 7 to 10 percent in the spine and 5 to 6 percent in the hip. Though neither study was designed to measure a decrease in fractures, the researchers analyzed the risk of fractures in pooled data.[6] They found that 3.2 percent of the women on Fosamax had vertebral fractures, compared with 6.2 percent in the women on a placebo. All this sounds good, but, as the drug companies admit in their ads in the journals on menopause, "Safety of treatment with Fosamax for longer than four years has not been studied: extensive studies are ongoing."

As this book was being completed, the first results of the Fracture Intervention Study were announced at the 1996 World Congress on Osteoporosis held in Amsterdam.[7] In the first of the randomized studies, 2,000 postmenopausal women who had suffered at least one spinal fracture were given either Fosamax (alendronate) or calcium. For the women treated with Fosamax, the risk of breaking a hip was reduced by 51 percent and the risk of breaking a wrist by 44 percent. Further fractures of the spine were 46 percent lower in this group as well. These results were considered so positive that the researchers concluded the study early so that all of the women could get the drug. Phase two of the study will look at the effect of Fosamax on over 4,000 women with low bone density who have not yet suffered a fracture of the spine. It should be completed in early 1997. These data are promising on two fronts. First, they indicate that osteoporosis can be treated and that further fractures can be prevented even if you wait until you actually have a problem. Second, they will answer the question of whether we need to use bisphosphonates for prevention in women with low bone density.

There are always some problems, however. Ever since Fosamax was approved by the FDA, there have been increasing reports of one particular side effect: Fosamax can cause severe ulcers of the esophagus if it's not taken in exactly the right way.[8] You have to take it with 6 to 8 ounces of plain water immediately after you wake up; studies suggest that the problem can occur if you don't swallow the pill completely—you should take it as soon as you're upright. Then, you shouldn't lie down for at least half an hour afterward. You shouldn't eat or drink anything for thirty minutes after you've taken Fosamax. This includes vitamins, calcium supplements, mineral water, coffee, tea, or juice. Although this doesn't sound too hard if it's helping you cure a disease, it's a bit much for prevention.

There are other, though rare, side effects as well—abdominal pain, nausea, heartburn, vomiting, difficulty swallowing, bloating, constipation, diarrhea, and gas. In addition, some patients have reported muscle pain, headache, and an altered sense of taste.

The ads for Fosamax mention that there are as yet no data on using it and estrogen together. They also caution against giving Fosamax to women with gastrointestinal problems, kidney disease, or low levels of calcium.

Although I think it's great that we have alternatives to estrogen that are specific for treating osteoporosis, I'd still be careful about using them purely for prevention at this stage. For now, Fosamax is probably best used by women who are five years out of menopause and have very low bone density or have already had a fracture.

Fluoride

Fluoride is the drug with the most potential, because it actually builds bone. It appears to affect osteoblast activity, not just slow down osteoclasts. The million-dollar question, however, is whether it will build good bone. Initial studies found that women on fluoride increased their bone density by 35 percent but had no decrease in fractures. This demonstrates that dense bone isn't enough—you need strong bone as well.[9] (It also points up a problem we discussed in Chapter 4—using intermediate endpoints such as bone density to predict the effect on fractures.)

Now there's a new slow-release formulation of fluoride that decreased the rate of fractures of the spine by 70 percent among the subjects in one study.[10] The study lasted fourteen months and compared women on fluoride with others on a placebo. The subjects were women ages fifty-six and fifty-eight with decreased bone density in the lumbar spine. The fluoride inhibited new vertebral fractures, though not recurrent ones. Another study found that women on fluoride increased their bone density by 20 percent over four years—far above the 5 to 10 percent reported for estrogen and bisphosphonates, or even for exercise. The side effects of fluoride are gastrointestinal. Its effects when taken with estrogen have not yet been determined. It's too soon to tell whether a perfect formulation of fluoride will be found, but this holds the best promise for building bone.

Ipriflavone

Ipriflavone, which is based on soy, is a variant on the bioflavinoids we mentioned in Chapter 13. It's been approved in Italy and Japan for the treatment of osteoporosis and has been found to increase bone density in the wrist and stabilize the lumbar spine after one year of treatment.[11] There's some preliminary evidence that it too may act to build bone rather than just stop resorption. It has very little in the way of side effects. Though it's too early to be certain of anything yet, this is a very promising drug.

When we talk about drugs meant to prevent something that won't happen for twenty to thirty years, it's important to realize that we'll probably have much better treatments by then. At the rate that pharmaceutical research is going, we should be able to rebuild your whole skeleton as well as identify the women destined by their genes to get into trouble, so we can head it off at the pass. So I worry about settling for the limited drugs we have now if you aren't definitely at serious risk.

DRUGS FOR HEART DISEASE

Cholesterol-Lowering Drugs

When diet, exercise, and other lifestyle changes aren't enough to keep your cholesterol down, or you find them too difficult or unpleasant to stick with, there are cholesterol-lowering medications you can take. These range from drugs that block cholesterol absorption to drugs that block the body's system for manufacturing cholesterol. When one drug alone doesn't work, you can take combinations.

Cholestyramine (Questran) and Colestipol

The treatment of high cholesterol usually begins with the drug that has the fewest side effects. Cholestyramine and colestipol bind bile in your intestine, making it harder for your body to absorb fat. The liver stores of cholesterol go down, and the liver takes some from the blood to make up for it. This lowers your LDL. It may also increase the good HDL and triglycerides. Initial doses have been found to decrease LDL cholesterol 10 to 15 percent; the highest doses reduce LDL 15 to 30 percent.[12] In addition, these drugs have been around long enough that we know they can reduce heart attacks.

Since these drugs aren't absorbed, their side effects are limited. Most of the side effects, not surprisingly, relate to the digestive system; they include constipation, bloating, stomach fullness, nausea, and gas. They can also interfere with the absorption of some medications and so should be taken one hour before, or three or four hours after, other drugs such as antibiotics, beta blockers, digosin, phenobarbital, thiazide diuretics, thyroid hormone, and coumadin. Long-term use can also interfere with the absorption of the fat-soluble vitamins A, C, and E.

The usual starting dose of cholestyramine is 4 grams once or twice a day with a maximal dose of 24 grams per day. It's available in a standard powder formula, a low-fat formula, and a flavored bar. Colestipol is a standard powder, usually given as 5 milligrams twice daily; the maximal dose is 30 grams.

This type of drug works best on women with moderately elevated LDL cholesterol and normal triglyceride levels.

Niacin

The other drug that has been proved to be both safe and effective in treating heart disease is niacin. (Although this is commonly thought of as a vitamin, at these dosages it is truly a drug.) It isn't clear how it works, but it has been shown to reduce LDL by 15 to 30 percent; it is available as 100-milligram and 500-milligram tablets as well as sustained-release formulas. The usual starting dose is 100 to 250 milligrams per day, with a gradual increase in the daily dose up to 1.5 grams per day. The maximum dose is 6 grams per day. It can't be used by women with ulcer disease, liver disease, or gout, and it should be used cautiously by women with diabetes. The main problem with niacin is its side effects, chief of which are flushing and itching—just what every perimenopausal woman needs. You can prevent the flushing by taking aspirin or nonsteroidal anti-inflammatory agents before you take the drug, by taking the drug with meals, or by using the more expensive sustained-release formula. The flushing generally stops after several weeks. You can treat dry skin and itching with moisturizers, and you can avoid gastrointestinal side effects by taking niacin with meals. The best thing about niacin is its low cost. It's the cheapest cholesterol-lowering drug available. It is the first-line drug for those with elevated LDL and low HDL or high triglycerides.

Hydroxymethylglutaryl Coenzyme A Reductase Inhibitors

These drugs are the newcomers on the block. They work by preventing the manufacture of the body's own cholesterol, which, as you'll remember from Chapter 6, is the source of most of the cholesterol in your blood. As a result, the liver pulls back some cholesterol that's already in the blood to shore up its stock, just as it does with cholestramine. These drugs include lovastatin (Mevacor), pravstatin, simvastatin (Zocor), and flurastatin. In women, lovastatin can decrease LDL cholesterol 24 to 40 percent as well as increase HDL slightly (7 to 9 percent) and decrease triglycerides somewhat more (9 to 18 percent).[13] The usual starting dose of lovastatin is 20 milligrams with dinner. If necessary, you can increase it to a maximum dose of 80 milligrams per day. With pravastatin, you start at 10 to 20 milligrams and go up to 40 milligrams. With simivastin, you start at 5 to 10 milligrams and go up to a daily dose of 40 milligrams. For flurastatin, you start at 20 milligrams and go up to 40 milligrams. These drugs are generally well tolerated. The side effects include some digestive problems, muscle aches, tiredness, headache, insomnia, and rash, although none of these effects are common.

This whole field got a tremendous boost recently when a large double-blind randomized prospective study in men and women with established coronary artery disease found that these drugs not only lowered cholesterol but also decreased the rate of heart attacks.[14] A second randomized controlled double-blind placebo study on lovastatin found that it appeared to widen arteries and seemed to prevent new lesions from appearing.[15] This was important because the only reason to bother about cholesterol is that it can cause heart disease. This second study looked only at men, however, so we can't be certain if the results will apply in the same way to women. Further, since both of these studies were done on people who already had heart disease, we don't have any idea whether lowering lipids in healthy women will have the same effect.

Gemfibrozil (Lopid)

This recently developed drug is especially good at decreasing high triglyceride levels and even increases HDL. In women with high triglycerides, it can reduce LDL by 10 to 15 percent. Researchers don't completely understand how it does this. The recommended dose is 600 milligrams twice daily one half hour before meals. It has few side effects. It does, however, increase the ability of the bile to form stones, and you should therefore not use it if you have gallbladder disease. It's the best drug for women and/or diabetics with high triglycerides.

There's been some concern that the cholesterol-lowering drugs have the potential to increase cancer. While this is still hypothetical, it points up the fact that we should use them only when nothing else works.

Aspirin

Aspirin doesn't lower cholesterol, but it seems to prevent heart attacks by decreasing the blood's ability to clot.[16] You should take aspirin for this purpose only under a doctor's supervision. Aspirin may be common, but it's still a drug, and it can have serious side effects when taken over the long term.

As with osteoporosis, I have confidence that we'll eventually have better and better ways to treat coronary heart disease and to predict which women are at risk. Only if you have heart disease or have very high cholesterol levels that don't respond to exercise or diet changes do you need to be on drugs.

CHAPTER 15

Hormones:
The Menu of Options

While other drugs are worth thinking about, the drugs most commonly taken to alleviate the symptoms of menopause are still hormones. They're also the drugs most commonly taken by women to prevent heart disease and osteoporosis.

You might wonder why I refer to hormones as *drugs* when they're made naturally by our bodies. The answer is that, first, it's not "natural" for us to have them in high levels after menopause; and, second, many of the hormones used in hormone therapy are not the ones our bodies make naturally, either before or after menopause. As I said earlier, calling hormones "replacement" therapy implies that we're just restoring something that's missing. The problem is that it's *not* what would be present, even if you were thirty-five; and when you're fifty-five, it's extra. And "extra" isn't always good.

Some of you may also be surprised to see "natural hormones" in this chapter, rather than in Chapter 11 or 12, where "alternative" approaches are discussed. But natural hormones (not to be confused with the phytoestrogens in some vegetables) are still hormones, and, as such, they're drugs.

HOW WE THINK HORMONES WORK

Hormones are powerful and complex, and we don't yet know nearly enough about how they work. For example (as noted in Chapter 7), we've known for a while that for a hormone to work, it needs a receptor to get into the cell.

This receptor is like a lock and the hormone is the key that fits it and opens the door. Researchers originally assumed that every drug that fit a given receptor would cause the same effect—open the same door. But further research has revealed that some drugs seem to fit a receptor (or lock) without opening the door. Instead, they block another hormone from getting in. These are antagonists or hormone blockers. Tamoxifen, which is used to treat breast cancer, is a good example, as is RU 486, which blocks progesterone in the uterus. So researchers refined their theory and came up with a nice simple model: drugs act either to cause an effect or to block it.

However, the more studies we did, the more complicated the model got. For example, our original assumption was that tamoxifen not only would block estrogen in the breast but would increase osteoporosis and heart disease by blocking estrogen everywhere. But it turned out that it didn't work that way. Much to our amazement, tamoxifen, though it does indeed block estrogen in the breast, acts *like* estrogen in the uterus, bones, and liver. It causes uterine cancer, and it prevents bone loss and high cholesterol, much the way estrogen does (though it doesn't work as well as estrogen in treating bone loss).[1] This isn't simply an either/or phenomenon, then, but something much more complicated.

So we've developed a new model to explain how hormones work. We now say that some drugs like tamoxifen are *selective estrogen receptor modulators* (SERMs).[2] It's likely that most of the phytoestrogens are SERMs as well. We're starting to figure out how SERMs work. It turns out that the locks aren't the same in every organ. Progesterone, for example, has two possible receptors. The receptor in the uterus is completely different from the one in the breast. So progesterone may block estrogen in the uterus and stimulate it in the breast.

In addition, some cells may have a double lock. And in that case it may matter which one you turn first. One drug may fit one lock or part of the receptor, causing one effect, while another may fit another area and have a completely different effect. Finally, some drugs will fit both spots and have a third effect. In fact, different drugs acting through the same receptor can induce different receptor conformations—that is, actually change the shape of the lock—and this results in different reactions.[3]

Are you totally confused? Good! You're starting to get my point—that none of this is simple and that we're only beginning to understand how all of these hormones work. We can't assume that natural progesterone and progestin, a synthetic cousin, act the same; and we can't assume that horse estrogen and synthetic estrogen act the same. Nor do we yet understand how a combination of hormones acts. Scientists are hoping to use some of this new information to design the perfect hormone: one that will protect the uterus and breast from cancer, stop hot flashes, and prevent osteoporosis and heart disease. It would be lovely—could it do housework too?—but I'm skeptical. It would still be a drug. And I have yet to see a drug that doesn't have some side effects. We'll see.

Meanwhile, I'm going to take you on a tour of the currently available hormones. If you decide to take hormones either to address symptoms you have right now or to prevent future disease, it's important that you explore the various possibilities. One size rarely fits all. Your decision should take into account your body and its metabolism, your lifestyle, and the reason you're taking these drugs.

The commonly used hormones are forms of estrogen, progesterone, and sometimes testosterone. These are often mixed and matched in a variety of ways and delivery systems. As I've pointed out, most of the studies on prevention have been done on Premarin, taken by mouth, without added progestin or testosterone. You have to be careful about extrapolating these data to all hormones or to all methods of taking them.

NATURAL VERSUS SYNTHETIC HORMONES

The word *natural* is fashionable. Somehow we think that anything is better and safer if it's natural. There are two ways to interpret this word with regard to hormones.

First, *natural* can mean that a hormone is most like the hormones we have in our bodies, either postmenopausally or premenopausally. With this interpretation, Premarin, which is made from the urine of pregnant mares and is in fact horse estrogen, isn't natural—unless you're a horse. Does this really matter? It's possible that the ingredient producing some of the observed effects of Premarin has nothing to do with horses. But on the other hand, these effects may have nothing to do with estrogen. The effects may come from some other, as yet unidentified, factor indigenous to horses. Maybe it's the soy the farmers are feeding them!

The other definition of *natural* is that a hormone is made from natural ingredients rather than in a laboratory. In this case, Premarin does qualify as natural, since horse urine isn't synthetic. But most other commercial hormones are made from progesterone, which is synthesized in a lab from diosgenin obtained from the wild yam or from soybeans. This includes progesterone that is "natural" in the first sense—in that it's the same as the progesterone our bodies make—and "unnatural": Provera.

Is a drug "natural" because it's made from a wild yam, or is it "unnatural" because it's then synthesized in a laboratory? The whole thing becomes ridiculous. It makes me laugh to see that the makers of estradiol are now advertising it as "plant-based estrogen." Needless to say, each pharmaceutical company is going to use the definition that allows it to call its own product "natural." Calling drugs "natural hormones" makes them sound less like drugs, doesn't it? Don't let anyone kid you—these are all drugs.

One very real problem with drugs that are "natural" in the first sense is that since they're just like the hormones that we have in our bodies, they can't be patented. Therefore, they're not available at the typical commercial pharmacy in the United States (although they're widely available in Europe and Canada). However, several pharmacies in the United States still compound their own drugs, as opposed to using only drugs made by large pharmaceutical companies. These pharmacies are able to make micronized progesterone, estradiol, or estriol to fill a doctor's prescription. They do much of their business by mail order. (A list can be found in Appendix 2.) With these pharmacies, you have less assurance of the quality and standardization of the product; still, many women swear by them.

DELIVERY SYSTEMS

How a drug is delivered to your bloodstream can vary. You can take a drug by mouth, through your skin, or through your vagina—even through your nose.

If you take it as a pill, it has to be digested before it reaches your bloodstream. Some drugs are better digested than others. Premarin probably works in part because it has to pass through your liver before it reaches the bloodstream. On the other hand, progesterone isn't very well digested, which means that you need very high doses to achieve adequate blood levels.

Any delivery other than the mouth is called *parenteral.* The skin is an excellent parenteral channel for absorbing a drug, and the drug then bypasses the digestive tract. Patches, creams, and gels applied to the skin go directly into the bloodstream. It's even easier to absorb drugs through mucus membranes (the wet linings of the different entrances to our bodies), so rectal suppositories and vaginal creams and suppositories are good ways to get hormones directly into the bloodstream (as are nasal sprays, such as the calcitonin spray we mentioned in Chapter 14). Finally, you can get a shot or have a drug implanted under your skin for delayed release.

Because there are so many different drugs and ways to deliver them, the choices for hormone therapy are like a restaurant menu (see Table 15.1). You can have one from column A and one from column B. Too often, a gynecologist will prescribe one drug or one combination as if that were the only choice. I'll try to sort out the most common types of drugs so that you at least feel you've seen the menu—and can insist that your "waiter" give you what you order.

TABLE 15.1 Common Menopausal Pharmaceutical Preparations

Brand name	Active ingredients	Size	Color	Dosage	Manu-facturer
Oral estrogens					
ESTRACE	Micronized estradiol	1 mg 2 mg	lavender turquoise	Initial 1 or 2 mg/day Maintenance 0.5–20 mg	Mead Johnson
ESTRATAB	Esterified estrogens	0.3 mg 0.625 mg 1.25 mg 2.5 mg	blue yellow red purple	Daily	Solvay
ESTROVIS	Quinestrol	0.1 mg	light blue	Once/day for seven days, discontinue one week, then once/week as maintenance	Parke-Davis
OGEN	Estropipate	0.625 mg 1.25 mg 2.5 mg	yellow peach gray	Twice daily	Abbott
ORTHO-EST	Estropipate	0.625 1.25	orange lavender	Cyclic (three weeks on, one week off)	Ortho
PREMARIN (package of 25)	Conjugated equine estrogens	0.3 mg 0.625 mg 0.9 mg 1.25 mg 2.5 mg	green maroon pink yellow purple	One daily for 25 days (cyclic) *or* one daily (continuous) with progestins	Wyeth-Ayerst
Patch					
CLIMARA	Transdermal estradiol (matrix)	0.5 mg 0.01 mg	clear	Once a week	Berlex
ESTRADERM (box of 8 patches)	Transdermal estradiol	0.05 mg/ day 0.1 mg/ day	10 cm² round 20 cm² oblong	Affix to abdomen. Change twice a week on same days every week. Take with a minimum of 10 days progestins, every month or 3 months, to protect uterus.	Ciba-Geigy
VIVELLE	Transdermal estradiol (matrix)	0.375 mg/day 0.05 mg/day 0.075 mg/day 0.1 mg/day	clear	Twice-weekly application	Ciba-Geigy
Progestogens (Progestins and Progesterone)					
AMEN	Medroxy-progesterone acetate	5 mg 10 mg	layered peach and white	5–10 mg/day for 5–10 days, beginning on 16th day of cycle. Bleeding starts 3rd to 7th day after stopping.	Carnick

TABLE 15.1   *(Continued)*

Brand name	Active ingredients	Size	Color	Dosage	Manu-facturer
AYGESTIN	Norethindrone acetate	5 mg	oblong white	2.5–10 mg for 5–10 days	Wyeth-Ayerst
CYCRIN	Medroxy-progesterone acetate	2.5 mg 5 mg 10 mg	white light purple peach	5–10 mg/day for 5–10 days, beginning on 16th day of cycle. Bleeding starts 3rd to 7th day after stopping.	Wyeth-Ayerst
MICRONIZED PROGESTERONE		25 mg 50 mg 100 mg 200 mg		Made up by pharmacist following physician's directions. 100 mg twice daily.	
NORLUTATE	Norethindrone acetate	5 mg	pink, cup-shaped	2.5–10 mg from 5th to 25th day of cycle	Parke-Davis
MEGACE	Megesterol acetate	20 mg	light blue	20 mg twice a day for hot flashes	Bristol-Myers
PROVERA	Medroxy-progesterone acetate	2.5 mg 5 mg 10 mg	orange hexagonal white round white	Daily continuously or twice a day cyclically. 5–10 mg/day for 10–12 days, beginning 13th or 15th day of cycle	Upjohn
Estrogen/progestin combinations					
PREMPRO	Conjugated equine estrogen Medroxypro-gesterone acetate	0.625 mg 2.5 mg	orange	Single tablet once a day	Wyeth-Ayerst
PREMPHASE	Conjugated equine estrogen Medroxypro-gesterone acetate	0.625 mg 2.5 mg		Single tablet once/day. Progesterone included only in 1st 2 weeks	Wyeth-Ayerst
Estrogen/androgen combinations					
ESTRATEST	Esterified estrogens Methyltestos-terone	1.25 mg 2.5 mg	dark green	One or two daily cyclically (three weeks on, one week off)	Solvay

TABLE 15.1   *(Continued)*

Brand name	Active ingredients	Size	Color	Dosage	Manu-facturer
ESTRATEST H.S.	Esterified estrogens Methyl-testosterone	0.625 mg 1.25 mg	light green	One or two daily cyclically	Solvay
PREMARIN with METHYL-TESTOSTERONE	Conjugated estrogens Methyl-testosterone	0.625 mg 5 mg 1.25 mg 10 mg	white yellow	One or two daily for three weeks on, one week off	Wyeth-Ayerst
Estrogen plus tranquilizers (oral)					
PMB 200	Conjugated estrogens Meprobamate	0.45 mg 200 mg	green	Three times daily cyclically	Wyeth-Ayerst
PMB 400	Conjugated estrogens Meprobamate	0.45 mg 400 mg	pink	Three times daily cyclically	Wyeth-Ayerst
*Estrogen vaginal creams**					
ESTRACE	Estradiol (17 beta-estradiol)	0.1 mg in 1 g cream		2–4 mg/day for 1–2 weeks, then reduce to ½ dosage for similar period. Maintenance at 1–3 g per week.	Mead Johnson
ESTRIOL CREAM	Estriol	0.1 mg per gram of cream		Available by prescription from some mail-order pharmacies; generic.	
OGEN	Estropipate	1.5 mg in 1 g cream		2–4 g/day	Abbott
ORTHO DIENESTROL	Dienestrol	0.01 percent		1–2 applicatorsful/day for 1–2 weeks; then ½ dosage for 1–2 wks. Maintenance at one applicatorful 1–3 times per week.	Ortho
PREMARIN	Conjugated estrogen	0.625 mg in 1 g cream		2–4 g cyclically to start	Ayerst

*Use a smaller amount than the dosages recommended by the pharmaceutical companies, as discussed in the text.

ESTROGEN

As we mentioned in Chapter 1, three main forms of estrogen occur naturally in our bodies, all made from cholesterol in the ovary and the adrenal gland. Estradiol predominates in premenopausal women. Estrone is the dominant estrogen postmenopausally. Estriol is a third, less potent, form, which is highest during pregnancy. Estradiol can be converted to estrone, and estrone can be converted back to estradiol. Estriol participates less in this interchange. All of them fit the estrogen receptor equally, but, as you might expect, they don't have the same effects. Estradiol is the most potent. Estrone and (as just noted) estriol are weaker. Because of this, high levels of estrone or estriol can bind with the receptor and have the potential to act as antiestrogens—to keep the more potent estradiol from binding.[4]

Oral Estrogen

Premarin

The most common method of taking estrogen is in a pill. Premarin, as I mentioned, is the most frequently used in the United States. Its "conjugated equine estrogens" are absorbed through the intestinal wall, where they begin to turn into estrone and estradiol. Then the compound continues on to the liver, as does everything you swallow. It reaches the liver at a very high concentration—much higher than the level of estrogen that the normal premenopausal ovary sends to the liver.

Not surprisingly, this super-high level of estrogen affects the liver. The estrogen stimulates some of the proteins that are made in the liver. This may be responsible for some of its good effects on cholesterol.

After the estrogen is metabolized, it's released into the bloodstream at a much lower level—more like the level found in a premenopausal woman (although there's still more estrone and less estradiol than a premenopausal woman would have).

As I said earlier, most of the studies on estrogen therapy in the United States have been done on Premarin, and mostly with women who have had hysterectomies. It's very good for hot flashes (although it may not eliminate them completely), and for many women it reduces insomnia. It also relieves vaginal dryness, although some women need to use a cream as well. It decreases bone loss, although this won't ensure that you won't get osteoporosis or fractures. It may have a beneficial effect on the heart, although this remains to be proven. It probably increases breast cancer risk and definitely increases endometrial cancer risk.

Problems with Premarin   The effects of Premarin on the liver don't appear to be limited to digestion. Even when it's given vaginally, which means that it avoids the digestive system, Premarin has more of an effect on the liver than non-horse estrogens do. There may be something else in the horse urine besides estrogen that causes some of this additional effect.

Another problem is that the level of estrogen produced in the blood of women on Premarin is probably much higher than normal. This is because Premarin consists of three major components. The first is estrone sulfate, which makes up 50 to 60 percent of the preparation. This is a hormone found in both horses and humans. Then there are two horse estrogens that aren't made by humans—equilin sulfate, which is 20 to 30 percent of the preparation; and 17 alpha dihydroequilin sulfate, which is 15 percent. The levels of the equilin estrogens in these pills are many times higher than our bodies' normal levels of estradiol or estrone.[5] What effect does that have? The pharmaceutical companies haven't told us that. And no one else has studied it. We simply don't know.

A third problem with Premarin is that you might not be comfortable with a medication based on the urine of pregnant mares. To begin with, it isn't a particularly appealing notion. As my coauthor exclaimed when she first learned of the derivation of Premarin, "You mean I'm swallowing horse piss every morning?" But there's also the more serious issue of the way the horses are treated. We've become increasingly aware in recent years of the moral issues raised by the abuse of animals in laboratories, at racetracks, and even in homes. For the reader who tries to buy "cruelty-free" products, the treatment of the animals used for her hormone pills might be of interest.

To get the urine needed to make Premarin, about 50,000 mares are impregnated each year. For seven months of her eleven-month pregnancy, each mare is kept in a tiny stall, barely large enough to hold her. She wears a harness with a device to collect her urine. In order to make the urine more concentrated, she is given only minimal water to drink.

The foals that are the offspring of these pregnancies are sold as pets, or kept to be used in their turn to produce more urine for Premarin, or—most commonly—slaughtered for their meat.

Most of the 480 Pregnant Mare Urine (PMU) farms are in Manitoba, Canada; a few are in other parts of Canada and in North Dakota. When a team from the World Society for the Protection of Animals (WSPA)—including Joe Silva from the Massachusetts Society for the Prevention of Cruelty to Animals—was invited to inspect 32 of the Manitoba farms, it found that the animals were given little to no exercise, had no space to lie down or move around, and were often neglected when they were ill.

When the company that produces Premarin, Wyeth-Ayerst, was confronted with the results of the WSPA inspection, it promised to make a few changes, but WSPA considered these inadequate and unconvincing.

Needless to say, the animal rights movement has taken the treatment of these horses on as a cause. It has called attention to the unpalatable ingredients in this popular pill by parodying a currently popular ad for milk: the anti-Premarin ad shows a cheery actress whose grin is capped with a yellow mustache.

On the other hand, a colleague of mine checked this matter out, and she reports that the mares are actually kept as well as any horses bred for uses other than racing or pleasure. Horses, my colleague points out, don't normally lie down. The mares do get out to exercise and are actually treated well, since each one is an important investment for the farmer.[6]

Although this controversy is unlikely to be settled soon, it is important to know about it as you look at your options.

How Much Premarin Should You Take?   Premarin comes in several different doses. The most common dose (typically, daily) is 0.625 milligram. A higher dose—1.25 milligrams—is sometimes prescribed, particularly for young women who have especially severe symptoms after hysterectomy. Since the risk of breast cancer is related to the strength of the dose as well as to how long estrogen is taken, this higher dose is probably the cause of some breast cancer. (It was also the dose used in the studies we mentioned earlier on men with heart disease.) A lower dose—0.3 milligram—is also available. A few studies have shown that it will prevent bone loss, but its effect on heart disease hasn't been studied.[7]

Almost all of the data we have are based on the 0.625-milligram dose. This is really quite amazing. It's almost certain that women's metabolism, their size, and the amount of their own hormones will make a difference in their absorption of the drug, and yet there's rarely any attempt to modify the dose to fit a particular woman's needs. (I guess that is just our fate as women . . . our clothes come in only a few set sizes as well.) I recommend that you take the lowest dose that will take care of the problem you want to treat. If it's symptoms or osteoporosis, this might be 0.3 milligram. (If your symptoms aren't decreasing enough, you can always increase the dose.) If that's not enough but 0.625 seems too high (for example, if you're experiencing breast tenderness), you can try 0.625 milligram of Premarin during the week but not on weekends. (This will often relieve you of breast tenderness.)

Many women start on Premarin after hysterectomies for relief of symptoms and just go on taking it for the rest of their lives. Others take it for a short time after the surgery, or until the normal age of menopause, to tide

them over, and then slowly taper off, mimicking a more natural menopause. If you've had a hysterectomy, you may not need to take any other
hormones. If you still have your uterus, on the other hand, you'll need to
consider taking a progestin or progesterone to protect it from cancer. (See
the section on progesterone later in this chapter.)

Side Effects of Premarin   The side effects of Premarin get very little press,
but they do exist. The most common are breast swelling and tenderness,
PMS, rash, increased growth of facial and body hair, intolerance of contact
lenses, migraine, dizziness, headache, depression, changes in libido, and
reduced tolerance of carbohydrates. (This last effect is a warning sign that
you're on your way to diabetes. Diabetics have problems with sugar, and
carbohydrates turn into sugar in the body.) Premarin doubles the risk of
gallbladder surgery. It also raises triglyceride levels. This could be a real
problem if you have a disease characterized by high triglyceride levels to
start with, since that is a serious risk for heart disease. Interestingly, the
package insert for Premarin also describes as a possible side effect blotchy
skin, especially on the face, which may be permanent. (So much for
enhancing your beauty!)

Women who are on Premarin alone won't get regular periods, but 25
percent will have some bleeding. There is a risk of endometrial hyperplasia, so any bleeding or spotting should be checked out immediately, and
you may need an endometrial biopsy to rule out any problems (see page
47). One study found that, compared with a woman who is not on estrogen, a woman who still has her uterus and takes estrogen alone has eight
times the chance of bleeding, a five times greater chance of having a D
and C, a 6.6 times greater chance of having a hysterectomy, and a seven
times greater likelihood of uterine cancer.[8] Nowadays, most women with
a uterus will be given a progesterone or progestin to prevent these problems.

Tapering Off Premarin   If you want to consider getting off Premarin at
any time, you should consider tapering off. (There's no medical problem
with stopping cold turkey, but you may experience severe withdrawal
symptoms.) This means alternating one pill with half a pill (or a pill of a
lower dosage) for two months, or taking a whole pill every other day. Then
go to half a pill (or reduced dosage) every day for two months. Then go to
half a pill every other day for two months. Finally, stop. (The pills aren't
scored, so you need to break them either with a sharp knife or an inexpensive pill-cutting tool that most pharmacies carry.) If at any time you experience severe symptoms, you're tapering off too fast and need to slow down.
Let your health care provider know if you decide to taper off.

Other Kinds of Oral Estrogen

One other form of oral estrogen is micronized estradiol (Estrace). This is "natural" in the sense that it's the same chemical formula as your own body's estradiol—the estrogen that's highest in premenopausal women. "Micronized" means that it's been suspended in very fine droplets to aid its absorption in the digestive tract. Other plant-based estrogens used in the United States include esterified estrogens (Estratab) and estropipate, or piperazine estrogen sulfate (Ogen). Any one of them will work. You may want to experiment with one of these other formulations. Everyone's body is different and responds differently to medications, so it's fortunate that there are options.

In Europe, the most commonly used oral estrogen is estradiol valerate (Progynon). Another form of oral estrogen used in Europe provides a combination of estrone, estradiol, and estriol. Estriol alone is also used in Europe for hormone therapy, and it's gained some popularity among alternative health care practitioners in the United States, since it's less potent than estradiol and estrone and may have some antiestrogenic effects. Some research done on rats and mice in the 1970s found that estriol protected them against breast cancer.[9] In addition, there are some epidemiological data suggesting that women in countries with higher rates of breast cancer have lower levels of estriol in their urine.[10] None of this is definitive, but it's extremely provocative.

Since estriol is the least potent of the estrogens, it has much less effect on the uterine lining, yet it can still reduce menopausal symptoms. Unfortunately, however, high doses (12 milligrams daily) of estriol are necessary to prevent osteoporosis. In one study of the effects of various compounds on lipids, estriol was found to have no effect on cholesterol.[11] Whether it has any direct beneficial effects on blood vessels remains to be seen. It therefore is a better choice for controlling symptoms than for prevention.

There are also synthetic oral estrogens. Their chemical structure is very different from that of human estrogen, but they have some estrogen effects. These include ethinyl estradiol (Estinyl), diethylstilbestrol (DES), and quinesterol (Estrovis). These are rarely used today.

The Estrogen Patch

Using the Patch

In the United States nearly everyone who takes estrogen takes it in the form of a pill, but in Europe the patch is far more common. Several types of patches are available in the United States, and they're growing in popularity. Estrogen delivered through the skin is absorbed better, since it doesn't have to go through the liver and intestine.

The most common patch is Estraderm. It releases 17 beta-estradiol, which is the estrogen our ovaries normally make before menopause. It consists of four layers. The first is a backing, which prevents evaporation, like a Band-Aid. The next layer is a little reservoir with the drug inside, suspended in alcohol, which carries the estrogen to the skin. The third layer is a membrane that controls how quickly it's released. The fourth layer is an adhesive that holds the patch on your skin.

The patch is about as big as a half dollar, though the sizes vary a little, depending on the dose. Usually you put it on a clean, dry area of your buttock or your abdomen. You don't want to put it on a breast, because absorbing very high doses of estrogen into the breast may be dangerous. And avoid the waistline—the patch will get rubbed if it's applied there. The patch stays on in the bath or shower, or when you go swimming.

With the patch, only about 10 percent of the drug is actually delivered, because by the end of four days, you run out of the alcohol that carries it to the skin. So about every four days, you have to change it.

The blood levels of estrogen you can get vary, but are usually similar to those of a premenopausal woman in the first half of her cycle. (This variability in blood levels bothers gynecologists, who like consistency.) The newer patches are a little stronger than the older ones.

The patches have about equal proportions of estrone and estradiol, replicating levels in a premenopausal woman. After the patch is applied, the estrogen levels gradually go up and then reach a steady state in about two hours. These levels last for a couple of days, then start to decline.

The patch may be perfect for women who have had hysterectomies, but for other women there's a problem, which is on the verge of being solved. The patch still stimulates cells in the endometrium, so you need to take some progestin to avoid uterine cancer or other problems. Right now, the best route is to use the patch for most of your cycle, and then take a progestin pill toward the end. This is, of course, less convenient than taking a single pill that gives you both estrogen and progestin. (Such a pill is now being used in the United States; see below.) There is now a combined patch called Estrogest that combines estrogen and norethindrone, a synthetic progesterone; it is available in Europe.

There are no long-term studies of the patch, so we don't know whether it can protect against heart disease. In the short term, we know that its effects on lipids are about the same as those of Premarin, at least after six months. (Your cholesterol may take a little longer to go down on the patch than on the pill, but it'll end up at the same place.) Like Premarin, the patch dilates the blood vessels. It has the same effect as oral estrogen on bone, hot flashes, and vaginal dryness.

The patch doesn't affect the liver, so it might be better for women with high blood pressure or a tendency toward blood clotting (thrombosis). It won't promote gallbladder disease or cause nausea, as Premarin some- times does. Thus for women who have gastrointestinal problems, gall- stones, or high triglycerides, the patch has some real advantages.

The most common and most severe side effect of the patch is skin irrita- tion, which is experienced by 5 to 30 percent of patients, depending on the climate they live in and the sensitivity of their skin. In one study,[12] 24 per- cent of the patients had a skin reaction, but only 4 percent discontinued the therapy because of it. So obviously it's not that bad. One of the things you can do for a skin irritation is put the patch on a different spot each time you use it. You can also wave it around for a few minutes before you apply it, to let some of the alcohol evaporate.

Like Premarin, the patch can cause breast tenderness, headache, migraine, dizziness, depression, an increase or decrease in weight, reduced tolerance of carbohydrates (which can be a precursor to diabetes), fluid retention, and change in libido.

There's now a new kind of patch, Climara. This is a matrix—a thin adhe- sive film with estradiol inside it under a transparent foil backing. It looks like a piece of clear plastic with a sticky side. Because it's a single layer, it doesn't have a fluid reservoir, so it's much less bulky and causes less skin irritation. It releases 5 micrograms of estradiol a day and has a surface area of 16 cubic centimeters—about the size of a half dollar, like the original patch. Once you remove it from the foil package, you need to apply it imme- diately. It lasts for seven days. Again, you can bathe, shower, or swim while wearing it.

Tapering Off the Patch

If you want to taper off the patch, the technique depends on the type you're using. If it's the reservoir type (thicker and translucent), you take a spot Band-Aid and cut out a quarter of it. Use the quarter to cover a quarter of the patch. After a couple of weeks cover half the patch, then three quar- ters, etc. If you prefer, you can cut the patch itself in half and seal the cut end with clear adhesive tape. (But don't cut it without sealing it; the alco- hol and estrogen will leak out.) If you have the newer matrix type (thin and clear), you can cut a quarter off the actual patch without sealing it, and use that dosage for a month, then cut it in half, then cut off three quarters, etc.

As with pills, if you experience withdrawal symptoms, you should go more slowly. Tell your health care provider you're tapering off.

Other Parenteral Methods of Estrogen Delivery

In countries other than the United States, an estrogen gel in an alcohol base is sometimes used; this is rubbed into the skin. You apply it over a large area of your abdomen and thighs and let it dry for two or three minutes before you put clothes on. It's odorless, and it isn't sticky. It's absorbed into your skin and gradually released into your body.

The gel is similar to the patch in that it uses estradiol (Oestrogel) and works by slow absorption. It's a bit trickier to use, though, because it's a little harder to be sure of the dose. The gel is absorbed fairly well, and like the patch, it doesn't go through the liver. It has slightly less effect on HDL and LDL, but it's basically just as good for protecting against osteoporosis. It doesn't irritate the skin as the patch can, because it doesn't contain any adhesives. Unfortunately, it's not yet available in the United States.

In the United Kingdom, Australia, and South Africa, women can use a crystalline implant of estradiol, both for prevention and for treatment. It works somewhat like the contraceptive Norplant. It's inserted under your skin in a minor surgical operation. Blood levels rise to a peak once a month, plateau for two to four months, and then decline. There are similar implants that add testosterone to the estrogen. The problem with implants is that they initially produce very high levels of estrogen, which can fall fairly rapidly, causing symptoms like hot flashes when they're first inserted. Since the pellets are under the skin, the dosage can't be changed until the next implant. But there are a number of advantages: an implant eliminates the inconvenience of taking a pill; over time, it produces more constant blood levels of hormone; and it produces stable changes in the lipids and bone.

Parenteral estrogen is easily absorbed. Since it doesn't go through the liver as a first step, the amount that eventually reaches your liver is similar to what would get there if your ovaries were making it. So it's more physiologic—more the way the body normally works. Parenteral estrogen doesn't cause an increase in your triglycerides, and it doesn't have as much effect as oral estrogen on lipids, LDL, or HDL, although there is some effect after six months to a year. It also results in a more stable level of hormones.

In general, the alternatives to oral estrogen, including the patch, deliver estrogen in a constant manner, produce higher physiologic estrone and estradiol levels than oral estrogens, and avoid the liver-protein effect. And the lower-dose vaginal methods (discussed on page 180) are certainly a good alternative if your only concern is vaginal atrophy (dryness). Unfortunately, they're more expensive.

So the effect of estrogen really depends a lot on the type, the dose, and how you take it. They're not all equivalent—the patch isn't equal to the Premarin, which isn't equal to vaginal estrogen. Which you choose to use depends very much on your own body and the reasons you're taking the drugs.

When You Shouldn't Take Estrogen

If you have undiagnosed vaginal bleeding, or if you might be pregnant, you absolutely shouldn't take estrogen. It's also a bad idea if you have a history of breast cancer, endometrial cancer, or ovarian cancer; a history of deep vein thrombophlebitis or pulmonary embolus; a blood-clotting disorder; or active liver or gallbladder disease.

TAMOXIFEN AND SERMS

Some doctors have suggested tamoxifen as an alternative to estrogen for preventing heart disease, osteoporosis, and recurrence of breast cancer. Initial data seemed to indicate that it decreased the incidence of heart attacks,[13] but that's been disproved by more recent studies.[14] It doesn't seem to have a bad effect on lipids, but that's a far cry from preventing heart attacks. When it's taken for a year, tamoxifen *increases* bone loss in premenopausal women, though it does prevent further loss in post-menopausal women. It causes uterine cancer as well. On top of that, it causes hot flashes.[15] Not exactly the ideal drug.

In addition, there is reason to believe that even tamoxifen's supposed role in preventing breast cancer should be questioned. Earlier studies had shown that when women who had had cancer in one breast took tamoxifen, it reduced the risk of cancer in the other breast by 30 to 50 percent.[16] A more recent randomized controlled study, however, showed that it had its maximum effect with women who took it for five years.[17] Taking it for five more years didn't offer any more protection, and may actually have caused more cancers. In other words, after a while the breast cells become resistant to tamoxifen and actually start to be fed by it.

This is a dramatic example of why you need good long-term studies. If we had based all of our recommendations on the five-year data without doing further studies, we would have had women taking tamoxifen forever. So convinced were we that tamoxifen was a wonder drug that the only reason researchers did the later study at all was to prove it. Luckily, we found out that we were wrong in time to prevent doing further damage. We have learned, not for the first time, that more isn't always better.

The new SERMs (selective estrogen receptor modulators), or designer estrogens, Raloxifene and Droloxifene, are modeled on tamoxifen, but they don't appear to cause cancer of the uterus. These aren't available as of this writing, though they will soon be appearing on the horizon. It is believed that they will protect against uterine cancer without a need for progesterone, while preventing osteoporosis, heart disease, and perhaps even breast cancer.[18, 19]

These drugs may simplify some of the conflicts we have over whether to take hormone therapy as it is currently used, but they're still drugs. Though having them will widen the range of a woman's options, the question remains whether everyone should take drugs for prevention. It's also crucial to remember that any study is only as good as the time frame it's investigating. Even if these new drugs turn out to do everything they are said to do, we won't be sure for thirty years what their thirty-year effect will be. Remember the study showing that tamoxifen taken for five years was better than tamoxifen for ten years, when it started to become stimulatory.

PROGESTERONE AND PROGESTINS

Progesterone is very different from estrogen, because your body produces almost all of its own progesterone only when you're premenopausal: it's produced by the corpus luteum after ovulation. The adrenal gland also produces a very small amount, but that's usually used as a building block for other hormones, such as testosterone. If you're not ovulating, then, you have virtually no progesterone.

Although natural progesterone—the form most like the hormone we produce naturally—is available, it's rarely used. It's plant-based and generic (like estriol), so it can't be patented. As I've said, if something can't be patented, manufacturers can't make as much money from producing it and have less incentive to study it. Therefore, progestins, which are molecules that have been changed a bit and can therefore be patented, are more commonly prescribed. The terms *progesterone* and *progestin* are often used interchangeably, but they shouldn't be, since the actions of progesterone and progestin can be very different.

As we discussed in Chapter 2, progesterone and progestins have only recently become part of "hormone replacement therapy." Initially, the only hormone "replaced" was estrogen. Then, when postmenopausal women on estrogen began to develop uterine cancer, progesterone and progestins came into the picture. Their addition to estrogen for a few days at the end of the cycle causes the uterine lining to be shed, preventing buildup and minimizing the risk of uterine cancer.

But progestins do other things as well. When added to estrogen, they can cause or intensify many symptoms of PMS: headaches, depression, irritability, bloating, fluid retention, abdominal cramping, and breast tenderness. In addition, progestins have their own effects on the liver and the blood vessels. In the liver, they lower triglycerides and block the helpful estrogen-derived increase in HDL. In the blood vessels, they block the helpful vasodilation of the coronary arteries induced by estrogen. Progestins may even counteract any potential benefit estrogen may have on libido. As of yet, we really don't have any long-term studies of progestin or progesterone, either alone or with estrogen. Therefore, we just can't assume that "HRT" is the same as "ERT."

Kinds of Progesterone and Progestins

As with estrogen, there are different forms of progesterone and progestins, and different methods of delivery, each of which influences its effects.

"Natural" progesterone isn't very well absorbed when taken by mouth (because it's broken down in the liver). Until recently, therefore, the only way it could be given was by vaginal suppository or by a skin cream. Vaginal suppositories allow progesterone to be absorbed without passing through the liver. It is a good delivery route but sometimes messy.

The skin creams have become somewhat controversial lately. There are a number of them on the market, claiming to contain progesterone and to decrease hot flashes and increase bone. Many of these actually have very little progesterone (see Table 15.2). The assumption is that because they're made from wild yam, they'll have the same effect as progesterone, which is also made from wild yam. Don't count on it.

A better development for advocates of progesterone is micronized progesterone, created by breaking progesterone up into very small pieces. Since it's taken orally, it's broken down by the liver. Thus in order to get blood levels of progesterone that were considered adequate, the original prescriptions called for high doses (200 milligrams), taken twice a day. But in the PEPI study (see Chapter 6), researchers decided to investigate whether 100 milligrams once a day of oral micronized progesterone added to estrogen would be adequate. They found that it was still effective at protecting the uterus and did not greatly interfere with the effect of estrogen on the lipids.[20] Other studies have shown that micronized progesterone is very good for preventing osteoporosis and may even build bone

TABLE 15.2   Percent of Progesterone Found in Commercially Available
"Natural" Progesterone Creams

Creams containing more than 400 mg progesterone per ounce of cream

Pro-Gest	Professional and Technical Services	Portland, OR
Pro-Oste-All	Saratl International	Pasadena, TX
Bio Balance	Elan Vitale	Scottsdale, AZ
OstaDerm	Bezwecken	Beaverton, OR
Progonol	Bezwecken	Beaverton, OR
PhytoGest	Karuna Corp.	Novato, CA
Edenn Cream	SNM	Norcross, GA
Equilibrium	Equilibrium Lab	Boca Raton, FL
Estro-All	Saratl International	Pasadena, TX
Femarone-17	Wise Essentials	Minneapolis, MN
Happy PMS	HM Enterprises, Inc.	Norcross, GA
NatraGest	Broadmoore Labs, Inc.	Ventura, CA
Pro-Alo	HealthWatchers System	Scottsdale, AZ
Pro-G	TriMedica	Scottsdale, AZ
ProBalance	Springboard	Monterey, CA
PROGEST-1 Complex	Kenogen	Eugene, OR
Angel Care	Angel Care	Atlanta, GA
Renewed Balance	American Image Marketing	Nampa, ID
Serenity	Health and Science	Crawfordvil, FL

Creams containing 5–20 mg progesterone per ounce of cream

Cielo	Transitions for Health	Portland, OR
EFX Wild Yam	Natural Efx, Inc.	Richardson, TX
Endocreme	Wuliton Labs	Palmyra, MO
Life Changes	MW Labs	Atlanta, GA
Novagest	Strate Dermatologics	Concord, CA
NUGESTRONE	Nutraceutics	Boca Raton, FL
PROGESTERONE plus	Professional Health Products	Sewickley, PA
Woman Wise	Jason Natural Cosmetics	Culver City, CA

Creams containing less than 5 mg progesterone per ounce of cream

Born Again	Alvin Last, Inc.	Yonkers, NY
Dioscorea Cream	Seroyal International, Inc.	Toronto, Canada
Nutrigest	NutriSupplies, Inc.	West Palm Beach, FL
Progerone	Nature's Nutrition Inc.	Vero Beach, FL
Progestone 10	Dixie Health, Inc.	Atlanta, GA
Progestone-HP	Dixie Health, Inc.	Atlanta, GA
Yamcon	Phillips Nutrition	Laguna Hill, CA

Note: The creams were obtained commercially and tested by a specific radioimmunoassay for progesterone after extraction and dilution.

Source: Prepared by Aeron Lifecycles (800-631-7900), September 16, 1996.

rather than just stop resorption.[21] It can also treat hot flashes without the use of estrogen.

Researchers have discovered that breast cell proliferation is higher in the second half of the menstrual cycle, when progesterone levels are higher.[22] This has led them to assume that progesterone stimulates breast tissue. To investigate this further, a study was done on women who were about to undergo breast-reduction surgery.[23] (This meant that the breast tissue removed in the operation could be examined afterward.) Each woman applied progesterone to one breast every day for two weeks. After the reduction surgery, the pathologists examined the breast tissue that had been removed and found that the progesterone had decreased cell division. This has been interpreted as demonstrating that progesterone prevents breast cancer. Again, though—as in the case of estriol—the data are provocative but not yet definitive. It would appear that a woman who has had breast cancer and needs to take some type of hormone might consider progesterone rather than any form of estrogen, especially if she's tried all non-drug possibilities and they haven't helped.

Micronized progesterone is available by prescription in Europe as Utrogestan and in Canada as Prometrium. It is also widely available from the alternative compounding pharmacies in the United States (see Appendix 2). Each pharmacy makes this form in its own way, so there are no standardized data on the levels that get delivered to the patient.

With regard to micronized progesterone, American gynecologists and their patients are caught in an economical and political bind. The reason gynecologists originally used progestins was that progesterone was not well absorbed orally. Now researchers have developed a "vehicle"—micronized progesterone—to deliver consistent blood levels of progesterone when given orally. A generous pharmaceutical company supplied micronized progesterone to the PEPI study but has not made its product commercially available in the United States. The progesterone compounded by mail-order companies hasn't been studied for its pharmacological characteristics because it's too expensive and it can't be patented. In one randomized controlled double-blind study, micronized progesterone had fewer side effects and a better effect on lipids and the endometrium than a progestin.[24] But as clinicians or consumers, we're stuck with a nonstandardized product or a possibly inferior standardized product because it's considered unprofitable to find out which is best for women.

It is for this reason that progestins are still more commonly used. Progestins are all related to androgens, the male hormones. Some of them have more of an androgenic effect than others. The two main types are C19 and C21 progestins. (The numbers relate to the chemical formula.)

C19 progestins tend to be more androgenic, so you're more likely to get acne, greasy hair, and greasy skin. They also tend to lower triglycerides, an effect that can be beneficial, since estrogens cause triglycerides to rise. Examples of C19 progestins include norethindrone and norethindrone acetate. Norethindrone is very potent, so you need smaller doses. It's used more frequently in Europe than in the United States.

C21 progestins are less androgenic. Provera (medroxyprogesterone acetate), the progestin most commonly used in the United States, is one of these. Provera is given in pill form, either continuously (see below) at a low dose or cyclically in the first half of the cycle. It has less effect on triglycerides than norethindrone or norethindrone acetate, and it blocks some, though not all, of the beneficial effects estrogen has on cholesterol. As discussed in Chapter 6, the PEPI study found that estrogen alone had the best effect on lipid levels, and estrogen with micronized progesterone was second. Provera was definitely third, although it didn't cancel out all of the beneficial effects of the estrogen.[25] Norethindrone is a reasonable alternative for women for whom Provera produces intolerable symptoms.

Ironically, the greatest advantage of the progestins is also the source of women's greatest complaints about them. As I discussed in Chapter 8, estrogen alone can cause endometrial cancer because it thickens the uterine lining over and over again. Progestins allow the body to slough off the lining; this helps ward off uterine cancer, but it means that you have to deal with menstrual bleeding. Twenty-five percent of women taking estrogen alone will have some bleeding, but 85 percent of women who take Premarin plus Provera will get periods again. These periods are usually light, predictable bleeding lasting four to five days every cycle. Even if you opt for the continuous approach described below, you could still get periods for six months to a year, though they should ultimately stop once your uterus becomes atrophic[26] (see the next section). This is the main reason most women don't stay on hormones. No one wants to be buying tampons or pads any longer than she has to. Sometimes, at my most cynical, I think it's all a plot by the manufacturers of menstrual products, who don't want to lose sales when all of us baby boomers stop bleeding.

ESTROGEN PLUS PROGESTERONE OR PROGESTIN

Cyclical versus Continuous Therapy

Estrogen and progesterone can be combined in various ways (see Table 15.3). In *cyclical therapy*, you take estrogen daily, add progestin for the first twelve days of the month, and then stop the progestin. You'll get a period as soon as the progestin is stopped.

TABLE 15.3   Ways of Taking Hormone Therapy

Day	Cyclical		Continuous	
	Estrogen	*Progestin*	*Estrogen*	*Progestin*
1	X	X	X	X
2	X	X	X	X
3	X	X	X	X
4	X	X	X	X
5	X	X	X	X
6	X	X	X	X
7	X	X	X	X
8	X	X	X	X
9	X	X	X	X
10	X	X	X	X
11	X	X	X	X
12	X	X	X	X
13	X		X	X
14	X		X	X
15	X		X	X
16	X		X	X
17	X		X	X
18	X		X	X
19	X		X	X
20	X		X	X
21	X		X	X
22	X		X	X
23	X		X	X
24	X		X	X
25	X		X	X
26	X		X	X
27	X		X	X
28	X		X	X
29*	X		X	X
30*	X		X	X
31*	X		X	X

*Depending on how many days there are in the month.

Because women were complaining about bleeding, doctors began experimenting with a new strategy, *continuous therapy.* In this kind of therapy, women take estrogen and progestin continuously, but use a lower dose of progestin. The hope is that the continuous level of progestin will be too low to cause bleeding but high enough to block the stimulating effects of the estrogen. This approach causes much less bleeding than the cyclical approach, but, as we've discussed, it doesn't wholly eliminate bleeding.

There's still a 60 to 70 percent chance that you'll have some breakthrough bleeding, or at least spotting. This wouldn't be too bad except for the fact that uterine cancer also shows up as breakthrough bleeding. This means that every time you bleed, you'll need an endometrial biopsy to be sure you don't have uterine cancer. On average, most women on continuous combined therapy have two to three endometrial biopsies. Even though the bleeding usually stops within six months to a year, some women continue to have periods. They then have to decide whether to stop hormone therapy completely or switch to just estrogen alone and take their chances. It's no wonder that gynecologists would rather take the bothersome, bleeding uterus out and be done with it—and that you end up with a hysterectomy you don't need.

It's important to note that the bleeding occurs only if you're also on estrogen. If you're taking progesterone or Provera alone, you usually won't bleed.

If you elect to take estrogen alone, you of course still need to have your endometrium monitored. (What you don't want to do is skip the Provera and *not* have your uterus monitored.) In the PEPI study discussed in Chapter 6, the women who took estrogen alone had a 30 percent chance over three years of developing endometrial hyperplasia, which was detected on routine endometrial biopsy. This means there is a 70 percent chance that it *won't* happen in the first three years. (We have no studies to determine what happens after that.) You may decide to see if you can tolerate estrogen alone and take progestins only if you develop hyperplasia—precancer. (If you've had a hysterectomy, you're already protected from endometrial cancer, since there are uterine cells only in the uterus itself, unlike the case with the breast and the ovary.) This approach is not currently recommended by most physicians, because of the chance of endometrial cancer; but only you can weigh the risks in your own case.

Progestocert

There's now an intrauterine device called Progestocert that gives out a very low, steady dose of progestin. Like the lower doses of the vaginal creams, it's not enough to be absorbed into the body as a whole. This is based on the very sensible idea that where you really want the progesterone is in the uterus, so that it can protect the endometrium. There isn't any known need for it in the rest of the body, so why not deliver it just where it's needed and avoid the side effects? This approach would eliminate the need for oral progestin. As currently designed, the device stops vaginal bleeding and works for five years, after which it would need to be replaced. As of yet we don't know what the long-term effects would be.

Prempro

A new pill that combines Premarin and Provera has just been approved in the United States. Called Prempro, it delivers continuous Premarin and progesterone in one pill much the way the oral contraceptive does. (In the cyclical form, it's called Premphase.) Wyeth-Ayerst is hoping to increase its market by making the combinations easier to take.

Notably, the small print in the ads for Prempro (as with advertisements for estrogen in the medical journals) includes much of the hedging we've discussed. It says some research has shown that taking estrogen without progestins might protect against heart disease, but that the studies aren't conclusive. The ads also mention that "the safety data regarding Prempro were obtained primarily from clinical trials and epidemiological studies of postmenopausal Caucasian women, who were generally [at] low risk for cardiovascular disease and higher than average risk for osteoporosis. The safety profile of Prempro derived from these study populations cannot necessarily be extrapolated to other populations of diverse racial and/or demographic compositions." The moral? Always read the small print in ads for prescription medications, or in the insert you get with a prescription. Although the ads you see or the inserts you get aren't always as detailed as what a doctor receives, they do provide have a lot of thought-provoking information—thoughts the pharmaceutical companies, required by law to supply this information, may not be all that eager to provoke.

TESTOSTERONE

Understanding Testosterone

As we've noted, the normal postmenopausal ovary produces testosterone as well as androstenedione and low levels of estrogen. It should come as no surprise that women whose ovaries have been surgically removed experience a rapid decline in testosterone levels. In addition, postmenopausal women who take estrogen seem to have lower testosterone levels.

The question is what effect these lower levels of testosterone have. How significant is this? There's some evidence that osteoporosis may be related to testosterone as well as estrogen. It's not clear what effect testosterone has on cholesterol.[27] In addition, there's conflicting evidence about the effects of testosterone on the libido (see Chapter 11).

Testosterone is rapidly metabolized to estrogen in the body by both fat and muscle, so it doesn't seem as if adding it would have much effect on your sex drive, although methyltestosterone (a variant of testosterone) isn't as easily converted. And it's important to note that testosterone appears to have effects only on women whose blood levels of testosterone are low to begin with. Nonetheless, there's a growing trend to add testosterone to the hormone mix in women who are complaining of inadequate libido.

The FDA has approved two combination pills of estrogen and testosterone. Estratest is a combination of estradiol and methyltestosterone and comes in two doses: regular and half strength. The other is Premarin plus methyltestosterone (the testosterone here is four times as strong in the Premarin version). In addition, you can get "natural" testosterone (like the kind in our bodies) or methyltestosterone in either a pill or cream, but it has to be made at one of the compounding pharmacies licensed to make drugs to specifications for individual physicians. By now you can guess that this is because it's not patentable.

Side Effects of Testosterone

As with progesterone, doctors too easily assume that this potent hormone will have no effects other than the desired ones. Some women on testosterone have complained of rages or anger, however. Other side effects include acne, facial hair, weight gain, and liver disease. In addition, there is evidence that testosterone counteracts the lipid changes estrogen can create. And it can compound the carcinogenic effect of estrogen on the breast and uterus. The Nurses' Health Study saw an increase in breast cancer in women taking androgens.[28]

In her popular book, *The Hormone of Desire*,[29] Susan Rako, a psychiatrist in Boston, suggests that there's a sensitive "window" of dosage that works best for women. In her own experience, she found that if the dose is too high, women may feel worse—agitated and depressed. On the other hand, on a much lower dose (one-quarter to one-half the dose of Estratest HS), they regain their sense of well-being and libido.

A recent ad for Estratest in the medical journals pictured a dejected-looking woman, while the copy described the new product as helping "where estrogen alone may not be enough" and "because she wants to feel like herself again." The implication is that this woman's libido is gone, and with it her sense of well-being. On the other side of the page, which reproduces the copy from the package insert, it says that the pill "should only be used for a short period of time because we don't know what the long-term effects are." But the implication of the ad itself belies this small-print message (which is there only because the law requires it). If you're taking this combination of estrogen and testosterone to increase your libido and sense of well-being, you're not just taking it for three months, unless you're planning one last desperate fling before settling into a life of loneliness and gloom. Presumably that's not what the Estratest manufacturers have in mind.

If you decide to take testosterone to increase your libido, you need to know that very little research has been done on it and that you may be risking serious side effects in the future.

DHEA has been touted in the popular press as the answer to aging. At this point there are no data to support this claim nor any safety information.

SALIVARY HORMONE TESTS

As I have mentioned, blood tests for hormones are notoriously unreliable. Because of this some labs will test hormone levels in the saliva. Although this is a good way to measure them, I don't know why you would want to. There is no *optimal* estrogen level—only the one which feels right for you. The dose of hormones you take should be balanced against your symptoms and not some arbitrary laboratory number determined in blood or saliva.

WHAT YOU REALLY WANT TO KNOW: WHAT'S BEST?

Is one form of estrogen better than the others? I doubt it. Is continuous combined hormone therapy better than cyclical therapy? If anything, it may be worse for heart disease, but it will produce less bleeding. Is it safe to take testosterone? We don't know. Some of these questions will be resolved by ongoing studies, and by the year 2008 we may have some answers. Meanwhile, any woman taking hormones has to realize that she's part of a large experiment.

CHAPTER 16

Decisions:
What Should *I* Do?

DECISION MAKING

So what now? You've got hot flashes and you can't decide whether to stock up on herbs, buy a bike, or take a pill. Or maybe you should do all three? Your doctor told you to go on hormones to prevent osteoporosis, but you're not sure whether or not you want to. You agree that menopause is just a normal phase in your life, but that doesn't mean it's comfortable. How are you going to "manage" it? It would be nice if you could just say, "Of course I'll take hormones" or "Of course I won't." But then you wouldn't be reading this book. As you've realized by now, it's not a simple decision. The ambivalence that women have toward hormones, as I said at the beginning of this book, is well warranted. Hormones can do a lot of good, and they can do a lot of harm.

I hope I've been able to help you clarify the various factors involved in the hormone dilemma. The major distinction I've been making throughout this book remains crucial. There are two very different reasons for considering menopausal hormone therapy. One reason is to treat the symptoms of perimenopause that are interfering with the quality of your life. These symptoms vary from woman to woman, so everyone needs to decide whether her own experience warrants treatment. Since the symptoms of perimenopause and early menopause are for the most part transient, women who take hormones for this reason alone will probably want to take them for four to five years at most and then taper off.

The other reason to consider menopausal hormone therapy is to treat or prevent heart disease or osteoporosis. When a woman's menopause is natural, we don't really know to what extent estrogen combined with progesterone can help accomplish such prevention. For women who take estrogen after surgical menopause it does appear that there is some benefit, at least in terms of the bone loss that sometimes occurs at menopause. It's more questionable whether estrogen will prevent heart disease, though if your cholesterol is high it might help control that, and the lowered cholesterol might in turn keep you from getting a heart attack. But we also know there's a cost for all women—an increased risk of breast cancer and possibly of ovarian and lung cancer.

We know that there are options other than hormone therapy, both for symptoms and for the prevention and treatment of heart disease and osteoporosis. In this chapter, I'll try to outline clearly the risks and benefits in a variety of situations and suggest ways to help you decide on the best approach for yourself.

Before you read any further, let me emphasize what may be the most crucial fact about this decision: *it's not a onetime deal.* You can always reevaluate your choice as your situation and your thinking change. In fact, you should *keep* reevaluating your decision, whatever it is. Set a certain time aside to do this, every September, maybe, or on your birthday. You don't want to be second-guessing yourself with every newspaper article, but you do want to recheck your decision periodically. Your health may change, and new information about hormones and other options will probably continue to come out. What makes sense for you today may not make sense five years from today—or even six months from today.

VALUES

Although we talk a lot about statistics and risks and benefits in this book, your decision always boils down to how you feel—how you feel physically and how you feel about the different approaches to dealing with menopause. You may have had strong feelings about whether or not to have natural childbirth, or whether or not to take birth control pills. Similarly, you may have strong feelings about how you want to approach menopause. It's those feelings we're after, because they're the most important factor in your decision. They're sometimes hard to sort out. You're exposed to so many *other* people's feelings, and when those people are health professionals, their feelings are often masked as objective truth. Any consultation with an expert—and that's what a doctor's appointment really is—involves an interaction between your feelings, your values, and those of the expert.

The Doctor's Values

When I was in medical school, we were told to put ourselves in the patient's position. What that really meant was to put the patient in our own, imaginary, position. That is, we were supposed to say, "If I were you, I would . . ." On the surface this sounds very kind and caring. In fact, it's very arrogant. If there's one thing I've learned in over twenty years as a doctor, it's that I'm not my patients. I don't know what I'd do if I were you, any more than you know what you'd do if you were me. Each of my patients is a unique individual, with her own beliefs, fears, hopes, and life history. When I'm lucky, I can tell her with accuracy what her particular medical situation is; what the available therapies are, if she needs any; and what those therapies can and can't do. In short, I can do, in a very specific way, what I'm trying to do more generally in this book—provide the best information I can so that my patient can make the best decision for herself.

Most doctors have their own biases, though we don't always admit that. To a large extent, both patients and doctors are caught up in a system that deifies doctors. We're not gods. At our best, we're highly trained professionals with a large but finite range of specialized knowledge. We don't know it all.

Also, we're subject to our own human frailties. We're often working long hours seeing patients, and we don't always have the time to critically review all of the literature. We're rarely educated on alternatives such as lifestyle changes, supplements, and other approaches to wellness. At the end of the day, we want to get home to our families and forget about our jobs for a few hours.

Too often, this can lead doctors to take shortcuts—especially when they're encouraged by their friendly pharmaceutical reps. The easiest way to deal with a patient is to prescribe a pill. It will take care of the patient's symptoms and prevent future illness to boot. What could go wrong? There's little incentive for doctors to question what they've been told about estrogen therapy or hormone therapy, because being able to prescribe these therapies makes their lives easier. So it just becomes automatic.

One of my friends is an epidemiologist who studies women's health. When she was in her early fifties, she went to the gynecologist for a routine checkup. She'd had an uneventful menopause and had no particular health problems. The gynecologist, a young woman, did the exam and then asked a couple of questions. "Does anyone in your family have heart disease?" Yes, my friend's mother had, but she'd been a smoker. "Anyone have breast cancer?" No. "Well, then, you should be on hormones," she said. "You're short and might get osteoporosis." My friend was never asked about her diet (vegetarian and low-fat) or exercise (she's been a runner all her life). She wasn't even asked about her cholesterol level. All of these are things a doctor should ask before even considering suggesting that a patient take hormones.

The young gynecologist's approach was not at all atypical. G. B. Holzman analyzed the prescribing practices of American physicians with regard to estrogen therapy and hormone therapy.[1] The study showed that most of them based their recommendations on an overall, quick assessment of symptoms and risks: hot flashes, vaginal changes, and cancer of the breast and endometrium. If the risk of symptoms was high and the risk of cancer low, then the patient was more likely to receive estrogen therapy or hormone therapy than if her symptoms were minimal and her risk of cancer was high. That's fine as far as it goes, but it doesn't go nearly far enough. Doctors rarely consider other risk factors, or what the patient's lifestyle is like and what she's willing or unwilling to do to change it.

Even when they do consider these other factors, doctors often hold us as patients to impossible standards. One popular book about menopause is very open-minded about hormone therapy: "Indeed the majority of menopausal women do perfectly well without hormone therapy provided they enter the menopause in optimal health and maintain good health throughout their postmenopausal years."[2] Unless you're the bionic woman, the chances are you won't live up to that requirement. While it's true you can do a lot to keep yourself in good shape, aging and the vicissitudes of life will cause some health problems for everyone.

I was recently interviewed in Toronto by a television reporter in her sixties, who told me her own story. Her gynecologist had said she needed to be on hormone therapy. She'd rather not, she said; she felt fine. The gynecologist was insistent. He asked her to take hormones for two months, keep a daily chart recording how she felt, and then come back to him. He was sure that she'd feel so much better that she'd never want to stop. Instead, she felt terrible. Her breasts hurt, she had headaches, she was retaining fluid, and she'd started bleeding again. She wanted to stop taking the pills. But he began to pressure her again. Since she was short and thin, he was sure she was at high risk of osteoporosis—she should have her bone density tested. She had the test and found out that her bone density was just fine. He finally gave in and stopped badgering her about hormones. (Ironically, his daily chart might be a good idea—if the doctor approaches it as a real learning tool instead of a propaganda device for hormone therapy. If you've already started taking hormones, keeping such a chart might help you decide whether you want to stop.)

Every time I get into an argument about hormone therapy with my colleagues (and, mind you, I get into a lot of these arguments), their parting shot is always: "Women feel so much better on hormones." How do they know? My guess is that they're talking about their own experience, or that of their mothers, wives, or girlfriends, rather than any actual study. Why is it that the vast majority of women who start on hormones stop within two years, if they feel so much better? Some women do indeed feel better, but some, like the reporter in Toronto, don't.

I think it does make the *doctors* feel better, however, when they can give you a pill to solve your problems—even your potential problems. That's the way we were trained in medical school. We don't want anyone to suffer, so if we can prevent suffering with a pill, we will. Further, even the most conscientious doctors are bound to develop biases based on the diseases they've treated. A cardiologist who sees people with heart disease all day long will lean more toward hormone therapy than a breast cancer surgeon such as myself. I fully admit that I'm scared of hormones because of my experiences treating women with breast cancer.

Too many doctors don't give patients credit for understanding this. We have a notion that if patients learn that their doctors aren't omniscient, they'll stop trusting us. In my own experience, however, it works the other way. If we make it clear that we're giving our best advice, based on what we know now, we're creating a framework for authentic trust, not blind obedience. Then, when our recommendations don't turn out to be magic cure-alls, we don't end up with alienated, disillusioned patients.

For example, in the 1950s, when doctors were offering DES to prevent miscarriages, wouldn't it have been wiser for them to have said, "We think this will work, but the studies aren't in yet. And we think that it's safe, but we don't know what it will do to the baby." Then the patient would have known she was taking a gamble; she could have decided whether or not it was worth it. If her daughter ended up getting cancer because of the drugs, it would still be devastating, of course, but at least she'd have understood her risk; she'd know that she hadn't been betrayed by her doctor.

This is terribly important in terms of hormone therapy. Doctors have been assuring women that it will make their lives much better but haven't been pointing out that we don't know the long-term dangers. Right now, more and more data are coming out that show very real dangers. And it's a moving target. Every day, new studies are published. The research continues, and we're constantly learning new things. So what the doctor may tell you today, in all good faith, may not be true tomorrow, or five years from now.

Your Values

There's one big advantage to the idea of the doctor as a god. You don't have to think for yourself. But even though figuring out what you really want to do and what you really think is best for you can be hard work, it's work worth doing.

Among the values you need to consider is what particular diseases frighten you the most. You may have seen your grandmother trapped for years in bed in a nursing home because of a broken hip. That picture scares you so much that you're willing to do whatever you can to avoid it. On the other hand, you may have lost three friends to breast cancer and be much more scared that this could happen to you. You shouldn't be completely driven by fear, but it certainly is a factor to consider.

Another factor to consider is the issue of animal rights mentioned in Chapter 15. Some women who want to take hormones may decide against taking Premarin because it comes from horse urine and decide instead to take a plant-based hormone such as Ogen or Estratab. For other women, this may not matter at all.

Another consideration is how you feel about discomfort. Do you find even mild hot flashes so embarrassing that you dread showing up at the office? Are you so uncomfortable with drugs that you'd rather put up with sleepless nights than take a pill you don't absolutely need?

Some women feel that they don't want to take medications their whole life and would rather rely on exercise and diet. Others feel that they're unlikely to ever start to exercise or eat a good diet and would rather take a pill. Still others prefer to do neither, and face whatever risks there are. There are many variations in between. My coauthor, for example, is probably at high risk for osteoporosis both because she periodically has to take corticosteroids and because she's had her ovaries removed. She hates exercise and loves fatty foods. She's on hormones now and is ambivalent about them—but she's equally ambivalent about exercise and giving up the foods she loves. As of this writing, she's leaning toward stopping the pills: she's increasing her exercise moderately and cutting back a little on her favorite foods—and possibly taking a chance on later health problems.

Personally, I decided some time ago not to take hormones unless I find myself having extremely debilitating symptoms—and then only temporarily. The research I've done for this book has strengthened my decision. My research has also made me stock up on herbs, reevaluate my diet, and pursue a regular exercise program.

It's important for you to realize that this isn't necessarily an either/or decision. You can take one route only, or combine more than one route, or do nothing at all.

In an attempt to help you sort out your own values, I've put together a pair of questionnaires to help you to think about treatments for symptoms and prevention in your own life. My questionnaires are not scientifically validated. Their purpose is to help you sort out your own thinking and feelings about these topics. Sometimes just doing this will make your decision clear to you. Remember, the questionnaires will not decide for you. Like medicine, like alternative treatments, like exercise and diet, a questionnaire is only a tool—to be used when it's helpful and discarded when it's not.

I've given you a way to score your responses and a way to interpret that score. I'm ambivalent about the scoring because while I want to help you clarify your thinking, I don't want you to get fixated on the score—one point more and you'll do *x*, one point less and you'll do *y*. Use your responses as a rough guide, not a mandate.

QUESTIONNAIRE PART ONE: SYMPTOMS

Perimenopausal Symptoms

Hot Flashes

- Once a day or less, and they're manageable. [1]
- More than once a day, and they occasionally interfere with my life. [2]
- Every fifteen minutes, and they're driving me crazy. [3]
- I could deal with them if I knew they were transient. [2]
- I have to do something to stop them. [3]

Night Sweats, Insomnia

- Occasionally I throw the covers off. [1]
- Most nights I wake up once drenched in sweat. [2]
- Every hour I wake up drenched in sweat and I have trouble falling asleep again. [3]
- I could manage if I didn't have to go to work. [2]
- I don't sleep as well as I used to. [1]
- I can't get back to sleep once I wake up. [2]
- I can't function unless I get a full night's sleep. [3]

Mood Swings

- I am more irritable than I used to be. [1]
- I have uncontrollable rages. [3]
- I have crying jags. [2]
- I just want to be alone. [2]
- I am fine one minute and then suddenly angry or depressed and then fine again. [3]
- I am driving my family crazy. [3]
- I haven't noticed any difference. [0]

Vaginal Dryness

- Intercourse is a little uncomfortable. [1]
- I can't even consider intercourse because of the pain involved. [3]
- I feel raw and sore all of the time. [3]
- I am uncomfortable during intercourse but fine otherwise. [2]
- I haven't noticed any change. [0]
- My partner and I are happy with nonpenetrating sex. [1]

Other Symptoms

- I have lost my interest in sex, and that devastates me. [3]
- I am not interested in sex, but I find that a relief. [1]
- I haven't noticed any change in my libido. [0]
- I urinate when I cough or laugh. [2]
- I have migraines that are getting worse. [1]
- I have gallstones. [1]
- I have had thrombophlebitis (clots in my veins). [1]
- My thinking seems fuzzy. [3]
- I can't concentrate. [3]

SCORING

0–12	*You have few symptoms.*
12–24	*You have moderate symptoms.*
24–36	*You have severe symptoms.*

Values

Lifestyle

- I hate pills and would rather tough it out. [1]
- I don't care what it takes, I just want it to get better, and fast. [3]
- I have always favored natural remedies. [2]
- I don't have time to exercise or change my diet—just give me a pill. [3]
- I have always thought that herbs were useless. [3]
- I go to the doctor because she or he is the expert, so I'll do what the doctor says. [3]
- It's important to me to be actively involved in all my own decisions about health care. [1]
- I am willing to experiment with other ways of seeking health care to get rid of my symptoms. [2]

- I am willing to experiment with different approaches to get rid of my symptoms. [2]
- I don't care what the studies say: women on hormones look younger to me. [3]
- I think menopause almost always includes unpleasant diseases that need treatment. [3]
- I can't let anyone at work know that I am old enough to be going through menopause. [3]
- I don't have time for menopause. [3]
- I couldn't take anything that came from horses' urine. [2]

SCORING

0–6   Low: You favor a lifestyle approach.
6–12   Moderate: You favor alternative approaches.
12–24   High: You favor hormone therapy.

DECISION 1: WHAT DO I DO FOR MY SYMPTOMS?

Part One of the questionnaire is designed to help you with decision 1: what to do about symptoms. When you've answered the questionnaire, you'll know that I'm not trying to trick you. If you have a high score in the section on perimenopausal symptoms, you have the most severe symptoms; and if you also score high in the section on values, you'll be most likely to want to take hormones. On the other hand, if you have low scores for symptoms and low scores for values, you'll be happy with lifestyle changes or with doing nothing. If you score in the middle for both symptoms and values, you're most likely to want to do something, but that something may not be drugs—you'll probably want to at least consider the alternative route.

If you're one of the above, your choices are easy. But, of course, most of us are mismatches. We have terrible symptoms but hate drugs, or our symptoms aren't that bad but are annoying enough that we like the idea of taking a pill to get rid of them. That's okay. If you have terrible symptoms but hate drugs, you'll be very motivated to try lifestyle changes and alternatives. If after several months they don't work, then you can reconsider drugs. And if you'd rather take a pill than put up with any degree of symptoms, you can do that and think about tapering off in a few years.

If you've had a premature menopause or a surgical menopause, either prematurely or not, you may want to take estrogen to tide you over what are usually more abrupt and severe symptoms. This doesn't mean you need to take them forever. (And taking hormones for long-term prevention is a separate decision.) Give yourself a year or two and then taper off gradually over another six months to a year. If you had a hysterectomy and ovary removal at a young age, you can consider taking hormones until around the natural age of menopause (about fifty) and then taper off. For those of you in this category, lifestyle changes are even more important to maintain your bones and heart in optimum condition. You might also want to start on some of the alternative regimens as you taper off your hormones.

If you've had breast cancer and are faced with sudden menopausal symptoms, you're in a different situation. One problem is that women who have been on hormone therapy are often diagnosed with breast cancer and then are told to stop their hormones cold turkey. This, needless to say, will cause your symptoms to come back with a vengeance. I suggest tapering off over at least four months if possible. The cancer has been there a long time, and I'm not sure that four months will make a difference. Discuss this with your doctor.

If you're a premenopausal woman with breast cancer who has undergone chemotherapy and has been abruptly put into menopause as a result, you can also have a lot of problems. There's a 30 percent chance that your periods will come back and the symptoms will go away. If they don't, the symptoms can be intense. (I think that young women who go through menopause abruptly, either surgically or because of drugs, tend to have more intense symptoms than older women, probably because the hormonal shifts are greater.) You might want to consider looking very seriously at lifestyle changes (most of which are also good for preventing a recurrence of breast cancer) and exploring some of the alternatives: paced respiration or acupuncture for hot flashes, nonestrogenic Chinese herbal formulas or vitamin E for vaginal dryness. If you're suffering so much that you feel that even if hormones will cause your cancer to come back, it's worth it, then I'd advise you to consider first the estrogenic herbs and then natural progesterone or estriol (or both) as less potent forms of hormones.

If breast cancer isn't a major concern and you decide to take hormones for symptoms, then you have to decide which ones and how to take them. This may be more complicated than it seems. In spite of their eagerness to have you take hormones, some gynecologists feel that you shouldn't take postmenopausal hormones until after you haven't had a period for a year, and so they suggest other, nonhormonal approaches. Others feel that it's better to start on hormone therapy as soon as you have symptoms. One approach is to take the birth control pill in this situation to "regulate your cycle." (Remember when they did that to many of us in puberty?) This approach makes sense because the dose of hormones in the current third-generation pill is still high enough to suppress your own hormonal flux, but there are no studies about it, and it does raise concerns about breast cancer. Another approach is to use progesterone or progestin to try to balance things out. (This is especially appropriate for heavy bleeding, as we discussed in Chapter 11.)

It's important to realize that any of these approaches could make you feel better or worse. Since you're taking these pills to control symptoms, for heaven's sake don't continue them if you're feeling worse.

If you decide to try hormone therapy and you still have your uterus, you'll probably want to take a progesterone or progestin along with an estrogen. This can be continuous or cyclical, patch or pill. Have a discussion with your health care provider, and together you can determine the best approach for you. If you feel that your doctor isn't listening to your concerns or doesn't have enough time for you, shop around. This is your body, and your choice. There is no right answer, and your doctor has to be willing to work with you on finding the best solution for you.

Once you've made your choice and found a clinician who'll work with you, it's a good idea to follow the example of the reporter in Toronto and keep a diary of how you feel on the hormone you're taking. This will clarify your symptoms and their timing and help you assess what you want to do. Sometimes you'll need to try several different approaches before you find what works for you. And by that time, your symptoms may even be gone— they're transient, remember. And remember that this decision may be good only for now: be ready to change when circumstances dictate.

DECISION 2: WHAT, IF ANYTHING, DO I WANT TO DO FOR PREVENTION?

Because taking hormones to prevent diseases is a different issue from taking them to treat symptoms, the decision-making process is different and your values may be different. You may decide that you need the help of hormones to get you through perimenopause but may not be sure that you want to take these drugs forever. Or you may have had very few symptoms but may be worried about your future health.

Comparative Risks and Benefits

There are many ways we could present the known data to help you get a clear sense of the risks and benefits for the general population of women— keeping in mind that your own situation may or may not fall into that category. One approach that can help you visualize the magnitude of the potential risk or benefit is to consider what's happening with a hypothetical group of 100 women at age fifty.[3]

The number of white women who would be expected to get hip fractures from osteoporosis over their lifetime is 15 out of 100 (see Figure 16.1). The number who would be spared a hip fracture if all 100 took estrogen from age fifty on is 2. The number who would be spared a hip fracture if they

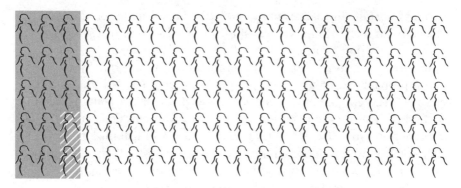

FIGURE 16.1   Hip fractures: White women.

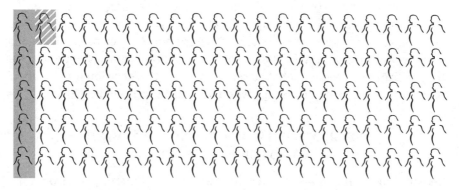

FIGURE 16.2   Hip fractures: African-American women.

Shaded area: Women with hip fractures
Striped shaded area: Decrease in hip fractures on estrogen

took estrogen and a progestin is about the same. Osteoporosis is one third as common in African-American women. Six out of 100 African-American women get hip fractures (see Figure 16.2). If all 100 of these women took estrogen postmenopausally, one woman would avoid a fracture—the total number of women with fractures would be 5 out of 100.[4]

As we've discussed, estrogen has its full effect on bones only while you are on it. So to get these benefits you'd need to take estrogen starting at age fifty and continue on well into your seventies to eighties—about twenty to thirty years. As we discussed in Chapter 5, it might make sense to start estrogen later, but unfortunately we really don't have enough data yet to know how effective that would be.

Of those same 100 white women, the number who would be expected to get heart disease is 46 (see Figure 16.3). If all of these 100 women took long-term estrogen to prevent heart disease and the most optimistic inter-

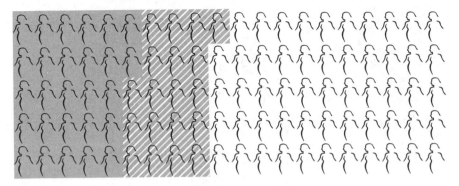

FIGURE 16.3   Heart disease.

Shaded area: Women with heart disease
Striped shaded area: Women whose heart disease would be prevented on estrogen

pretation of the studies were true, 19 would avoid heart disease while 27 would still get it. As I've said, adding progestin to the estrogen might lower the benefit. As with osteoporosis, it's the women who are currently on estrogen who seem to have the most benefit in avoiding heart disease. This too may mean taking estrogen for twenty to thirty years. As we discussed in Chapter 6, if you're not at risk, it seems likely that you could save yourself from heart disease and fractures in your old age by starting hormones at age sixty-five rather than at fifty. The studies are new, so there's no definitive proof, but this is worth seriously considering.

Ten out of these same 100 women would normally get breast cancer. (This isn't the familiar one-in-eight chance over your *lifetime* you're used to

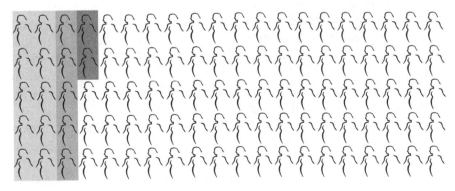

FIGURE 16.4   Breast cancer.

Light area: Women with breast cancer
Darker area: Additional cases of breast cancer in women on estrogen
Darkest area: Additional cases of breast cancer in women on estrogen plus progestin

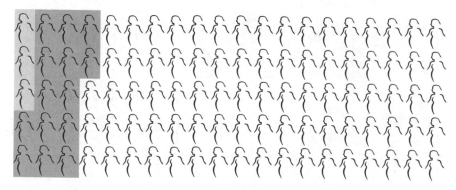

FIGURE 16.5   Endometrial cancer.

Light area: Women with endometrial cancer
Dark area: Women with endometrial cancer on estrogen

hearing, but the number of women out of 100 fifty-year-olds.) The number who would get breast cancer if all 100 of these women had taken estrogen for at least ten years is 13 to 15 (see Figure 16.4). (That is, 3 to 5 more women would get breast cancer.) If those same 100 women also took pro-gestin, 15 to 17 of them would get breast cancer (5 to 7 more than the orig-inal 10). Thirty percent of women with breast cancer will die of it.

Finally, the number of women who would naturally get endometrial can-cer is 3 out of 100 (see Figure 16.5). If these 100 women took estrogen alone for more than five years, 22 of them would get endometrial cancer—19 extra cases. If the 100 women took both estrogen and progestin, only 3 of them would get endometrial cancer.

From our earlier discussions, you'll realize that these estimates are based on limited data. If you have risk factors for heart disease or osteoporosis, your benefit from hormones may be slightly higher, although that hasn't been studied directly. For example, the lifetime probability that a white woman at risk for coronary heart disease will get the disease is 71 out of 100. If all 100 women took estrogen, that number would decrease to 60. In other words, 11 women would avoid heart disease, and the life expectancy of our fifty-year-old would go from 79.6 years to 81.1. For white women at high risk for osteoporosis, the risk of hip fracture is 36 out of 100. Taking estrogen or estrogen and progestin would reduce that to 31 out of 100, or prevent 5 hip fractures.[5]

But just as the benefit grows for women whom estrogen may help, the dan-ger grows for women it can harm. For a white woman at risk for breast can-cer, the chance of getting it is 19 out of 100. If all 100 women took estrogen alone, that risk would increase to 24, or add 5 cases. If progestin were to increase the risk, one estimate is that there would be 16 additional cases.

But this information by itself is incomplete. You also need to look at the ages at which the diseases affected by hormone therapy typically occur. The average age at which heart disease is diagnosed is seventy-four. The average age at which osteoporotic hip fracture is diagnosed is seventy-nine. The average age at which breast cancer is diagnosed is sixty-nine. Although heart disease is definitely more common than breast cancer, it's more a disease of old age. Below age seventy-five there are three times as many deaths from breast cancer as from heart disease. And if you exclude smokers— who make up the majority of early deaths from heart disease—there are six times as many deaths from breast cancer as heart disease. As you've probably noticed, you're more likely to know women your own age with breast cancer than with heart disease.

Finally, it's important to look at what the overall impact on your longevity will be. That is, if you balance out the potential protection from heart disease and the risk of breast cancer, and season it with a little benefit in terms of osteoporosis, you'll find that, on average, a fifty-year-old white woman with no risk factors and an intact uterus will add a little less than a year to her life expectancy by taking estrogen and progestin. If her uterus is gone, she'll add a year. If she's at risk for heart disease, she can add 1.5 years. If she actually has heart disease, this will go up to 2.1 years. If she's at risk for breast cancer, overall she'll add eight months. If she's at risk for hip fracture, she'll add one year. (Keep in mind that these are only averages. One individual might live much longer, while another may not gain any time.)

For some people, those added months can be precious. For others, they may only prolong the agony of whatever disease they're dying from. I've seen ninety-year-olds so hale and hearty that their granddaughters envy them. But I've also seen many others lying in hospitals or nursing homes, hooked up to IVs that only slightly lessen their pain, and long past any ability to relate to the world around them. Eight months of extra life might be a blessing or a torment—and there's no way to know in advance which it will be.

Comparisons with Other Options

I've presented these numbers as if your options for prevention were hormone therapy versus nothing. But you need to consider the "competition" when looking at hormone therapy. Hormones aren't the only tools available. What effect would lifestyle changes such as diet, exercise, weight loss, stress reduction, and quitting smoking have on these same diseases? I decided to make two tables directly comparing lifestyle and alternative therapies with hormones. I thought it would be a few hours' work—just find the medical literature where the comparisons existed, make sure that among them they had all the elements I wanted, and then make up my table. I was amazed at how hard it was to find anything. Although some data on lifestyle changes are available (nearly none are available on alternatives), it's almost impossible to convert these data to exactly the same type of numbers. The reports often compare apples and oranges. Therefore, I've made tables that compare generally the effects of a number of interventions on both intermediate risk factors (cholesterol and bone mineral density) and endpoints such as the number of fractures and of deaths from heart disease. These interventions include estrogen and hormone therapy, other drugs, exercise, diet, soy consumption. I've put soy in its own category, even though it's part of one's diet, because its qualities are so important and because most Americans don't usually eat soy foods (see Table 16.1). (A "+" means a positive change; a "++" indicates a very positive change. A "−" means a negative change. A "=" means no change.)

TABLE 16.1   Comparing the Various Approaches to
Preventing Cardiovascular Disease

Approach	Cholesterol	LDL	HDL	Triglycerides	Mortality
ERT[6,7]	−	−(5–15%)	+(10–16%)	++(20–24%)	−
HRT[8]	−(2–7%)	−(10–13%)	+(3–12%)	++(17–22%)	
Tamoxifen[9]	−(12%)	−(20%)	=		
Lovastatin[10]	−−(32%)	−(22%)	+(1%)		
Diet[11]	−(19%)	−(24.3%)	−(19.7%)	+(10.9%)	
Soy[12]	−(9.3%)	−(12.9%)	+(2.4%)	−(10.5%)	
Exercise[13]	−	−	+	−	

You might be surprised to find that eating the right diet does more for your lipids than estrogen therapy and that soy is as good as estrogen in its direct effect on coronary blood vessels. Although these percentages seem low, for every 1 mg/dl increase in HDL, the risk of fatal coronary vascular disease goes down 3 percent (for LDL it's a 2 percent lower risk for every 1 mg/dl decrease). The benefits of any of these approaches to cardiovascular disease appear to be strongest in women who already have heart disease or who have very high risk factors. How much LDL cholesterol decreases with estrogen therapy is directly related to how high it was to start with.

The major effect of estrogen is that it increases HDL and dilates coronary blood vessels while it also lowers LDL and increases triglycerides. Soy protein has the same effect on lowering LDL, not as much an effect on HDL, but an equal effect on blood vessels; and it lowers triglycerides to boot. The only other way to increase HDL is exercise. The best way to decrease your cho-lesterol is to take a cholesterol-lowering drug, although diet comes close.

TABLE 16.2   Comparing the Various Approaches to Preventing Osteoporosis

	BMD spine	BMD hip	BMD wrist	Fracture hip
ERT and HRT[14,15]	+(3–8%)	+(1.4–11%)	+(4–18%)	–(50%)
Bisphosphonates[16]	+(8.8%)	+(5.9%)		–(48%)
Exercise[17,18]	+(3–6.1%)	+(3.1%)		
Soy[19]	=		+	
Tamoxifen[20]	+(1.17%)	+(1.81%)		

For osteoporosis, again it's rather startling to see how little bone density goes up with estrogen therapy—or with any other intervention, for that matter. It's important to remember, however, that for every 1 percent decrease in the level of bone mineral density (BMD), the risk of fracture increases 2.6 times. And the bone is actually decreasing in bone mineral density, about 3 to 5 percent a year. Bisphosphonates and estrogen do about the same job as exercise when it comes to increasing bone density. Tamoxifen really doesn't do a very good job, although it does prevent fur-ther bone loss. Are these effects additive? We really don't know. There are some data suggesting that taking estrogen, getting enough calcium, and exercising are better than any one approach alone, but so far there are no definitive studies to prove it.

In addition, I've made a summary of the effects of estrogen therapy on your chance of dying at an early age and compared them with the effects of physical fitness (see Table 16.3). Note that physical fitness is as good as estrogen in helping you live longer. Steven Blair of the Cooper Institute, who determined the estimates for physical fitness, defines the amount of physical fitness needed as a brisk thirty-to-sixty-minute walk each day.[21]

TABLE 16.3   Effect on Various Approaches on Overall Mortality

	Number of people studied	Duration of study	Mortality
ERT[22]	490	>10 years	decreased 46%
Physical Fitness[23]	3120	8 years	decreased 50%

You can change your mortality statistics by changing your lifestyle. If you're a smoker and you quit, you can add 11.5 percent to your life expectancy. Lower your cholesterol, and you'll move into a group whose mortality rate is 40.5 percent lower. Lower your blood pressure, and you'll move into a group whose mortality rate is 55.1 percent lower. If you can avoid non-insulin-dependent diabetes (by weight control), you'll be in a group whose mortality rate is 70 percent lower.[24]

As you look at the tables, you begin to realize how right the physical fitness gurus have been all along. Lifestyle changes can be as effective as drugs, and sometimes even more effective. Both soy and exercise are beneficial for fighting osteoporosis, heart disease, and breast cancer. They're a little closer to the "designer drugs" the pharmaceutical companies are looking for, but far less expensive.

Making Decision 2

Looking at numbers is all well and good, but you're an individual, not a number. We often act as though statistics were objective information—a sacred truth. But how statistics are presented will affect your opinion of them. It's the old story: Is the glass half full or half empty? It's important that you recognize the biases of the medical profession in the way data are presented to you. Making this decision depends a lot on your own values.

Part Two of our questionnaire will help you sort out your own feelings, risk factors, values, and habits. As with Part One, there's a general score. But don't take it too seriously; just because your score is high doesn't mean that you have to take hormones, and a low score doesn't imply that you can't. Use this questionnaire simply as another tool to help you sort out where you are right now.

QUESTIONNAIRE PART TWO: PREVENTION

Risk Factors for Future Disease

Osteoporosis

- I have had a fracture after age fifty. [3]
- My mother has severe osteoporosis. [3]
- I have lost more than an inch in height. [3]
- I spent most of my life dieting. [2]
- I had anorexia nervosa when I was younger. [2]
- I have been an athlete or ballet dancer and lost my period for a while. [2]
- I have taken cortisone or corticosteroids (such as prednisone) for more than five years. [2]

- I have taken thyroid replacement for most of my life. [2]
- I had a hysterectomy and my ovaries out before age forty. [2]
- I had chemotherapy and stopped menstruating before age forty. [2]
- I smoke cigarettes. [2]
- I take medication for seizures. [2]
- I was an athlete as a child and a teenager. [1]
- I exercise at least three times a week. [1]
- I have big bones. [1]
- I have always eaten a high-calcium diet. [1]
- I am overweight. [1]
- I am African American. [1]
- I am Asian. [1]
- I am Caucasian. [3]

Heart Disease

- My mother had a heart attack before age sixty-five. [3]
- My father had a heart attack before age fifty-five. [3]
- I have had a heart attack. [3]
- I have high blood pressure. [2]
- I have a cholesterol count between 230 and 300. [2]
- I have a cholesterol count over 300. [3]
- I have chest pain (angina). [3]
- I am more than twenty pounds overweight. [2]
- I am a couch potato. [2]
- I have a high-stress job, and it's driving me crazy. [2]
- I have diabetes. [2]
- I smoke cigarettes. [2]
- I eat mostly junk food and am unlikely to stop. [2]
- I went through menopause naturally before age forty. [2]
- I had a surgical menopause before age forty. [2]
- I had menopause caused by chemotherapy before age forty. [2]
- I exercise at least three times a week. [1]
- My cholesterol is less than 200. [1]
- I eat a low-fat diet. [1]
- I drink a cocktail or glass of wine a night. [1]

Breast Cancer

- I have had breast cancer or precancer. [1]
- My mother, sister, or daughter has had breast cancer. [1]

- There is breast cancer on my father's side of the family. [1]
- There is colon cancer in my family. [2]
- There is uterine or ovarian cancer in my family. [2]
- I took DES during a pregnancy. [2]
- My first full-term pregnancy was before age thirty. [3]
- My first full-term pregnancy was after thirty-five. [2]
- I have never had children. [2]
- I took birth control pills for more than ten years. [2]
- I am Caucasian. [2]
- I had radiation treatment for acne, or to shrink my thymus gland, or for Hodgkin's disease. [2]
- I received a lot of X rays as a teenager for TB, scoliosis, or chest problems. [2]
- I drink more than three alcoholic drinks a week. [1]
- I rarely drink alcohol. [2]
- I had my first period before age thirteen. [2]
- I had my menopause after age fifty. [2]
- I had my menopause before age forty-five and did not take hormones. [3]
- I exercised more than three times a week when I was premenopausal. [3]
- I was an athlete as a teenager and a young adult. [3]
- I rarely exercised as a child or a young adult. [1]
- I have been exercising for the past five years or more. [2]

Endometrial cancer

- My mother had endometrial cancer. [1]
- I am overweight. [2]
- I have more than three alcoholic drinks a week. [2]
- I almost never drink alcohol. [3]

Other

- I have fibroids. [1]
- I have endometriosis. [1]
- I have sore breasts. [1]
- I have lumpy breasts. [1]
- I have gallbladder problems. [1]
- I have or had phlebitis. [1]
- I have high triglycerides. [1]
- I have lupus. [1]
- I have asthma. [1]
- I have liver disease. [1]

SCORING:

0–30	*You are at risk of diseases related to hormones.*
30–60	*You are at moderate risk for diseases related to hormones and diseases helped by hormones.*
60–100	*You are at risk of diseases which could be helped by hormones.*

<hr>

Values

Fears

- I am particularly afraid of breast cancer. [1]
- I am particularly afraid of endometrial cancer. [1]
- I am particularly afraid of heart disease. [3]
- I am particularly afraid of osteoporosis. [3]
- I am particularly afraid of taking drugs. [1]
- I do not believe in using drugs to deal with a natural life process. [1]
- I believe in taking medications to relieve discomfort, regardless of whether it comes from a disease or from a natural life process. [3]
- I don't want to take a drug made from horse urine. [2]

Habits

- I love junk food. [3]
- I buy vegetables, but they rot in my refrigerator. [3]
- I have never in my life been able to stick to a diet. [3]
- I have never been able to stick to my New Year's resolutions. [3]
- I hate taking vitamins or supplements. [3]
- I think that herbs are worthless. [3]
- I'm willing to try "health foods" if I can find creative, tasty ways to cook them. [1]
- Once I set my mind to do something, I always succeed. [1]
- My family sabotages me every time I try to change. [3]
- I will never quit smoking. [3]
- I drink a glass or more of wine a night and am not about to change now. [3]
- I rarely drink alcohol. [1]
- I have never been able to keep up an exercise program for more than two weeks. [3]
- My stationary bike is a clothes hanger. [3]
- I have never been able to find a sport I like doing. [3]
- I have no time for lifestyle changes. [3]

- I have lost the same twenty pounds fifty times. [3]
- My weight is stable. [1]
- I have never been on a diet. [1]
- I have never been able to take a pill (even for birth control) every day—I always forget. [1]
- I am extremely reliable and will take any medication exactly as directed. [3]
- I always trust my doctor and think he or she knows best. [3]
- My mother went through menopause without drugs and is fine. [1]

Side effects

- I believe hormones will make me feel young. [3]
- I don't mind if I continue bleeding on hormones; it's better than a hip fracture. [3]
- I can't wait to stop bleeding and don't want to take anything that will make me start again. [1]
- I can put up with some bleeding as long as I know it will stop. [3]
- I don't want to be running to the doctor for an endometrial biopsy every time I have bleeding. [1]
- I don't mind taking a pill, but a patch is weird. [3]
- I can't remember to take a pill and would rather use a patch. [3]
- I'd rather do the least I can to get me over the hump. [1]

SCORING

0–15	*You favor lifestyle approaches.*
15–30	*You could consider alternatives.*
30–80	*You may prefer hormones.*

A high score for any one disease means you're at higher risk. Don't take this too seriously either, because these risk factors don't necessarily add up. As I said in an earlier chapter, some of them are like concurrent life sentences. But generally, the more risk factors you have, the greater your chance of getting the disease in question. In the section on values and habits, the higher your score, the more likely you are to lean toward hormones for prevention. The lower your score, the more likely you are to want to explore lifestyle changes and alternatives.

As with symptoms, those of you whose scores match perfectly—high risk of heart disease and osteoporosis and unlikely to exercise—are easy. It's those of you who are at equal risk for both osteoporosis and breast cancer who may have a problem. That's when you need to look at your values. Which scares you more? If it's breast cancer, try the lifestyle and alternative route. If it's osteoporosis, and changing your lifestyle is unrealistic, consider hormones. (Remember, there are no guarantees with any of this. You can take hormones and still get a hip fracture. You can stay away from them and still get breast cancer. You can eat well and exercise and still get all of these diseases, or you can smoke, drink, and eat cheesecake every day and live to ninety. We're looking at odds, not certainties.)

If You Decide to Take Preventive Hormones

A critical question—if you decide to take hormones as a preventive—is: When is it best to start estrogen therapy or hormone therapy? Although the current trend is to put all women on hormones at menopause and have them keep taking hormones for life, this isn't the only choice. Since the greatest effect on decreasing mortality from heart disease seems to be in those women currently on hormones, it may make sense to wait until you're in your sixties or seventies. If it turns out that hormones work because they dilate blood vessels, then you'd want to be on hormones when a heart attack happens. On the other hand, there are data suggesting that you need to start estrogen right at menopause to prevent the bone loss of osteoporosis. What is best? At the moment, we have no answers to these questions.

If you decide to take hormones for prevention, you can take conjugated equine estrogen (Premarin), estradiol (Estrace) or estrone (Ogen), a patch or a pill. If you have a uterus, you'll need to take progesterone or a progestin, in addition to estrogen.

Prevention of Heart Disease

Lifestyle: *exercise; low-fat, low-cholesterol diet; stress reduction; high-soy diet*
Supplements: *garlic, bioflavinoids*
Drugs: *Lovostatin, blood-pressure-lowering drugs, aspirin, estrogen therapy (?), hormone therapy (?)*

For those of you taking hormones chiefly to prevent heart disease or to lower your cholesterol, it would appear that you're better off with micronized progesterone if you can get it, as it will have the least harmful effect on your cholesterol. Premarin may help your lipid levels slightly more than other formulations of estrogen, because it passes through the liver.

Prevention of Osteoporosis

Lifestyle: *exercise, low-protein diet, high-soy diet*
Supplements: *vitamin D, calcium, magnesium, oatstraw, bioflavinoids*
Drugs: *natural progesterone, estrogen therapy, hormone therapy, Fosamax, calcitonin, fluoride*

For those with a family history of osteoporosis, there's good news. In a study of women whose mothers had osteoporosis, the women who exercised and took calcium had higher bone densities.[25] You *can* overcome your genes. If you're going to take hormones for osteoporosis, the good news is that you don't have to worry about the offsetting effects of progesterone or progestins. It doesn't seem to have much deleterious effect. But as we said, you do have to take the estrogen right away and for the rest of your life to get the full effect.

Prevention of Breast Cancer

Lifestyle: *exercise, low-fat and high-soy diet with abundant fruits and vegetables, stress reduction*
Supplements: *vitamins E, A, and C*
Drugs: *tamoxifen (?)*

For women who have had breast cancer, the issue is more complex. Although there's a growing trend toward putting women who have had breast cancer on hormone therapy, it scares me a lot. There really are no data confirming its safety. In addition, even if your first cancer is cured (or estrogen-receptor-negative), the possibility of a second tumor in the other breast caused by the hormones overshadows any possible protection they might offer against osteoporosis or heart disease. If you're also at very high risk for osteoporosis, you might consider Fosamax, but, as we mentioned in Chapter 14, no long-term studies have been done on it. For now I'd stick to lifestyle changes. If you really feel you must take hormones regardless of the risk, I'd lean toward micronized progesterone for your bones rather than estrogen.

If You're Undecided

If you are still undecided about preventive hormones, you may want to consider a bone-density test. If knowing that your bone density is low—or, for that matter, high—will help you decide, the test might be worth doing. Those of you who have taken steroids or thyroid medication (Synthroid) or dilantin, and thus who are at potentially greater risk of osteoporosis, might find the information helpful in making your decision. Of course, you need to consider all the problems with the test mentioned in Chapter 5. Also, it's not worth taking the test if you've already decided that you will or won't take hormones.

Just as this book was going to press, there was news from the no-free-lunch department. The study of osteoporotic fractures demonstrated a direct relationship between bone density and breast cancer risk. Women who have a low bone density have a lower risk for breast cancer; women with a high bone density have 2.0 to 2.5 times the risk for developing breast cancer. In other words, if your own estrogen levels are low, you are more at risk for osteoporosis but less at risk for breast cancer.[26]

You should also know your cholesterol and blood pressure. Get a mammogram, too. If you're at very high risk for breast cancer, you can consider being tested for the breast cancer gene. (I would do this only in a research setting, however, because right now women who turn out to have the gene could face discrimination by insurance companies, in custody battles, and in employment.) All of these pieces of data may help you decide.

Finally, if you're still not sure, I would suggest that you volunteer for the Women's Health Initiative (see Appendix 6). This study will randomly decide, by computer, whether you will or won't take hormones. The information from this study might ensure that our daughters won't be faced with this dilemma. I can't recommend it too highly. By the year 2008, we'll have some answers because of the women who volunteer.

STOPPING HORMONES

Tapering Off

What if you've been on hormones for several years and you decide to get off? Be sure to taper off slowly, over six to twelve months, rather than quitting abruptly (see Chapter 15). Remember that if you go off and do nothing additional, your cholesterol will probably go up and your bone density will start to go down. A friend of mine told me that she stopped taking Premarin and was surprised to find that her cholesterol was the same as it had been before she had started. So if you're worried about cholesterol, when you stop hormones you should probably change your diet, or exercise, and if your cholesterol is dangerously high, consider specific cholesterol-lowering drugs.

What Do I Tell My Doctor?

A friend of mine, a professor of public health, knowing that I was writing this book, said to me, "Whatever else you talk about, be sure you tell your readers how to tell your doctor or provider if you decide to stop taking hormones." She admitted that, for all of her professional success, she was afraid to tell her gynecologist that she wanted to go off hormones after ten years.

Her fear reflects a sad reality, both about doctors' attitudes toward patients and about the pressure on doctors to prescribe hormones. When a woman chooses not to follow her doctors' advice, the medical profession calls it a "compliance problem." Doctors ask themselves: Why can't we get these women to do what we want? It's an appalling attitude, but most women, whether they want to be or not, are intimidated by it. And most women would much rather have a partnership with their doctor. The best way to do this is to come well prepared.

First, call ahead and let your provider know that you want to have a discussion about menopause and hormones. Trying to have this discussion in the middle of a routine yearly visit can be frustrating to both provider and patient. With advance warning, your provider can make sure there's enough time scheduled. Before you go, marshal all of your questions and arguments. Write down your points. Bring a friend with you to the appointment for moral support if you need to. It's often helpful to bring a tape recorder as well. When you're nervous, it can be hard to hear what the doctor is actually saying. And often providers will be more circumspect about what they say when they're being recorded. If your provider has an opinion, ask why, and what data she or he is basing it on. It's important to feel that your provider is a partner you can work with to find the right approach to fit your life and values. If it doesn't feel right, it probably isn't—and you should see someone else. Don't forget other options—an herbalist, a traditional Chinese doctor, a homeopath. Remember: This isn't a disease you're treating; it is a normal part of life.

A FINAL THOUGHT: YOU ARE THE EXPERT

For some of you, taking hormones—short-term or long-term, for symptoms or for prevention—will be the right decision. For others, it won't. There are lots of options open to you, and there will always be different options you can consider, at any time. I've tried in this book to give you as much information as possible, so that you'll have some tools to help you make your decision. But the most important tool is one I can't give you—self-knowledge. In the final analysis, it isn't me, or your doctor, or anyone else, who knows what's best for you. For that knowledge, you and you alone are the expert.

How to Find a Practitioner

Menopause in General

American Board of Obstetrics and Gynecology
4225 Roosevelt Way NE, Suite 305
Seattle, WA 98105
206-547-4884
This board certifies doctors. You can call to find out if someone is certified.

American College of Obstetrics and Gynecology (ACOG)
409 12 Street SW
Washington, DC 20024
202-638-5577
ACOG can give you a list of board-certified physicians. It also publishes pamphlets and reports. Generally its bias is toward HRT.

Alternative Approaches

Naturopathy and Herbs

American Association of Naturopathic Physicians
2366 Eastlake Avenue, Suite 322
Seattle, WA 98102
206-323-7610
Can provide referrals to naturopaths; also publishes a quarterly newsletter.

National College of Naturopathic Medicine
11231 Southeast Market Street
Portland, OR 97216
503-255-4860
This college offers a degree in naturopathic medicine and provides referrals.

North Eastern Herbal Association
PO Box 146
Marshfield, VT 05658
802-456-1402
An association of practicing herbalists, growers of herbs, and students. It has a newsletter and a directory of herbalists in the Northeast.

Traditional Chinese

New England School of Acupuncture
30 Common Street
Watertown, MA 02172
617-926-1788
This school offers a master's-level training in acupuncture and Chinese medicine. It also offers a three-year herbal medicine program.

American College of Traditional Chinese Medicine
455 Arkansas Street
San Francisco, CA 94107
415-282-7600
This college offers a master of science degree in traditional Chinese medicine. Contact for information and referrals to local professional associations and practitioners.

National Council of Acupuncture Schools and Colleges
PO Box 954
Columbia, MD 21044
301-997-4888
Oversees and regulates the quality of training and education.

National Commission for the Certification of Acupuncturists
1424 16 Street NW, Suite 105
Washington, DC 20036
202-232-1404
Ensures minimal entry-level professional competence.

American Association of Acupuncture and Oriental Medicine
433 Front Street
Catasaugua, PA 18032-2506
610-433-2448

National Acupuncture and Oriental Medicine Alliance
638 Prospect Avenue
Hartford, CT 06105-4298
203-586-7509

In states where acupuncture is licensed and state regulated, you can find the names of local practitioners in the yellow pages or by contacting the Department of Health, Board of Medical Examiners, or Department of Licensing. In states without licensing, seek out practitioners who are nationally board certified and have Dipl. Ac. (for Diplomate of Acupuncture) after their names.

No license is required to practice Chinese herbal medicine. Ask practitioners what their training was and where they went to school. Ask for references from previous patients. Make sure that you can communicate with them. A professional practitioner of Chinese medicine should be able and willing to give a written traditional Chinese diagnosis of the case. Practitioners also should belong to local and national Chinese medicine-acupuncture professional associations.

Homeopathy

International Foundation for Homeopathy
2366 Eastlake Avenue East, Suite 301
Seattle, WA 98102
206-324-8230
This group sponsors courses and has a directory of their students.

National Center for Homeopathy
801 North Fairfax Street, Suite 306
Alexandria, VA 22314
703-548-7790
Maintains a directory of homeopaths with a wide range of training and education.

Homeopathic Academy of Naturopathic Physicians
14653 South Graves Road
Mulino, OR 97042
503-829-7326
This is a rigorous homeopathic training program and has a listing of its alumni.

Other: Biofeedback

Association for Applied Psychophysiology and Biofeedback
10200 West 44 Avenue, Suite 304
Wheat Ridge, CO 80033
303-422-8436
Its affiliate trains and certifies biofeedback practitioners.

Other: Massage

American Massage Therapy Association
820 Davis Street, Suite 100
Evanston, IL 60201
847-864-0123
847-864-1178
Members must pass a certification exam or graduate from a massage therapy program approved or accredited by an AMTA commission on massage training.

Lifestyle Changes

Support

American Psychological Association
750 First Street NE
Washington, DC 20002-4242
202-336-5500
Publishes a short book called Women and Depression: Risk Factors and Treatment. *Also issues a pamphlet, "Choosing a Psychotherapist."*

American Association for Marital and Family Therapists
1100 17 Street NW, 10th Floor
Washington, DC 20036
800-374-2638
Will provide you with a list of certified marital or family therapists in your area.

National Mental Health Association
Information Center
1021 Prince Street
Alexandria, VA 22314-2971
703-684-7722 or 800-969-6642
Will give referrals, support, and information

American Association of Sex Educators, Counselors and Therapists
435 N Michigan Avenue, Suite 1717
Chicago, IL 60611
312-644-0828
Has a referral service that will help you find a reputable sex therapist.

Meditation and Hypnosis

Maharishi International University
1000 North Fourth Street
Fairfield, IA 52556
515-472-5031
Can provide information about local teachers of Transcendental Meditation.

Guided Imagery

Academy of Guided Imagery
PO Box 2070
Mill Valley, CA 94942
800-726-2070
Has a 150-hour training program for health care professionals and publishes a directory of trained imagery practitioners.

Hypnosis

National Guild of Hypnotists
PO Box 308
Merrimack, NH 03054
603-429-9438
Offers training and certification programs.

American Institute of Hypnotherapy
16842 Von Karman Avenue, Suite 475
Irvine, CA 92714
800-872-9996
Offers a doctoral program in hypnotherapy.

American Society of Clinical Hypnosis
2200 East Devon Avenue, Suite 291
Des Plaines, IL 60018
708-297-3317
Will provide a list of medical doctors and dentists who also do hypnosis.

How to Find Remedies: Drugs, Mail Order

Pharmacies (Mail-order pharmacies that can compound prescriptions for "natural" hormones)

Bajamar Women's Healthcare Pharmacy
800-255-8025

Belmar Pharmacy
800-525-9473

Delk Pharmacy
1602 Hatcher Lane
Columbia, TN 38401
615-388-3952

Health Watchers Systems
13402 N Scottsdale Road, Suite B 150
Scottsdale, AZ 85254
800-321-6917

Professional and Technical Services, Inc.
621 SW Alder, Suite 900
Portland, OR 97205-3627
503-226-1010; fax 503-226-6455
Toll-free 800-888-6814 (regular
    customers) and 800-866-9085
    (professionals)

Women's Health America Group
(formerly Madison Pharmacy
    Associates)
Pharmacy: 800-222-4767

Women's International Pharmacy
5708 Monona Drive
Madison, WI 53716-3152
608-221-7800; toll-free 800-279-5708

Mail-Order Herbs

Amrita Herbals
Route 1, Box 737
Floyd, VA 24380

Avena Botanicals
PO Box 365
West Rockport, ME 04865

Blessed Herbs
Route 5, Box 1042
Ava, MO 65608

Ryan Drum
Waldron Island, WA 98297

Green Terrestrial
Route 9W, Box 41
Milton, NY 12547

Herb Pharmacy
Box 116
Williams, OR 97544

Wish Garden Herbs
PO Box 1304
Boulder, CO 80306

Nutrition (Soy Products)

Betsy's Tempeh
S&P Farm
14780 Beardslee Road
Perry, MI 48872
517-675-5213
Offers free recipe brochure.

Reduced Fat Tofu
White Wave Soy Foods
Boulder, CO 80301
To locate nearest vendor in your area, call 800-488-9283.

Vitasoy
800-VITASOY
Offers recipes and information for soymilk products.

APPENDIX 3

Books, Videos, Pamphlets, and the Internet

GENERAL BOOKS ABOUT MENOPAUSE

Menopause in General

Janine O'Leary Cobb. *Understanding Menopause: Answers and Advice for Women in the Prime of Life*. New York: Penguin, 1993. *A very good and friendly book by the editor of the newsletter "A Friend Indeed."*

Paula Brown Doress, Diana Laskin Siegal (and the Midlife and Older Women Book Project). *Ourselves Growing Older*. New York: Simon and Schuster, 1987. *Very good overview of the second half of life.*

Paula Dranov. *Estrogen: Is It Right for You? A thorough factual guide to help you decide.* New York: Simon and Schuster, 1993. *A short, balanced book on the pros and cons of hormone therapy.*

Carol Landau, Ph.D., Michele G. Cyr, M.D., and Anne W. Moulton, M.D. *The Complete Book of Menopause*. New York: Berkley, 1992. *Written by two gynecologists and a psychologist, this book is a good overall guide to menopause in all of its aspects. It sticks to traditional medicine and lifestyle issues and doesn't discuss alternative approaches.*

Susan Perry and Katherine A. O'Hanlan, M.D. *Natural Menopause: The Complete Guide to a Woman's Most Misunderstood Passage*. Reading, Mass.: Addison-Wesley, 1992. *A good guide to all of the aspects of menopause from a friendly balanced approach (does not include alternatives).*

Ann Voda, Margaret Dinnerstein, and S. R. O'Donnell. *Changing Perspective on Menopause*. Austin: University of Texas Press, 1982. *Menopause from an anthropological, literary, psychological, and physiological perspective.*

Menopause with a slant toward drugs

Lila Nachtigall, M.D., and Joan Rattner Heilman. *Estrogen: A Complete Guide to Reversing the Effects of Menopause Using Hormone Replacement Therapy.* New York: HarperCollins, 1991. *Listed in the interest of fair play; this is a book which is very pro hormone therapy.*

Morris Notelovitz, M.D., and Diana Tonnessen. *Menopause & Midlife Health.* New York: St. Martin's, 1993. *A good overall look at midlife, with hints for lifestyle change.*

Menopause with a slant toward natural approaches

Ellen Brown and Lynne Walker. *Breezing Through the Change.* Berkeley, Calif.: Frog, 1994. *An alternative book about menopause.*

Sadja Greenwood, M.D. *Menopause, Naturally: Preparing for the Second Half of Life.* Volcano, Calif.: Volcano, 1996. *A wonderful overview of all the aspects of menopause. To order call 800-879-9636.*

Dee Ito. *Without Estrogen: Natural Remedies for Menopause and Beyond.* New York: Random House, 1994. *A wonderful tour of the alternative approaches to menopause complete with examples of how women incorporate them into their lives.*

Susan M. Lark, M.D. *The Estrogen Decision.* Los Altos, Calif.: Westchester, 1994. *Covers hormone therapy and its alternatives. Especially good chapters on yoga and acupressure for menopause. Can be ordered at 415-941-5784.*

Christiane Northrup, M.D. *Women's Bodies, Women's Wisdom: Creating Physical and Emotional Health and Healing.* New York: Bantam Books, 1994. *Women's health with a strong holistic philosophy.*

Linda Ojeda, Ph.D. *Menopause Without Medicine.* Alameda, Calif.: Hunter House, 1995. *A good overall book on alternatives to hormones.*

Textbooks

Karen J. Carlson, M.D., Stephanie A. Eisenstat, M.D., Fredric Frigoletto, Jr., M.D., and Isaac Schiff, M.D. *Primary Care of Women.* Mosby Mo., 1995. *A multiauthored textbook about primary care of women's health.*

Phyllis L. Carr, M.D., Karen M. Freund, M.D., and Sujata Somani, M.D. *The Medical Care of Women.* Philadelphia, Pa.: Saunders, 1995. *A multiauthor textbook from Harvard on all of women's health issues.*

Bernard Eskin, M.D. *The Menopause: Comprehensive Management.* New York: McGraw-Hill, 1994. *One of the first textbooks on menopause and therefore one of the most traditional.*

Rogerio A. Lobo, M.D. *Treatment of the Postmenopausal Woman: Basic and Clinical Aspects.* New York: Raven, 1994. *A multiauthor textbook for physicians. One of the more balanced ones as regards hormone therapy.*

Menopause culture and stories

Germaine Greer. *The Change: Women, Aging and the Menopause.* New York: Ballantine, 1993. *A classic.*

Gail Sheehy. *The Silent Passage: Menopause*. New York: Random House, 1992. *The book that started women talking.*

Dena Taylor and Amber Coverdale Sumrall, eds. *Women of the 14th Moon: Writings on Menopause*. Capitola, Calif.: Crossing, 1991. *An anthology of women's experiences.*

Robert A. Wilson. *Feminine Forever*. New York: Evans, 1966. *This is the original and worth a read if you can find it tucked away in the library. He is truly an evangelist for estrogen.*

Menopause Cross-Culturally

Y. Beyene. *From Menarche to Menopause: Reproductive Lives of Peasant Women in Two Cultures*. State University of New York Press, 1989. *An anthropological comparison of menopause among the Mayans in southern Mexico and rural Greek islanders.*

Margaret Lock. *Encounters with Aging: Mythologies of Menopause in Japan and North America*. University of California Press, 1993. *Results of twenty years of study of menopause in Japan and North America.*

The Business of Menopause

Sandra Coney. *The Menopause Industry: How the Medical Establishment Exploits Women*. Alameda, Calif.: Hunter House, 1994. *One of the first books to look at the business side of menopause. The pictures of the old ads for hormones alone are worth the price of the book. Can be ordered by calling 800-266-5592.*

Barbara Seaman and Gideon Seaman. *Women and the Crisis in Sex Hormones*. New York: Rawson, 1977. *One of the first books to look at the widespread use of sex hormones in normal women.*

Symptoms and Their Treatment

Ann Voda. "Menopause, Me and You" (pamphlet). Available by writing to Dr. Ann Voda, College of Nursing, 25 South Medical Drive, Salt Lake City, UT 84112 ($5.95) *Excellent information about hot flashes from one of the main researchers on the subject.*

Heart Disease

Dean Ornish, M.D. *Dr. Dean Ornish's Program for Reversing Heart Disease*. New York: Random House, 1990. *The lifestyle approach to preventing and reversing heart disease. It works.*

Women and Heart Disease: The Silent Epidemic. Videotape and brochure from American Heart Association (Pamphlet and Video). Order from 7320 Greenville Avenue, Dallas TX 75231.

Breast Cancer

Susan Love, M.D. *Dr. Susan Love's Breast Book*. Reading, Mass.: Addison-Wesley, 1995. *Everything you want or need to know about benign and malignant breast disease. Women tell me it's the bible.*

Susun S. Weed. *Breast Cancer? Breast Health: The Wise Woman Way*. Woodstock, N.Y.: Ash Tree, 1996. *The herbal approach to breast problems.*

Incontinence

K. Burgio. *Staying Dry: A Practical Guide to Bladder Control*. Baltimore and London: Johns Hopkins University Press, 1989. *A best-selling book explaining incontinence; gives an action plan that helps 90 percent of the people who try it.*

R. Chalker. *Overcoming Bladder Disorders*. New York: Harper and Row, 1990. *An excellent book by a woman urologist.*

Lifestyle Changes

Nutrition

Mark Messina. *The Simple Soybean and Your Health*. Wayne, N.J.: Avery, 1994. *An authoritative book by one of the world's experts.*

Earl Mindell. *Earl Mindell's Soy Miracle*. New York: Simon and Schuster, 1995. *Good source of information and recipes.*

Dean Ornish. *Everyday Cooking*. New York: HarperCollins, 1996.

Harriet Roth. *Deliciously Simple*. New York: Penguin, 1986.

Nina Shandler. *Estrogen: The Natural Way—Over 250 Easy and Delicious Recipes for Menopause*. New York: Villard, 1997.

Marcia S. Williams. *No Apologies Cookbook*. Freedom, Calif.: Crossing, 1986.

Marcia S. Williams. *More Healthy Cooking*. Freedom, Calif.: Crossing, 1991.

Exercise

B. Anderson, E. Burke, and B. Pearl. *Getting in Shape*. Bolinas, Calif.: Shelter, 1994. *Programs for stretching, muscle-building, and aerobic exercises; PO Box 279, Bolinas, CA 94924.*

Collage Video. *The Complete Guide to Exercise Videos*. Catalogue of over 300 exercise workout tapes. Order from 5390 Main St. NE, Dept. 1, Minneapolis, MN 55421 (800-433-6769).

Bob Greene and Oprah Winfrey. *Make the Connection*. New York: Hyperion, 1996.

Casey Meyers. *Walking: A Complete Guide to the Complete Exercise*. New York: Random House, 1992.

Leora Myers. *Menopause and Beyond: A Fitness Plan for Life*. San Francisco, Calif.: Adelaide, 1995. *Guides you in fitness: stretching, weight training, aerobics, and more.*

Staff and Researchers of Melpomene Institute for Women's Health Research. *The Bodywise Woman*. Champaign, Ill.: Human Kinetics, 1990. *Reliable information about physical activity and health. Order from PO Box 5076, 61825-5076 (800-747-4457).*

Meditation

Herbert Benson. *The Relaxation Response*. New York: Avon, 1975. *Classic book about this deceptively simple technique.*

Joan Borysenko. *Minding the Body, Mending the Mind.* New York: Bantam Books, 1988. *Best-selling book discussing mind-body healing techniques.*

Lawrence LeShan. *How to Meditate.* New York: Bantam, 1974. *Classic book on meditation.*

Support

Lonnie Barbach. *For Each Other: Sharing Sexual Intimacy.* New York: Signet Penguin, 1984. Also: *The Pause: Positive Approaches to Menopause.*

Karen Johnson, M.D. *Trusting Ourselves: The Complete Guide to Emotional Well-Being for Women.* New York: Atlantic Monthly, 1991. *This book addresses stress, anxiety, depression, and relaxation.*

Quit Smoking

T. Ferguson. *The Smoker's Book of Health.* New York: Putnam, 1987. *How to quit when you are ready and decrease the consequences until you are.*

Alternative Approaches

Craig Clayton and Virginia McCullough. *A Consumer's Guide to Alternative Health Care.* Holbrook, Mass.: Adams, 1995. *A survey of all the alternatives out there.*

Michael Lerner. *Choices in Healing: Integrating the Best of Conventional and Complementary Approaches to Cancer.* Boston: MIT Press, 1994. *A wonderful book on ways to integrate alternative approaches and traditional medicine.*

Alternative and Complementary Medicine Resources on the Internet:

Rosenthal Center
http://cpmcnet.columbia.edu/dept/rosenthal/

Herbs

German Commission E Monograph. Translated and made available by the American Botanical Council. $149. PO Box 201660, Austin, TX 78720. This is the German government's analysis of indication and safety of commonly used herbs.

Michael T. Murray, ND. *The Healing Power of Herbs: The Enlightened Person's Guide to the Wonders of Medicinal Plants.* Rocklin, Calif.: Prima, 1995. *Careful look at selected herbs. Can be ordered by calling 916-632-4400.*

Varro E. Tyler. *The Honest Herbal: A Sensible Guide to the Use of Herbs and Related Remedies.* Binghamton, N.Y.: Haworth, 1993.

Susun Weed. *Menopausal Years: The Wise Woman Way.* Woodstock, N.Y.: Ash Tree, 1992. *A description of a natural approach to menopause. Includes how to identify and prepare herbs. Send $9.95 plus $4.00 postage and handling to PO Box 64, Woodstock, NY 12498. Phone and fax 914-246-8081.*

Michael A. Weiner, Ph.D., and Janet Weiner. *Herbs That Heal.* Mill Valley, Calif.: Quantum, 1994. *A good compendium of herbs in general with reviews of the most recent articles.*

Herbal information on the Internet:
American Botanical Council/HerbalGram
http://www.herbalgram.org

Herbal Research Foundation
http://sunsite.unc.edu/herbs/hrfinfo.html

IBIS, Interactive BodyMind Information System
http://www.teleport.com/~ibis/
Everything you want to know about all of the alternative options for any one disease.

Traditional Chinese

John Boik. *Cancer and Natural Medicine: A Textbook of Basic Science and Clinical Research.* Princeton, Minn.: Oregon Medical Press, 1996. *This is a wonderfully researched medical book on herbs and how they relate to cancer treatment. It leans toward traditional Chinese herbs.*

Honora Lee Wolfe. *Menopause: A Second Spring.* Boulder, Colo.: Blue Poppy, 1995. *A good overview of traditional Chinese medicine and how it views menopause.*

Ted Kaptchuk. *The Web That Has No Weaver.* New York: Congdon and Weed, 1983. *Said to be the best introduction for anyone interested in exploring Chinese medicine and its theories.*

Bob Flaws. *Imperial Secrets of Health and Longevity.* Boulder, Colo.: Blue Poppy, 1994. *An introduction to the theories and practices which support longevity and health according to traditional Chinese medicine.*

Mind-Body

Deepak Chopra, M.D. *Perfect Health: The Complete Mind/Body Guide.* New York: Harmony, 1991. *Nearly everything you need to know to adopt an Ayurvedic lifestyle.*

Alice D. Domar, Ph.D., and Henry Dreher. *Healing Mind, Healthy Woman: Using the Mind-Body Connection to Manage Stress and Take Control of Your Health.* New York: Holt, 1996. *A book applying the principles of the mind-body connection to women's lives.*

M. Rossman. *Healing Yourself: A Step-by-Step Program for Better Health Through Imagery.* New York: Walker, 1987.

Homeopathy

Trevor Smith. *Homeopathy for the Menopause.* Worthing, England: Insight, 1994.

Supplements

Sherry W. Sultenfuss and Thomas Sultenfuss. *A Woman's Guide to Vitamins and Minerals.* Chicago, Ill.: Contemporary, 1995.

Drugs

John Lee and Virginia Hopkins. *What Your Doctor May Not Tell You About Menopause: The Breakthrough Book on Natural Progesterone.* New York: Warner, 1996. *A critical evaluation of the current use of estrogen. Lee is an evangelist for "natural progesterone," however. As I mention in this book, some of the data are provocative, but we aren't quite there yet.*

Susan Rako, M.D. *The Hormone of Desire: The Truth About Sexuality, Menopause, and Testosterone.* New York: Harmony, 1996. *Provocative look at some women's apparent need for testosterone. More conjecture than science at this point.*

On the Internet:
Doctor's Guide to Menopause Information and Resources
http://www.pslgroup.com/MENOPAUSE.HTM
A lot of up-to-date information; it is, however, sponsored by the pharmaceuticals industry.

Surgery

Winifred Berg Cutler. *Hysterectomy: Before and After.* New York: Harper and Row, 1988. *A comprehensive book on this often unnecessary surgery.*

William Parker. *A Gynecologist's Second Opinion.* New York: Plume, 1996. *Good descriptions of alternative procedures to hysterectomy.*

Decision Making

Foundation for Informed Medical Decision Making. *Hormone Replacement Therapy: A Shared Decision Making Program.* Videotape, 1995. *A good review of the issues, although a little weak on the alternatives. Order from PO Box 5457, Hanover, NH 03755-5457 (603-650-1107).*

Harvard Health Publications Special Report: "Postmenopausal Hormone-Replacement Therapy" (pamphlet). Boston: Harvard Women's Health Watch, 1996. To order, write to Harvard Medical School, Health Publications Group, department HRT-Rep, PO Box 380, Boston, MA 02117. *A very good overview of the issues.* ($16.00.)

National Women's Health Network "Taking Hormones and Women's Health: Choices, Risks and Benefits" (pamphlet). Washington, D.C., 1325 G Street NW, 1989. *A careful review of the issues.* ($7.50 and $1.50 postage.)

Office of Technology Assessment (U.S. Congress). "Menopause, Hormone Therapy and Women's Health" (pamphlet). Washington, D.C.: U.S. Government Printing Office, 1992 (OTA-BP-BA-88). Fax orders to 202-512-2250. *A well-balanced report prepared at the request of Congress.* ($6.00.)

Newsletters and Journals

Menopause in General

A Friend Indeed
Box 515
Place du Parc Station
Montreal, Canada H2W 2 P1
514-843-5730
or PO Box 1710
Champlain, NY 12919-1710
This newsletter is published by Janine O'Leary Cobb ten times a year. It is chock-full of good information and provides a forum for women to exchange their experiences. $30 a year.

Harvard Women's Health Watch
PO Box 420234
Palm Court, FL 32142-0234
A very open-minded and balanced view of women's health.

Hot Flash: Newsletter for Midlife and Older Women
National Action Forum for Midlife and Older Women
Box 816
Stony Brook, NY 11790-0609
212-725-8625
A quarterly newsletter providing information on political and social issues related to menopause. $25 a year.

Menopause News
2074 Union Street
San Francisco, CA 94123
Published six times a year, it provides medical and psychological information.

Women's Health Advocate Newsletter
PO Box 420235
Palm Coast, FL 32142-0235
A good look at women's health issues.

Lifestyle Changes—*Nutrition*

Nutrition Action Healthletter
Center for Science in the Public Interest, Suite 300
1875 Connecticut Avenue NW
Washington, DC 20009-5728

Soy Connection—Health and Nutrition News About Soy
10525 NW Ambassador Drive, Suite 202
Kansas City, MO 64153

Tuft's University Diet and Nutrition Letter
PO Box 57857
Boulder, CO 8032-7857
Published monthly by Tuft's University Diet and Nutrition. $20 a year.

Alternative Approaches—*Herbs*

Herbal Gram
American Botanical Council and Herb Research Foundation
Box 2016600
Austin, TX 78720
A source of information about herbs. $35 a year, published quarterly.

Drugs
(The following are drug companies' publications.)

Wyeth-Ayerst Laboratories
PO Box 9251
Garden City, NY 11530-9836
The makers of Premarin publish a series of pamphlets called "Life After 45" on menopause and aging, with a bias (surprise) toward HRT. They also publish Seasons Magazine, *which is free and has articles about menopause, aging, etc.*

CIBA Pharmaceutical Company
Division of CIBA-GEIGY Corporation
5566 Morris Avenue
Summit, NJ 07901
Puts out a booklet on menopause called "Midlife: No Crisis," focusing on estrogen therapy.

Mead Johnson Laboratories
Bristol Myers Squibb Company
PO Box 4000
Princeton, NJ 08543-4000
Makers of estradiol, they put out "For the Woman Approaching Menopause."

Organizations

Menopause in General

National Women's Health Network
514 10th Street NW, Suite 400
Washington, DC 20004
202-347-1140
*This is a national public-interest organiza-
tion dedicated to women's health issues.
It has a booklet on menopause and a
newsletter: The Network News.*

National Black Woman's Health
   Project
1211 Connecticut Avenue NW,
   Suite 310
Washington, DC 20036
202-835-0117
202-833-8790 fax
email NBWHPDC@aol.com
An advocacy and support group.

International Menopause Society
8 Avenue Don Bosco
1150 Brussels
Belgium
*Primarily a group of gynecologists promot-
ing the study of medical intervention in
menopause.*

Older Women's League
666 11th Street NW, Suite 700
Washington, DC 20001
202-783-6686
*An advocacy organization which focuses on
issues of concern to middle-age and older
women.*

Society for Menstrual Cycle Research
c/o Mary Anna Friederich, MD
10559 N 104 Place
Scottsdale, AZ 85258
*Membership is $20 a year and includes a
quarterly newsletter.*

Boston Health Book Collective
240A Elm Street
Somerville, MA 02144
617-625-0271
The collective publishes Our Bodies, Ourselves *and* Ourselves, Growing Older.

Osteoporosis

National Osteoporosis Foundation
2100 M Street NW, Suite 602
Washington, DC 20037
202-223-2226

Heart Disease

American Heart Association
7320 Greenville Avenue
Dallas, TX 75231
214-373-6300

Breast Cancer

National Breast Cancer Coalition
1707 L Street NW, Suite 1060
Washington, DC 20036
202-296-7477

Y-Me National Breast Cancer
  Organization
212 West Van Buren Street
Chicago, IL 60607
312-986-8228
Toll free hotline 800-221-2141

Cancer in General

Commonweal Cancer Help Program
PO Box 316
Bolinas, CA 94924
415-868-0970
*Holds retreats for individuals with
  cancer.*

National Coalition for Cancer
  Survivorship
1010 Wayne Avenue, 5th Floor
Silver Spring, MD 20910
301-585-2616

Wellness Community
2200 Colorado Avenue
Santa Monica, CA 90404
310-453-2200
Free support groups.

Other: Lupus

Lupus
The Lupus Foundation of America
1717 Massachusetts Avenue NW
Washington, DC 20026
800-558-0121

Other: Incontinence

Help for Incontinent People (HIP)
Box 544
Union, SC 29379
802-579-7900
*$15 membership fee; free quarterly
  newsletter and a Resource Guide of
  Continence Aids and Services ($10).*

Lifestyle Changes
Exercise

Melpomene Institute for Women's
  Health Research
1010 University Avenue
St. Paul, MN 55104
612-642-1951
*This group has been studying the relation-
  ship between women's health and physical activity since 1981. It publishes the
  Melpomene Journal three times a year.*

Prevention Walking Club
Rodale Press
Box 6099
Emmaus, PA 18099
800-441-7761
*A $9.97 membership includes a quarterly
  newsletter and an annual magazine about
  various aspects of walking.*

Support

Self-Help Clearinghouse
St. Clares-Riverside Medical Center
25 Pocono Road
Denville, NJ 07834
201-625-7101
*This group has information about support
  groups for various illnesses.*

Stop Smoking

American Lung Association
1740 Broadway
New York, NY 10019-4374
212-315-8700
Information about quitting smoking.

Alternative Approaches

Herbs

Herbal Research Foundation
1007 Pearl Street, Suite 200
Boulder, CO 80302
303-449-2265
303-449-7849
HRF is a clearinghouse for information about herbalism, and especially new research. It is a membership-based organization.

California School of Herbal Studies
PO Box 39
Forestville, CA 95436
707-887-7457
A school offering a nine-month program in Western herbalism.

Mind-Body

Mind/Body Medical Institute
Deaconess Hospital
1 Deaconess Road
Boston, MA 02215
A good source of relaxation tapes.

Mind-Body Health Sciences, Inc.
393 Dixon Road
Boulder, CO 80302

Drugs

American College of Obstetricians and
Gynecologists Resource Center
409 12th Street NW
Washington, DC 20024-2188
202-638-3577

Surgery

Hysterectomy Educational Resources
and Services (HERS Foundation)
422 Bryn Mawr Avenue
Bala Cynwyd, PA 19004
610-667-7757

Women's Health Initiative Research Centers

You can call 800-54-WOMEN and be connected to the center nearest you or call directly one of the centers listed below.

Birmingham, Alabama
University of Alabama, Birmingham
205-975-7575

Tucson, Arizona
University of Arizona at Tucson
(satellite center in Phoenix)
602-321-7440; 800-341-7672

Los Angeles, California
University of California, Los Angeles
310-825-7755

Oakland, California
Kaiser Foundation Research Institute
800-304-3879

Orange, California
University of California, Irvine
714-456-7241

Palo Alto, California
The Leland Stanford Junior University
415-725-5013

Sacramento/Davis, California
University of California, Davis
916-734-0130

San Diego, California
University of California, San Diego
619-622-5770 (La Jolla)
619-498-4980 (Chula Vista)

Torrance, California
Harbor-UCLA Research
   and Education Institute
310-222-8171

Washington, D.C.
George Washington University
202-676-5150

Washington, D.C.
Medlantic Research Institute
202-877-6301

Gainesville, Florida
University of Florida
904-376-1611 ext. 6324

Miami, Florida
University of Miami
305-548-4800 (English);
305-548-4805 (Español)

Atlanta, Georgia
Emory University School of
  Medicine
404-473-8600

Honolulu, Hawaii
University of Hawaii
808-547-7283

Chicago, Illinois
Northwestern Univ. Medical School
312-908-0895

Chicago, Illinois
Rush-Presbyterian-St. Luke's
  Medical Center
312-942-4464

Iowa City, Iowa
University of Iowa at Iowa City
(satellite center in Bettendorf)
319-335-6628 or 800-348-4692

Boston, Massachusetts
Brigham and Women's Hospital
617-278-0782

Worcester, Massachusetts
University of Massachusetts
  Medical Center
508-856-2316

Detroit, Michigan
Wayne State University
313-745-7615

Minneapolis, Minnesota
Univ. of Minnesota Medical Center
612-336-5743

Reno, Nevada
University of Nevada, Reno
702-784-4906

Newark, New Jersey
University of Medicine and
  Dentistry of New Jersey
201-982-4001 or 800-WOMEN-10

Bronx, New York
Albert Einstein College of Medicine
718-430-8788 (English);
718-430-8701 (Español)

Buffalo, New York
State University of New York, Buffalo
716-829-3128

Stony Brook, New York
Research Foundation of SUNY
516-444-3905

Chapel Hill, North Carolina
University of North Carolina,
Chapel Hill
919-966-4215

Winston-Salem, North Carolina
Bowman Gray School of Medicine
919-272-0455
800-644-9448

Cincinnati, Ohio
Univ. of Cincinnati Medical Center
513-558-6061

Columbus, Ohio
Ohio State University Research
  Foundation
614-293-8092

Portland, Oregon
Kaiser Foundation Research Institute
503-335-6747

Pittsburgh, Pennsylvania
University of Pittsburgh
412-624-6926

Pawtucket, Rhode Island
The Memorial Hospital
800-742-3446

Memphis, Tennessee
University of Tennessee, Memphis
901-767-4200

Houston, Texas
Baylor College of Medicine
713-798-8310

San Antonio, Texas
University of Texas Health
   Science Center, San Antonio
210-567-4930

Seattle, Washington
Fred Hutchinson Cancer Research Center
206-667-6550

Madison, Wisconsin
University of Wisconsin
608-263-1201 or 608-263-7713

Milwaukee, Wisconsin
Medical College of Wisconsin
414-456-4700

Notes

Chapter 1   What Is Menopause?

1. Neugarten, B. L., and Kraines, R. J. "Menopausal symptoms in women of various ages." *Psychosomatic Medicine* 1965; 27: 266–273.
2. Sherman, B. M., and Korenman, S. G. "Hormonal characteristics of the human menstrual cycle throughout reproductive life." *Journal of Clinical Investigation* 1975; 55: 699–706.
3. Shideler, S. E., DeVane, G. W., Kalra, P. S., Benirschke, K., and Lasley, B. I. "Ovarian-pituitary hormone interactions during the perimenopause." *Maturitas* 1989; 11(4): 331–339.
4. Burger, H. G. "The menopause: When it is all over or is it?" *Australian New Zealand Journal Obstetrics and Gynaecology* 1994; 34(3): 293–295.
5. New England Research, Inc. *Women and Their Health in Massachusetts: Final Report 1991.* Watertown, Mass.: New England Research Institute, 1991.
6. Yen, S. C., and Jaffe, R. B. *Reproductive Endocrinology.* Philadelphia: Saunders, 1991, p. 392.
7. Sluijmer, A. V., Heineman, M. J., De Jong, F. H., and Evers, J. L. "Endocrine activity of the postmenopausal ovary: The effects of pituitary down-regulation and oophorectomy." *Journal of Clinical Endocrinology and Metabolism* 1995; 80: 2163–2167.
8. Ushiroyama, T., and Sugimoto, O. "Endocrine function of the peri- and postmenopausal ovary." *Hormone Research* 1995; 44: 64–68.
9. Hreshchyshyn, M. M., Hopkins, A., Zylstra, S., and Anbar, M. "Effects of natural menopause, hysterectomy, and oophorectomy on lumbar spine and femoral neck bone densities." *Obstetrics and Gynecology* 1988; 72: 631.
10. Cauley, J. A., Gutal, J. P., Kuller, L. H., LeDonne, D., and Powell, J. G. "The epidemiology of serum sex hormones in postmenopausal women." *American Journal of Epidemiology* 1989; 129(6): 1120–1131.
11. Yen and Jaffe, op. cit., p. 585.
12. Hreshchyshyn, op. cit.
13. Stone, L. *The Family, Sex, and Marriage.* New York: Harper and Row, 1979, p. 67.

14. Hale, J. R. *Renaissance Europe.* Berkeley: University of California Press, 1971, p. 15.
15. Fraser, A. *The Weaker Vessel.* New York: Vintage, 1984, p. 101.
16. Utian, W. "Overview on menopause." *American Journal of Obstetrics and Gynecology* 1987; 156(5): 1280–1283.
17. Lock, M. "Menopause: Lessons from anthropology." Presentation at annual meeting, North American Menopause Society, San Francisco, Sept. 21–23, 1995.
18. Diamond, J. "Why Women Change." *Discover* 1996; July: 131–137.
19. Weed, S. *The Menopausal Years: The Wise Woman Way.* Woodstock, N.Y.: Ash Tree, 1992.
20. Quoted in Gray, F. D. "The Third Age." *The New Yorker* (Special Women's Issue), Feb. 26/March 4, 1996: 191.
21. Quoted ibid.

Chapter 2   The Medicalization of Menopause

1. Coney, S. *The Menopause Industry.* Alameda, Calif.: Hunter House, 1994, p. 67.
2. Utian, W. H. "Overview on menopause." *American Journal of Obstetrics and Gynecology* 1987; 156: 1280–1283.
3. Ibid., p. 1280.
4. Wilson, R. *Feminine Forever.* New York: Evans, 1966.
5. Rhoades, F. P. "Minimizing the menopause." *Journal of the American Geriatric Society* 1967; 15(4): 346–354.
6. Utian, op. cit., p. 1281.
7. Ibid., p. 1283.
8. Barrett-Connor, E., and Miller, V. "Estrogens, lipids, and heart disease." *Clinics in Geriatric Medicine* 1993(9): 57–67.
9. McCullough, M. "Hope or Hype?" *The Philadelphia Inquirer,* May 13, 1996.
10. Pike, M. C., Pike, A., Rude, R., Shoupe, D., and Richardson, J. "Pilot trial of a gonadotropin hormone agonist with replacement hormones as a prototype contraceptive to prevent breast cancer." *Contraception* 1993; 47(5): 427–444.
11. Van Keep, P. A. "The history and rationale of hormone replacement therapy." *Maturitas* 1990; 12: 163–170.
12. Ibid., p. 167.
13. Leiblum, S. R., and Swartzman, L. C. "Women's attitudes toward the menopause: An update." *Maturitas* 1986; 8(1): 47–56.
14. Lock, M., Kaufert, P., and Gilbert, P. "Cultural construction of the menopausal syndrome: The Japanese case." *Maturitas* 1988; 10: 317–332.
15. Lock, M. "Menopause in cultural context." *Experimental Gerontology* 1994; 29(3/4): 307–317.
16. Ibid., p. 313.
17. Flint, M., and Samil, R. S. "Cultural and subcultural meanings of the menopause." In *Multidisciplinary Perspectives on Menopause,* Flint, M., Kronenberg, F., and Utian, W. (eds.). *Annals of New York Academy of Sciences,* 1990, pp. 134–148.
18. Martin, M. C., Block, J. E., Sanchez, S. D., Arnaud, C. D., and Beyene, Y. "Menopause without symptoms: The endocrinology of menopause among rural Mayan Indians." *American Journal of Obstetrics and Gynecology* 1993; 168(6): 1839–1845.
19. Flint, M., and Samil, R. S. "Cultural and subcultural meanings of the menopause." *Annals of New York Academy of Sciences* 1990; 592: 134–148; (discussion) 185–192.
20. Beyene, Y. "Cultural significance and physiological manifestation of menopause: A biocultural analysis." *Culture, Medicine, and Psychiatry* 1986; 10: 47–71.
21. Chirawitkul, T., and Manderson, L. "Perception of menopause in Northeast Thailand: Contested meaning and practice." *Social Science Medicine* 1994; 39(11): 1545–1554.
22. Ibid., p. 1546.

23. Cooper, W. *No Change: A Biological Revolution for Women.* London: Arrow, 1983.
24. Hunt, K. "Perceived value of treatment among a group of long-term users of hormone replacement therapy." *Journal of the Royal College of General Practitioners* 1988; 38: 398–401.
25. Ibid., pp. 399–400.
26. Hunter, M. S., and Liao, K. L. "Intentions to use hormone replacement therapy in a community sample of 45 year old women." *Maturitas* 1994; 20: 13–23.
27. Doress-Worters, P. B. Preface to Coney, op. cit., p. 9.
28. Wilson, op. cit., pp. 18ff.
29. Cyran, W. "Estrogen replacement therapy and publicity." In *Aging and Estrogens. Frontiers of Hormone Research,* Vol. 2, Lauritzen, C., and van Keep, P. A. (eds.). Basel: Karger, 1973, p. 152.
30. Lee, J. R. *What Your Doctor May Not Tell You About Menopause.* New York: Warner, 1996.
31. Seaman, B., and Seaman, G. *Women and the Crisis in Sex Hormones.* New York: Bantam, 1977.
32. Wilson, op. cit., p. 97.
33. Hemminki, E., and Sihvo, S. "A review of postmenopausal hormone therapy recommendations: Potential for selection bias." *Obstetrics and Gynecology* 1993; 82(6): 1021–1028.
34. Coronary Drug Project Research Group. "The Coronary Drug Project: Initial findings leading to modifications of its research protocol." *Journal of the American Medical Association* 1970; 214: 1303–1313.
35. Ziel, H. K., and Finkle, W. D. "Increased risk of endometrial carcinoma among users of conjugated estrogens." *New England Journal of Medicine* 1970; 293: 1167–1170.
36. *The Wall Street Journal,* June 15, 1995: 5.
37. Hemminki and Sihvo, op. cit.
38. Meyers, J. H. *The U. S. Retail Prescription Market Year in Review.* Boca Raton, Fla.: CPSNET, 1966.
39. Bowman, M. A., and Pearle, D. L. "Changes in drug prescribing patterns related to commercial company funding of continuing medical education." *Journal of Continuing Education of the Health Professions* 1988; 8(1): 13–20.
40. Tanouye, E. "Estrogen study shifts ground for women and for drug firms." *The Wall Street Journal,* June 15, 1995: A5.
41. Utian, W. "Nonhormonal medication." In *Modern Approach to the Menopausal Years,* Greenblatt, Robert (ed.). Berlin, N.Y.: DeGruyter, 1986, pp. 117–125.
42. Prior, J. "One voice on menopause." *Journal of the American Women's Association* 1994 (Jan.-Feb.); 49(1):27–29.
43. Seaman and Seaman, op. cit., pp. 6–7.
44. *Osteoporosis Report* 1995; 11(3): 7.

Chapter 3   "What Does It Feel Like?"

1. Cobb, J. O. *Understanding Menopause.* New York: Plume, 1993.
2. New England Research Institute, Inc. *Women and Their Health in Massachusetts: Final Report.* Watertown, Mass.: 1991.
3. Bungay, G. T., Vessey, M. P., and McPherson, C. K. "Study of symptoms in middle life with special reference to the menopause." *British Medical Journal* 1980; 281(6234): 181–183.
4. Gambone, J., Meldrum, D. R., Laufer, L., Chang, R. J., Lu, J. K. H., and Judd, H. L. "Further delineation of hypothalamic dysfunction responsible for menopausal hot flashes." *Journal of Clinical Endocrinology Metabolism* 1984; 59: 1097.
5. New England Research Institute, op. cit.

6. Judd, H. L. "The pathophysiology of menopausal hot flushes." In *Neuroendocrinology of Aging*, Meites, J. (ed.). New York: Plenum, 1983, pp. 173–202.

7. Voda, A. "Climacteric hot flashes." *Maturitas* 1981; 3: 73–90.

8. Weed, S. *The Menopausal Years: The Wise Woman Way*. Woodstock, N.Y.: Ash Tree, 1992.

9. Greenwood, S. *Menopause Naturally*. Volcano, Calif.: Volcano, 1996, p. 32.

10. Holte, A. "Influences of natural menopause on health complaints: A prospective study of healthy Norwegian women." *Maturitas* 1992; 14: 127–141.

11. Kaufert, P. A., Gilbert, P., and Tate, R. "The Manitoba Project: A reexamination of the link between menopause and depression." *Maturitas* 1992; 14: 143–155.

12. New England Research Institute, op. cit.

13. Greene, J. G., and Cooke, D. J. "Life stress and symptoms at the climacterium." *British Journal of Psychiatry* 1980; 136: 486–491.

14. New England Research Institute, op. cit.

15. Yesavage, J. A., and Sheikh, J. I. "Nonpharmacologic treatment of age-associated memory impairment." *Compr Ther* 1988; 14(6): 44–46.

16. Sherwin, B. B. "Estrogenic effects on memory in women." *Annals of New York Academy of Sciences* 1994; 14(743): 213–230.

17. Sherwin, B. B. "Estrogen and/or androgen replacement therapy and cognitive functioning in surgically menopausal women." *Psychoneuroendocrinology* 1988; 10: 325–335.

18. Barrett-Connor, E., and Kritz-Silverstein, D. "Estrogen replacement therapy and cognitive function in older women." *Journal of the American Medical Association* 1993; 260: 2637–2641.

19. Robinson, D., Friedman, L., Marcus, R., Tinklenberg, J., and Yesavage, J. "Estrogen replacement therapy and memory in older women." *Journal of the American Geriatric Society* 1994; 42(9): 919–922.

20. Voytko, M. L. "Estrogen effects on cognition in brain biology." Presentation at IBC Menopause Conference, Philadelphia, Pa., May 9–10, 1996.

21. New England Research Institute, op. cit.

22. Hunter, M., Battersby, R., and Whitehead, M. "Relationships between psychological symptoms, somatic complaints, and menopausal status." *Maturitas* 1986 (8): 217–228.

23. Ibid.

24. Castelo-Branco, C., Duran, M., and Gonzalez-Merlo, J. "Skin collagen changes related to age and hormone replacement therapy." *Maturitas* 1992; 15: 113–119.

25. Savas, M., Bishop, J., Laurent, G., Watson, N., and Studd, J. "Type III collagen content in the skin of postmenopausal women receiving oestradiol and testosterone implants." *British Journal of Obstetrics and Gynaecology* 1993; 100(2): 154–156.

26. Holland, E. F., Studd, J. W., Mansell, J. P., Leather, A. T., and Bailey, A. J. "Changes in collagen composition and cross-links in bone and skin of osteoporotic postmenopausal women treated with percutaneous estradiol implants." *Obstetrics and Gynecology* 1994; 83 (2): 180–183.

27. Grady, Deborah. Personal communication.

28. Pfeiffer, E., and Davis, G. C. "Determinants of sexual behavior in middle and old age." *Journal of the American Geriatric Society* 1972; 20(4): 151–158.

29. Sarrel, P. M., and Whitehead, M. I. "Sex and menopause: Defining the issues. *Maturitas* 1985; 7(3): 217–224.

30. McCoy, N., and Davidson, J. M. "A longitudinal study of the effects of menopause on sexuality." *Maturitas* 1985; 7(3): 203–210.

31. Chirawitkul, T., and Manderson, L. "Perception of menopause in Northeast Thailand: Contested meaning and practice." *Social Science Medicine* 1994; 39(11): 1545–1554.

32. Michael, R. P., and Keverne, E. B. "A male sex-attractant on rhesus monkey vaginal secretions." *Journal of Endocrinology* 1970; 46(2): xx-xxi.

33. Sherwin, B. B. "Changes in sexual behavior as a function of plasma sex steroid levels in post-menopausal women." *Maturitas* 1985; 7: 225–233.

34. Rako, S. *The Hormone of Desire.* New York: Harmony, 1996.

Chapter 4   Prevention and Risk: Understanding Research

1. Stampfer, M. J., Colditz, G. A., Willett, W. C., Manson, J. E., Rosner, B., Speizer, F. E., and Hennekens, C. H. "Postmenopausal estrogen therapy and cardiovascular disease: Ten year follow up from the Nurses' Health Study." *New England Journal of Medicine* 1991; 325: 756–762.

2. Coronary Drug Project Research Group. "The Coronary Drug Project: Initial findings leading to modifications of its research protocol." *Journal of the American Medical Association* 1970; 214: 1303–1313.

3. Matthews, K. A., Kuller, L. H., Wing, R. R., Meilahn, E. N., and Plantinga, P. "Health prior to use of estrogen replacement therapy: Are users healthier than nonusers?" *American Journal of Epidemiology* 1996; 143: 971–978.

4. Matthews, K. A., Kuller, L. H., Wing, R. R., Meilahn, E. N., and Plantinga, P. "Health prior to hormone use: Matthews et al. reply to Grodstein." *American Journal of Epidemiology* 1996; 143: 983–984.

5. Petitti, D. B. "Coronary heart disease and estrogen replacement therapy: Can compliance bias explain the results of observational studies?" *Annals of Epidemiology* 1994; 4: 115–118.

6. Matthews et al., " . . . Reply to Grodstein."

7. Colditz, G. A., Hankinson, S. E., Hunter, D. J., Wilett, W. C., Manson, J. E., Stampfer, M. J., Hennekens, C., Rosner, B., and Speizer, F. E. "The use of estrogens and progestins and the risk of breast cancer in postmenopausal women." *New England Journal of Medicine* 1995; 332: 1589–1593.

8. Stanford, J. L., Weiss, N. S., Voight, L. F., Daling, J. R., Habel, L. A., and Rosing, M. "Combined estrogen and progestin hormone replacement therapy in relation to risk of breast cancer." *Journal of the American Medical Association* 1995; 274: 37–142.

9. Adami, H. O., and Persson, I. "Hormone replacement and breast cancer: A remaining controversy?" *Journal of the American Medical Association* 1995; 274: 178–179.

Chapter 5   Osteoporosis: Are We All Going to Crumble?

1. Tenenhouse, A. "Epidemiology of osteoporosis." *First McGill International Symposium on Recent Advances in Infertility and Reproductive Endocrinology Pre IX World Congress on Human Reproduction Symposium,* May 28, 1996.

2. Seeman, E. "The dilemma of osteoporosis in men." *American Journal of Medicine* 1995; 98(Supp. l2A): 2A/76S–2A/88S.

3. Pocock, N. A., Eisman, J. A., Hopper, J. L., Yeates, M. G., Sambrook, P. N., and Eberl, S. "Genetic determinants of bone mass in adults: A twin study." *Journal of Clinical Investigations* 1987; 80: 706–710.

4. Conference Report Consensus Development Conference. "Prophylaxis and treatment of osteoporosis." *American Journal of Medicine* 1991; 90: 107–110.

5. Morrison, N. A., Cheng, Q. I. J., Tokita, A., et al. "Prediction of bone density from vitamin D receptor alleles." *Nature* 1994; 367: 284–287.

6. Cauley, J. A., Cummings, S. R., Black, D. M., Mascioli, S. R., and Seeley, D. G. "Prevalence and determinants of estrogen replacement therapy in elderly women." *American Journal of Obstetrics and Gynecology* 1990; 163(5, Part 1): 1438–1444.

7. Baran, D. T. "Quantitative ultrasound: A technique to target women with low bone mass for preventative therapy." *American Journal of Medicine* 1995; 98 (Supp. 2A): 2A/48S–2A/51S.

8. Kanis, J. A., Melton, J., Christiansen, C., Johnston, C. C., and Khaltaev, N. "The diagnosis of osteoporosis." *Journal of Bone and Mineral Research* 1994; 9: 1137–1141.

9. Ibid., p. 1138.

10. Melton L. J., Chrischilles, E. A., Cooper, C., Lane, A. W., and Riggs, B. L. "How many women have osteoporosis?" *Journal of Bone and Mineral Research* 1992; 9: 1005–1009.

11. Tobias, J. H., Cook, D. G., Chambers, T. J., and Dalsell, N. "A comparison of bone mineral density between Caucasian, Asian and Afro-Caribbean women." *Clinical Science* 1994; 87: 587–591.

12. Prior, J. C., Vigna, Y. M., Barr, S. I., Kennedy, S., Schulzer, M., and Li, D. K. B. "Ovulatory premenopausal women lose cancellous spinal bone: A five year prospective study." *Bone* 1996; 18: 261–267.

13. Riis, B. J. "The role of bone loss." *American Journal of Medicine* 1995; 98(Supp. l2A): 2A/29S–2A/32S.

14. Clements, D., Compston, J. E., Evans, C., and Evans, W. D. "Bone loss in normal British women: A 5 year follow up." *British Journal of Radiology* 1993; 66; 1134–1137.

15. Kanis, J. A., and Adami, S. "Bone loss in the elderly." *Osteoporosis International* 1994; Supp. 1: S59–65.

16. Pansini, F., Bagni, B., Bonaccorsi, G., Albertazzi, P., Zanotti, L., Farina, A., Campobasso, C., Orlandi, R., and Mollica, G. "Oophorectomy and spine bone density: Evidence of a higher rate of bone loss in surgical compared with spontaneous menopause." *Menopause: Journal of the North American Menopause Society* 1995; 2(2): 109–115.

17. Bruns, M. E., Overpeck, J. G., Smith, G. C., Hirsch, G. N., Mills, S. E., and Bruns, D. E. "Vitamin D dependent calcium binding protein in rat uterus: Differential effects of estrogen, tamoxifen, progesterons, and pregnancy on accumulation and cellular localization." *Endocrinology* 1988; 122(6): 2371–2378.

18. Martin, M. C., Block, J. E., Sanchez, S. D., Arnaud, C. D., and Beyene, Y. "Menopause without symptoms: The endocrinology of menopause among rural Mayan Indians." *American Journal of Obstetrics and Gynecology* 1993; 168(6): 1839–1845.

19. Siddle, N., Sarrel, P., and Whitehead, M. "The effect of hysterectomy on the age at ovarian failure: Identification of a subgroup of women with premature loss of ovarian function and literature reviews." *Fertility and Sterility* 1987; 47(1):94–100.

20. Pike, M. C., Pike, A., Rude, R., Shoupe, D., and Richardson J. "Pilot trial of a gonadotropin hormone agonist with replacement hormones as a prototype contraceptive to prevent breast cancer." *Contraception* 1993; 47(5): 427–444.

21. Prior, J. C. "Progesterone as a bone-trophic hormone." *Endocrine Reviews* 1990; (11): 386–398.

22. Seeman, E., Hopper, J. L., Bach, L. A., Cooper, M. E., Parkinson, E., McKay, J., and Jerums, G. "Reduced bone mass in daughters of women with osteoporosis." *New England Journal of Medicine* 1989; 20(9): 554–558.

23. Cummings, S. R., Nevitt, M. C., Browner, W. S., Stone, K., Fox, K. M., Ensrud, K. E., Cauley, J., Black, D., and Vogt, T. M. "Risk factors for hip fracture in white women." *New England Journal of Medicine* 1995; 332: 767–773.

24. Kanis et al., op. cit.

25. Chrischilles, E. A., Butler, D., Cavis, C. S., and Wallace, R. B. "A model of lifetime osteoporosis impact." *Archives of Internal Medicine* 1991; 151: 2026–2032.

26. Owen, R. A., Melton, L. J., Johnson, K. A., Ilstrup, D. M., and Riggs, B, L. "Incidence of Colles' fracture in a North American community." *American Journal of Public Health* 1982; 72: 605–607.

27. Jensen, G. F., Christiansen, C., Boesen, J., Hegedus, V., and Transbol, I. "Relationship between bone and mineral content and frequency of postmenopausal fractures." *Acta Medica Scandinavia* 1983; 213: 61–63.
28. Melton, L. J. "Epidemiology of fractures." In *Osteoporosis: Etiology, Diagnosis, and Management*, Riggs, B. L., and Melton, L. J. (eds.). New York: Raven, 1988, pp. 133–154.
29. Jensen et al., op. cit.
30. Chrischilles et al., op. cit.
31. Ibid.
32. Clements et al. op. cit.
33. Melton, L. J., Eddy, D. M., and Johnston, C. C. "Screening for osteoporosis." *Annals of Internal Medicine* 1990; 112(7): 516–528.
34. Torgerson, D. J., Donaldson, C., Russell, I. T., and Reid, D. M. "Hormone replacement therapy: Compliance and cost after screening for osteoporosis." *European Journal of Obstetrics, Gynecology, and Reproductive Biology* 1995; 59(1): 57–60.
35. Merck and Company, Inc. "Maximizing sales growth." Annual Report. Whitehouse Station, N.J., 1995.
36. Ettinger, B., Genant, H. K., and Cann, C. E. "Long term estrogen replacement therapy prevents bone loss and fractures." *Annals of Internal Medicine* 1985; 102: 319–324.
37. Lee, J. R. *Natural Progesterone*. Sebastopol, Calif.: BLL, 1993.
38. Ibid., pp. 53–58.
39. Ettinger, B., and Grady, D. "The waning effect of postmenopausal estrogen on osteoporosis." *New England Journal of Medicine* 1993; 329: 1192–1193.
40. Sowers, M., Clark, M., Hollis, B., Wallace, R., and Jannausch, M. "Radial bone mineral density in pre- and perimenopasual women: A prospective study of rates and risk factors." *Journal of Bone and Mineral Research* 1992; 7: 647–657.
41. Pouilles, J. M., Tremollieres, F., and Ribbot, C. "The effects of menopause on longitudinal bone loss from the spine." *Calcified Tissue International* 1993; 52: 340–343.
42. Geelhoed, E., Harris, A., and Prince, R. "Cost-effectiveness analysis of hormone replacement therapy and lifestyle intervention for hip fracture." *Australian Journal of Public Health* 1994; 18: 153–160.
43. Ensrud, K. E., Palermo, L., Black, D. M., et al. "Hip bone loss increases with advancing age: Longitudinal results from the study of osteoporotic fractures." In *Sixteenth Annual Meeting of the American Society for Bone and Mineral Research*, Raisz, L. G. (ed.). Kansas City, Mo.: Liebert, 1994, S153.
44. Black, D. "Alendronate prevents hip and other fractures in some osteoporosis patients." Presentation at 1996 World Conference on Osteoporosis. Amsterdam, Netherlands, May 1996.
45. Black D. M. "Why elderly women should be screened and treated to prevent osteoporosis." *American Journal of Medicine* 1995; 98(Supp. 12A): 2A/67S–2A/75S.

Chapter 6 Heart Disease: What's Your Real Risk?

1. Bush, T. L. "The epidemiology of cardiovascular disease in postmenopausal women." *Annals of New York Academy of Sciences* 1990; 592: 263–271; (discussion) 334–345.
2. Berliner, J. A., Navab, M., Fogelman, A. M., Frank, J. S., Demer, L. L., Edwards, P. A., Watson, A. D., and Lusis, A. J. "Atherosclerosis: Basic mechanisms. Oxidation, inflammation, and genetics." *Circulation* 1995; 91(9): 2488–2496.
3. Williams, R. *The Trusting Heart*. New York: Washington Square, 1985.
4. Scherwitz, L., McKelvain, R., Laman, C., et al. "Type A behavior, self-involvement, and coronary atherosclerosis." *Psychosomatic Medicine* 1983; 45(1): 45–57.
5. Clarkson, T. B., Adams, M. R., Kaplan, J. R., Shively, C. A., and Koritnik, D. R. "From menarche to menopause: Coronary artery atherosclerosis and protection in

cynomolgus monkeys." *American Journal of Obstetrics and Gynecology* 1989; 160(5): 1280–1285.

6. Haertel, U., Heiss, G., Filipiak, B., and Doering, A. "Cross-sectional and longitudinal associations between high density lipoprotein cholesterol and women's employment." *American Journal of Epidemiology* 1992; 135: 68–78.

7. Haynes, S. G., and Feinleib, M. "Women, work and coronary heart disease: Prospective findings from the Framingham heart study." *American Journal of Public Health* 1980; 70(2): 133–141.

8. Grady, D., Rubin, S. M., Petitti, D. B., et al. "Hormone therapy to prevent disease and prolong life in postmenopausal women." *Annals of Internal Medicine* 1992; 117: 1016–1037.

9. Greenland, P., Reicher-Reiss, H., Goldbourt, U., et al. "In hospital and 1 year mortality in 1524 women after myocardial infarction." *Circulation* 1991; 83: 484.

10. Barrett-Connor, E., and Goodman-Gruen, D. "Prospective study of endogenous sex hormones and fatal cardiovascular disease in postmenopausal women." *British Medical Journal* 1995; 311: 1193–1196.

11. Coronary Drug Project Research Group. "The Coronary Drug Project: Findings leading to discontinuation of the 2.5 mg/day estrogen arm." *Journal of the American Medical Association* 1973; 226: 652–657.

12. Nachtigall, L. E., Nachtigall, R., Nachtigall, R. D., and Beckman, E. M. "Estrogen replacement therapy II: A prospective study in the relationship to carcinoma and cardiovascular and metabolic problems." *Obstetrics and Gynecology* 1979; 54(1): 74–79.

13. Bush, T. L., Barrett-Connor, E., Cowan, L. D., Criqui, M. H., Wallace, R. B., Suchindran, C. M., Tyroler, H. A., and Rifkind, B. M. "Cardiovascular mortality and noncontraceptive use of estrogen in women: Results from the Lipid Research Clinics Program Follow-up Study." *Circulation* 1987; 75: 1102–1109.

14. Stampfer, M. J., and Colditz, G. A. "Estrogen replacement therapy and coronary heart disease: A quantitative assessment of the epidemiologic evidence." *Preventive Medicine* 1991; 20: 47–63.

15. Grodstein, F., Stampfer, M. J., Manson, J. E., Colditz, G. A., Willett, W. C., Rosner, B., Speizer, F. E., and Hennekens, C. H. "Postmenopausal estrogen and progestin use: The risk of cardiovascular disease." *New England Journal of Medicine* 1996; 335.

16. Colditz, G. A. "The Nurses' Health Study: Findings during 10 years of follow-up of a cohort of U.S. women." *Current Problems in Obstetrics and Gynecology Fertility* 1990; 13: 129–174.

17. Paganini-Hill, A. "The risks and benefits of estrogen replacement therapy: Leisure World." *Journal of Fertility and Menopausal Studies* 1995; 40 (Supp. 1): 54–62.

18. Barrett-Connor, E. "Postmenopausal estrogen and prevention bias." *Annals of Internal Medicine* 1991; 115: 455–456.

19. Matthews, K. A., Kuller, L. H., Wing, R. R., Meilahn, E. N., and Plantinga, P. "Prior to use of estrogen replacement therapy, are users healthier than nonusers?" *American Journal of Epidemiology* 1996; 143: 971–978.

20. Petitti, D. B. "Coronary heart disease and estrogen replacement therapy: Can compliance bias explain the results of observational studies?" *Annals of Epidemiology* 1994; 4: 115–118.

21. LaCroix, A. Z. "Psychosocial factors and risk of coronary heart disease in women: An epidemiologic perspective." *Fertility and Sterility* 1994; 62: 133S–139S.

22. Correspondence between Kriegsmann, Barbara (Executive Director of Marketing, Wyeth-Ayerst), and Lipner, Robyn (professional staff member, Committee on Labor and Human Resources, United States Senate), April 16, 1991.

23. Haarbo, J., Nielsin, L. B., Stender, S., and Christiansen, C. "Aortic permeability to LDL during estrogen therapy." *Arteriosclerosis and Thrombosis* 1994; 14(2): 243–247.

24. Writing Group for the PEPI Trial. "Effects of estrogen or estrogen/progestin regimens on heart disease risk factors in postmenopausal women: The postmenopausal estrogen/progestin interventions (PEPI) trial." *Journal of the American Medical Association* 1995; 272(3): 199–208.
25. Ibid.
26. Sullivan, J. M. "Coronary arteriography in estrogen-treated postmenopausal women." *Progress in Cardiovascular Diseases* 1995; 38(3): 211–222.
27. Williams, J., Honore, E. K., Washburn, S. A., and Clarkson, T. B. "Effects of hormone replacement therapy on reactivity of atherosclerotic coronary arteries in cynomolgous monkeys." *Journal of American Cell Cardiology* 1994; 24: 1757–1761.
28. Barnes, S. Presentation at Menopause Conference: Advances in Hormone Replacement and Alternative Therapeutic Strategies. Philadelphia, Pa.: May 9–10, 1996.
29. Sullivan, J. M., Shala Bashar, A., Miller, L. A., Lerner, J. L., and McBrayer, J. D. "Progestin enhances vasoconstrictor responses in postmenopausal women receiving estrogen replacement." *Menopause: Journal of the North American Menopause Society* 1995; 2(4): 193–199.
30. Grodstein, F., Stampfer, M. I., Manson, I. E., Colditz, G. A., Willett, W. C., Rosner, B., Speizer, F. E., and Hennekens, C. H. "Postmenopausal estrogen and progestin use and the risk of cardiovascular disease." *New England Journal of Medicine* 1996; 335(7): 453–461.
31. Sherwin, B. B, Gelfand, M. M., Schucher, R., and Gabor, J. "Postmenopausal estrogen and androgen replacement and lipoprotein lipid concentrations." *American Journal of Obstetrics and Gynecology* 1987; 156: 414–419.
32. Barrett-Connor, E., and Miller, V. "Estrogens, lipids, and heart disease: Care of the older woman." *Clinics in Geriatric Medicine* 1993; 1(9): 57–67.

Chapter 7   Breast Cancer: Every Woman's Fear?

1. Horwitz, K. B., Sartorius, C. A., Hovland, A. R., Jackson, T. A., Groshong, S. D., Tung, L., and Takimoto, G. S. "Surprises with antiprogestins: Novel mechanisms of progesterone receptor action." *Ciba Foundation Symposium* 1995; 191: 235–249; (discussion) 250–253.
2. Pike, M., Spicer, D. V., Dahmoush, L., and Press, M. F. "Estrogens, progestogens, normal breast cell proliferation, and breast cancer risk." *Epidemiologic Reviews* 1993; 15(1): 17–35.
3. Feinleib, M. "Breast cancer and artificial menopause: A cohort study." *Journal of the National Cancer Institute* 1968; 41: 315–329.
4. Hoffman, D. A., Lonstein, J. E., Morin, M. M., et al. "Breast cancer in women with scoliosis exposed to multiple diagnostic X rays." *Journal of the National Cancer Institute* 1989; 81: 1307.
5. Bernstein, L., Hanisch, R., Sullivan-Halley, J., and Ross, R. K. "Treatment with human chorionic gonadotropin and risk of breast cancer." *Cancer Epidemiology Biomarkers and Prevention* 1995; 4: 437–440.
6. Wolff, M. S., Toniolo, P. G., Lee, E. W., Rivera, M., and Dubin, N. "Blood levels of organochlorine residues and risk of breast cancer." *Journal of the National Cancer Institute* 1993; 85: 648.
7. Barnes, S., Peterson, T. G., and Coward, L. "Rationale for the use of genistein-containing soy matrices in chemoprevention trials for breast and prostate cancer." *Journal of Cellular Biochemistry* 1995; Supp. 22: 181–187.
8. Peterson, G., and Barnes, S. "Genistein inhibition of the growth of human breast cancer cells: Independence from estrogen receptors and the multidrug resistance gene." *Biochemistry, Biophysics Research Community* 1991; 179(1): 661.

9. Berrino, F., Muti, P., Micheli, A., Bolelli, G., Krogh, V., Sciajno, R., Pisani, P., Panico, S., and Secreto, G. "Serum sex hormone levels after menopause and subsequent breast cancer." *Journal of the National Cancer Institute* 1996; 88(5): 291–296.

10. Greenberg, E. R., Barnes, A. B., Resseguie, L., et al. "Breast cancer in mothers given diethylstilbesterol in pregnancy." *New England Journal of Medicine* 1984; 311: 1393.

11. Rookus, M. A., and van Leeuwen, F. E. "Oral contraceptives and risk of breast cancer in women aged 20–54 years." *Lancet* 1994; 344: 844–851.

12. Steinberg, K. K., Thacker, S. B., Smith, J., Stroup, D. F., Zack, M. M., Flanders, D., and Berkelman, R. L. "A meta-analysis of the effect of estrogen replacement therapy on the risk of breast cancer." *Journal of the American Medical Association* 1991; 265: 1985–1990.

13. Yang, C. P., Daling, J. R., Band, P. R., Gallagher, R. P., White, E., and Weiss, N. S. "Noncontraceptive hormone use and the risk of breast cancer." *Cancer Causes and Control* 1992; 3: 475–479.

14. Schairer, C., Byrne, C., Keyl, P. M., Brinton, L. A., Sturgeon, S. R., and Hoover, R. N. "Menopausal estrogen and estrogen-progestin replacement therapy and risk of breast cancer (United States)." *Cancer Causes and Control* 1994; 5(6): 491–500.

15. Colditz, G. A., Hankinson, S. E., Hunter, D. J., Wilett, W. C., Manson, J. E., Stampfer, M. J., Hennekens, C., Rosner, B., and Speizer, F. E. "The use of estrogens and progestins and the risk of breast cancer in postmenopausal women." *New England Journal of Medicine* 1995; 332: 1589–1993.

16. Stanford, J. L., Weiss, N. S., Voight, L. F., Daling, J. R., Habel, L. A., and Rosing, M. "Combined estrogen and progestin hormone replacement therapy in relation to risk of breast cancer." *Journal of the American Medical Association* 1995; 274: 37–142.

17. Chang, K. J., Fournier, S., Lee, D. E., Lignieres, B., and Linares-Cruz, G. "Influences of percutaneous administration of estrodiol and progesterone on human breast epithelial cell cycle in vivo." *Fertility and Sterility* 1995; 63(4): 785–791.

18. Bergkvist, L., Adami, H. O., Persson, I., Bergstrom, R., and Krusemo, U. B. "Prognosis after breast cancer diagnosis in women exposed to estrogen and estrogen-progestin replacement therapy." *American Journal of Epidemiology* 1989; 130(2): 221–227.

19. Colditz et al., op. cit.

20. Stomper, P. C., Van Voorhis, B. J., Ravnikar, V. A., and Meyer, J. E. "Mammographic changes associated with postmenopausal hormone replacement therapy: A longitudinal study." *Radiology* 1990; 174: 487–490.

21. Laya, M. B., Gallagher, J. C., Schreiman, J. S., Larson, E. B., Watson, P., and Weinstein, L. "Effect of postmenopausal hormone replacement therapy on mammographic density and parenchymal pattern." *Radiology* 1995; 196: 433–437.

22. Fletcher, S. W., Black, W., Harris, R., Rimer, B. K., and Shapiro, S. "Report of the International Workshop on Screening for Breast Cancer." *Journal of the National Cancer Institute* 1993; 85: 1644–1656.

23. Byrne, C., Schairer, C., Wolfe, J., Parekh, N., Salane, M., Brinton, L., Hoover, R., and Haile, R. "Mammographic features and breast cancer risk: Effects with time, age, and menopause status." *Journal of the National Cancer Institute* 1995; 87: 1622–1629.

24. Grady, D., Rubin, S. M., Petitti, D. B., et al. "Hormone therapy to prevent disease and prolong life in postmenopausal women." *Annals of Internal Medicine* 1992; 117: 1016–1037.

25. Shi, Y. E., Liu, Y. E., Lippman, M. E., and Dickson, R. B. "Progestins and antiprogestins in mammary tumour growth and metastasis." *Human Reproduction* 1994; 9(Supp. 1): 162–170.

26. Dhodapkar, M. V., Ingle, J. N., and Ahmann, D. L. "Estrogen replacement therapy withdrawal and regression of metastatic breast cancer." *Cancer* 1995; 75: 43–46.

27. Spicer, D., Pike, M. C., and Henderson, B. E. "The questions of estrogen replacement therapy in patients with a prior diagnosis of breast cancer." *Oncology* 1990; 4(12): 49–62.

28. Ganz, P. A., Greendale, G., Kahn, B., and O'Leary, J. F. "Are breast cancer survivors willing to take hormone replacement therapy?" *Proceedings of American Society of Clinical Oncology Meeting* 1996; 15: 109.

29. Peters, M. "The effect of pregnancy in breast cancer." *Prognostic Factors in Breast Cancer* 1968; 65.

30. Guinee, V. F., Olsson, H., Moller, T., et al. "Effect of pregnancy on prognosis for young women with breast cancer." *Lancet* 1994; 343: 1587.

31. Lambe, M., Hsieh, C.-C., Trichopoulos, D., Ekbom, A., Pavia, M., and Adami, H.-O. "Transient increase in the risk of breast cancer after giving birth." *New England Journal of Medicine* 1994; 331(1): 5.

32. Anonymous. "Systemic treatment of early breast cancer by hormonal, cytotoxic, or immune therapy: 133 randomised trials involving 31,000 recurrences and 24,000 deaths among 75,000 women. Early Breast Cancer Trialists' Collaborative Group." *Lancet* 1992; 339(8784): 1–15 (see comments).

33. DiSaia, P. J., Grosen, E. Q., Odicino, F., Cowan, B., Pecorelli, S., Wile, A., and Creasman, W. T. "Replacement therapy for breast cancer survivors: A pilot study." *Cancer* 1995; 76: 2075–2078.

34. Eden, J. A., Bush, T., Nand, S, and Wren, B. G. "A case-control study of combined continuous estrogen-progestin replacement therapy among women with a personal history of breast cancer." *Menopause* 1995; 2(2): 67–72.

35. Couzi, R. J., Helzsouer, K. J., and Fetting, J. H. "Prevalence of menopausal symptoms among women with a history of breast cancer and attitudes toward estrogen replacement therapy." *Journal of Clinical Oncology* 1995; 13: 2737–2744.

Chapter 8   Endometrial Cancer:
The First Problem with Estrogen

1. Kurman, R., Kaminski, P. F., and Norris, H. J. "The behavior of endometrial hyperplasia: A long term study on 'untreated' hyperplasia in 170 patients." *Cancer* 1985; 56: 403–412.

2. Grady, D., Gebretsadik, T., Kerlikowske, K., Ernster, V., and Petitti, D. "Hormone replacement therapy and endometrial cancer risk: A meta-analysis." *Obstetrics and Gynecology* 1995; 85(2): 304–313.

3. Grady, D., Rubin, S. M., Petitti, D. B., Fox, C. S., Black, D., Ettinger, B., Ernster, V. L., and Cummings, S. R. "Hormone therapy to prevent disease and prolong life in postmenopausal women." *Annals of Internal Medicine* 1992; 117(12): 1016–1037.

4. Greendale, G. A., and Judd, H. L. "Hormone therapy in the menopause." In *The Medical Care of Women*, Carr, P. T., Freund, K. M., and Somani, S. (eds.). New York: Saunders, 1995, pp. 635–642.

5. Writing Group for the PEPI Trial. "Effects of estrogen or estrogen/progestin regimens on heart disease risk factors in postmenopausal women." *Journal of the American Medical Association* 1994; 273(3): 199–208.

Chapter 9   For Better or Worse:
Hormone Therapy and Other Diseases

1. Hebert, L. E., Scherr, P. A., Beckett, L. A., Albert, M. S., Pilgrim, D. M., Chown, M. J., Funkenstein, H. H., and Evans, D. A. "Age-specific incidence of Alzheimer's disease in a community population." *Journal of the American Medical Association* 1995; 273(17): 1354–1359.

2. Paganini-Hill, A., and Henderson, V. W. "Estrogen deficiency and risk of Alzheimer's disease in women." *American Journal of Epidemiology* 1994; 140(3): 256–261.

3. Henderson, V. W., Paganini-Hill, A., Emanuel, C. K., Dunn, M. E., and Buckwalter, J. G. "Estrogen replacement therapy in older women. Comparisons between Alzheimer's disease cases and nondemented control subjects." *Archives of Neurology* 1994; 51(9): 896–900.

4. Brenner, D. E., Kukull, W. A., Stergachis, A., van Belle, G., Bowen, J. D., McCormick, W. C., Teri, L., and Larson, E. B. "Postmenopausal estrogen replacement therapy and the risk of Alzheimer's disease: A population-based case-control study." *American Journal of Epidemiology* 1994; 140(3): 262–267.

5. Fillitt, H., Weinreb, H., Cholst, I., Luine, V., McEwen, B., Amador, R., and Zabriskie, J. "Observations in a preliminary open trial of estradiol therapy for senile dementia-Alzheimer's type." *Psychoneuroendocrinology* 1986; 11(3): 337–345.

6. Tang, M. X., Jacobs, D., Stern, Y., Marder, K., Schofield, P., Gurland, B., Andrews, H., and Mayeux, R. "Effect of oestrogen during menopause on risk and age at onset of Alzheimer's disease." *Lancet* 1996; 348(9025): 429–432 (see comments).

7. Quoted in Brody, J. E. "Tantalizing data suggest estrogen may prevent or delay Alzheimer's." *The New York Times,* July 31, 1996: C7.

8. Gast, M. Presentation at Menopause Conference: Advances in Hormone Replacement and Alternative Therapeutic Strategies. Philadelphia, Pa.: May 9–10, 1996.

9. Henderson, V. W. "Alzheimer's disease in women: Is there a role for estrogen replacement therapy?" *Menopause Management* 1995; 4(6): 10–14.

10. Paganini-Hill, A., Ross, R. K., and Henderson, B. E. "Postmenopausal oestrogen treatment and stroke: A prospective study." *British Medical Journal* 1988; 297(20–27): 519–522.

11. Thompson, S. G., Meade, T. W., and Greenberg G. "The use of hormonal replacement therapy and the risk of stroke and myocardial infarction in women." *Journal of Epidemiology and Community Health* 1989; 43(2): 173–178.

12. Paganini-Hill, A. "Estrogen replacement therapy and stroke." *Progress in Cardiovascular Diseases* 1995; 38(3): 223–242.

13. Calle E. E., Miracle-McMahill, H. L., Thun, M. J., and Heath, C. W., Jr. "Estrogen replacement therapy and risk of fatal colon cancer in a prospective cohort of postmenopausal women." *Journal of the National Cancer Institute* 1995; 87(7): 517–523.

14. Giovannucci, E., Egan, K. M., Hunter, D. J., Stampfer, M. J., Colditz, G. A., Willett, W. C., and Speizer, F. E. "Aspirin and the risk of colorectal cancer in women." *New England Journal of Medicine* 1995; 333(10): 609–614.

15. Schoen, R. E., Weissfeld, J. L., and Kuller, L. H. "Are women with breast, endometrial, or ovarian cancer at increased risk for colorectal cancer?" *American Journal of Gastroenterology* 1994; 89(6): 835–842.

16. Broeders, M. J., Lambe, M., Baron, J. A., and Leon, D. A. "History of childbearing and colorectal cancer risk in women aged less than 60: An analysis of Swedish routine registry data 1960–1984." *International Journal of Cancer* 1996; 66(2): 170–175.

17. Chute, C. G., Willett, W. C., Colditz, G. A., Stampfer, M. J., Rosner, B., and Speiz, F. E. "A prospective study of reproductive history and exogenous estrogens on the risk of colorectal cancer in women." *Epidemiology* 1991; 2(3): 201–207.

18. Wu, A. H., Paganini-Hill, A., Ross, R. K., et al. "Alcohol, physical activity, and other risk factors for colorectal cancer: A prospective study." *British Journal of Cancer* 1987; 55: 687–694.

19. Newcomb, P. A., and Storer, B. E. "Postmenopausal hormone use and risk of large-bowel cancer." *Journal of the National Cancer Institute* 1995; 87(18): 1416.

20. MacLennan, S. C., MacLennan, A. H., and Ryan, P. "Colorectal cancer and oestrogen replacement therapy. A meta-analysis of epidemiological studies." *Medical Journal of Australia* 1995; 162(9): 491–493.
21. Nevitt, M. C., Cummings, S. R., Lane, N. E., Hochberg, M. C., Scott, J. C., Pressman, A. R., Genant, H. K., and Cauley, J. A. for the Study of Osteoporotic Fractures Research Group. "Association of estrogen replacement therapy with the risk of osteoarthritis of the hip in elderly white women." *Archives of Internal Medicine* 1996; 156: 2073–2080.
22. Kerlikowske, K., Brown, J. S., and Grady, D. G. "Should women with familial ovarian cancer undergo prophylactic oophorectomy?" *Obstetrics and Gynecology* 1992; 80(4): 700–707.
23. Kaufman, S. C., Spiritas, R., Alexander, N. J. "Do fertility drugs cause ovarian tumors?" *Journal of Women's Health* 1995; 4(3): 241–259.
24. Hartge, P., Hoover, R., McGowan, L., Lesher, L., and Norris, H. J. "Menopause and ovarian cancer." *American Journal of Epidemiology* 1988; 127: 990–998.
25. Rodriguez, C., Calle, E. E., Coates, R. J., Miracle-McMahill, H. L., Thun, M. J., and Heath, C. W., Jr. "Estrogen replacement therapy and fatal ovarian cancer." *American Journal of Epidemiology* 1995; 141(9): 828–835.
26. Grodstein, F., Colditz, G. A., and Stampfer, M. J. "Postmenopausal hormone use and colecystectomy in a large prospective study." *Obstetrics and Gynecology* 1994; 83(1): 5–11.
27. Craft, P., and Hannaford, P. C. "Risk factors for acute myocardial infarction in women: Evidence from the Royal College of General Practitioners' oral contraception study." *British Medical Journal* 1989; 298: 165–168.
28. Report from the Boston Collaborative Drug Surveillance Program, Boston University Medical Center. "Surgically confirmed gallbladder disease, venous thromboembolism, and breast tumors in relation to postmenopausal estrogen therapy." *New England Journal of Medicine* 1974; 290(1): 15–19.
29. Daly, E., Vessey, M. P., Hawkins, M. M., Carson, J. L., Gough, P., and Marsh, S. "Risk of venous thromboembolism in users of hormone replacement therapy." *Lancet* 1996; 348: 977–980.
30. Jick, H., Derby, L. E., Myers, M. W., Vasilakis, C., and Newton, K. M. "Risk of hospital admission for idiopathic venous thromboembolism among users of postmenopausal oestrogens." *Lancet* 1996; 348: 981–983.
31. Grodstein, F., Stampfer, M. J., Goldhaber, S. Z., Manson, J. E., Colditz, G. A., Speizer, F. E., Willett, W. C., and Hennekens, C. H. "Prospective study of exogenous hormones and risk of pulmonary embolism in women." *Lancet* 1996; 348: 983–987.
32. Akkad, A. A., Habiba, M. A., Ismail, N., Abrams, K., and al-Azzawi, F. "Abnormal uterine bleeding on hormone replacement: The importance of intrauterine structural abnormalities." *Obstetrics and Gynecology* 1995; 86(3): 330–334.
33. Sener, A. B., Seckin, N. C., Ozmen, S., Gokmen, O., Dogu, N., and Ekici, E. "The effects of hormone replacement therapy on uterine fibroids in postmenopausal women." *Fertility and Sterility* 1996; 65(2): 354–357.
34. Namnoum, A. B., Hickman, T. N., Goodman, S. B., Gehlbach, D. L., and Rock, J. A. "Incidence of symptoms recurrence after hysterectomy for endometriosis." *Fertility and Sterility* 1995; 64(5): 898–902.
35. Goh, J. T., and Hall, B. A. "Postmenopausal endometrioma and hormonal replacement therapy." *Australia New Zealand Journal of Obstetrics and Gynaecology* 1992; 32(4): 384–385.
36. Sanchez-Guerrero, J., Liang, M. H., Karlson, E. W., Hunter, D. J., and Colditz, G. A. "Postmenopausal estrogen therapy and the risk for developing systemic lupus erythematosus." *Annals of Internal Medicine* 1995; 122(6): 430–433.

37. Troisi, R. J., Speizer, F. E., Willett, W. C., Trichopoulos, D., and Rosner, B. "Menopause, postmenopausal estrogen preparations, and the risk of adult-onset asthma. A prospective cohort study." *American Journal of Respiratory and Critical Care Medicine* 1995; 152(Part 1): 1183–1188.

38. Adami, H. O., Persson, I., Hoover, R., Schairer, C., and Bergkvist, L. "Risk of cancer in women receiving hormone replacement therapy." *International Journal of Cancer* 1989; 44(5): 833–839.

39. Zang, E. A., and Wynder, E. L. "Differences in lung cancer risk between men and women: Examination of the evidence." *Journal of the National Cancer Institute* 1996; 88(3/4): 183–192.

Chapter 10   What Are My Options
for Feeling Better Right Now?

1. Anonymous. "Complementing mainstream medicine." *Nature Medicine* 1996; 2(6): 619.

2. Duda, R. B., Kessel, B., Curtin, M., Goodman, D., Kessel, M., Eisenberg, D., Colditz, G., Prouty, J., and Bookman, L. "The use of herbal remedies and alternative therapies by breast cancer patients." *Proceedings of Annual Meeting of the American Society of Clinical Oncology* 1995; 14: A70.

3. Dickstein, E. S., and Kunkel, F. W. "Foxglove tea poisoning." *American Journal of Medicine* 1980; 9(1): 167–169.

4. Weed, S. *Wise Woman Herbal Healing.* Woodstock, N.Y.: Ash Tree, 1989.

5. McCaleb, R. S. "Food ingredient safety evaluation." *Food Drug Law Journal* 1992; 47: 657–665.

6. Cargill, Marie. Personal conversation, November 1995.

7. Elghamry, M. I., and Shihata, I. M. "Biological activity of phytoestrogens." *Planta Medica* 1965; 13: 352–357.

8. Komori, A., Yatsunami, J., Okabe, S., et al. "Anticarcinogenic activity of green tea polyphenols." *Japanese Journal of Clinical Oncology* 1993; 23(3): 186–190.

9. Usuki, S. "Effects of hachimijiogan, tokishakuyakusan, kei-shibukuryogan, ninjinto, and unkeito on estrogen and progesterone secretion in preovulatory follicles incubated in vitro." *American Journal of Chinese Medicine* 1991; 19(1): 65–71.

10. Dwyer, J. T. "Dietary fat and breast cancer: Testing interventions to reduce risks." In *Exercise, Calories, Fat, and Cancer,* Jacobs, M. M. (ed.). New York: Plenum, 1992.

11. Heber, D., Ashley, J. M., Leaf, D. A., et al. "Reduction of serum estradiol in postmenopausal women given free access to low fat high carbohydrate diet." *Nutrition* 1991; 7: 137.

12. Rose, D. "Diet, hormones and cancer." *Annual Review of Public Health* 1993; 14: 1–17.

13. Clifford, C., and Kramer, B. "Diet as a risk and therapy for cancer." *Clinical Nutrition* 1993; 77(4): 725–740.

14. Aldercreutz, H., Markkanen, H., and Watanabe, S. "Plasma concentrations of phyto-oestrogens in Japanese men." *Lancet* 1993; 342 (8881): 1209–1210.

15. Aldercreutz, H., Mousavi, Y., Clark, J., Hockerstedt, K., et al. "Dietary phytoestrogens and cancer in vitro and in vivo studies." *Journal of Steroid Biochemisty and Molecular Biology* 1992; 41(3–8): 331–337.

16. Sakamoto, S., Yoshino, H., Shirahata, Y., Shimodairo, K., and Okamoto, R. "Pharmacotherapeutic effects of kuei-chih-fu-ling-wan (keishu-bukuryo-gan) on human uterine myomas." *American Journal of Chinese Medicine* 1992; 20(3): 313–317. Also--Sakamoto, S., Kudo, H., Kawasaki, T., Kuwa, K., et al. "Effects of a Chinese herbal medicine, keishi-bukuryo-gan, on the gonadal system of rats." *Journal of Ethnopharmacology* 1988; 23(2–3): 151–158. Also Usuki, op. cit.

17. Okamoto, R., and Kumai, A. "Antigonadotropic activity of hop extract." *Acta Endocrinology* (Copenhagen) 1992; 127(4): 371–377.
18. Serraino, M., and Thompson, L. "The effect of flaxseed supplementation on the initiation and promotional stages of mammary tumorogenesis." *Nutrition and Cancer* 1992; 3930; 253–260.
19. Messina, M., and Barnes S. "The role of soy products in reducing risk of cancer." *Journal of the National Cancer Institute* 1991; 83(8): 541–546.
20. Barnes, S., Grubbs, C., Setchell, K. D. R., et al. "Soybeans inhibit mammary tumors in models of breast cancer." In *Mutagens and Carcinogens in the Diet*, Pariza, M. (ed.). New York: Wiley-Liss, 1990, pp. 239–253.
21. Zhang, G. L. "Treatment of breast proliferation disease with modified xiao yao san and er chen decoction." *Chung His I Chieh Ho Tsa Chih* 1991; 11(7): 400–402.
22. Albert-Puleo, M. "Fennel and anise as estrogenic agents." *Journal Ethnopharmacology* 1980; 2(4): 337–344.
23. Takeuchi, T., Nishii, O., Okamura, T., and Yaginuma, T. "Effects of paeoniflorin, glycyrrhizin, and glycyrrhetic acid on ovarian androgen production." *American Journal of Chinese Medicine* 1991; 19(1): 73–78. Also—Takeuchi, T., Nishii, O., Okamura, T., and Yaginuma, T. "Effect of traditional herbal medicine, shakuyaku-kanzo-to on total and free serum testosterone levels." *American Journal of Chinese Medicine* 1989; 17(1–2): 35–44. Also—Ota, H., Fukushima, M., and Maki, M. "Stimulatory action of shakuyaku on aromatase activity in culuted rat follicles." *Nippon Sanka Fujinka Gakkai Zasshi* 1989; 41(5): 525–529. Also—Kato, T., and Okamoto, R. "Effect of shakuyaku-kanzo-to on serum estrogen levels and adrenal gland cells in ovariectomized rats." *Nippon Sanka Fujinka Gakkai Zasshi* 1992; 44(4): 433–439. Also—Takahashi, K., and Kitao, M. "Effect of TJ-68 (shakuyaku-kanzo-to) on polycystic ovarian disease." *International Journal Fertility and Menopausal Studies* 1994; 39(2): 69–76.
24. Zhang, J. P., and Zhou, D. J. "Changes in leucocytic estrogen receptor levels in patients with climacteric syndrome and therapeutic effect of luiwei dihuang pills." *Chung Hsi I Chieh Ho Tsa Chih* 1991; 11(9): 521–523, 515. Also—Zhu, X. Y., He, S. Z., Zhong, Z. H., Zhang, F. Y., et al. "Effects of liuwei dihuang granules, pills and decoction on contents of cAMP E2, T, Zn and Cu in plasma of renal yin deficient patients." *Chung Kuo Chung Yao Tsa Chih* 1993; 18(8): 503–504.
25. Albert-Puleo, op. cit.
26. Li, W., Zhou, C. H., and Li, Q. L. "Effects of Chinese materia medica in activating blood stimulating menstrual flow on the endocrine function of ovary-uterus and its mechanisms." *Chung Kuo Chung Hsi I Chieh Ho Tsa Chih* 1992; 12(3): 165–168.
27. Cargill, op. cit.
28. Walach, H. "Does a highly diluted homeopathic drug act as a placebo in healthy volunteers? Experimental study of belladonna 30c in double blind crossover design—A pilot study." *Journal of Psychosomatic Research* 1993; 37(8): 851–860.

Chapter 11 From Flashes to Fuzzy Thinking: What You Can Do Right Now

1. Kronenberg, F., and Barnard, R. M. "Modulation of menopausal hot flashes by ambient temperature." *Journal of Therm Biology* 1992; 17: 43–49.
2. Kronenberg, F. "Hot flashes: Epidemiology and physiology." *Annals of the New York Academy of Sciences* 1990; 592: 52–86.
3. Hammar, M., Berg, G., and Lindgren, R. "Does physical exercise influence the frequency of postmenopausal hot flushes?" *Acta Obstetrica et Gynecologica Scandinavica* 1990; 69: 409–412.

4. Notelovitz, M., and Tonnessen, D. *Menopause and Midlife Health.* New York: St. Martin's, 1993, p. 244.
5. Murkies, A. L., and Lombard, C. "Dietary flour supplementation decreases post-menopausal hot flushes: Effect of soy and wheat." *Maturitas* 1950; 21: 189–195.
6. Freedman, R. R., and Woodard, S. "Behavioral treatment of menopausal hot flushes: Evaluation by ambulatory monitoring." *American Journal of Obstetrics and Gynecology* 1992; 167: 436–439.
7. Irvin, J. H., Domar, A., Clark, C., Zuttermeister. P. C., and Friedman, R. "The effects of relaxation response training on menopausal symptoms." Paper presented at the Annual Meeting of the Society of Behavioral Medicine. Boston: April 13–16, 1994.
8. Wyon, Y., Lingrem, T., Lundeberg, T., and Hammar, M. "Effects of acupuncture on climacteric vasomotor symptoms, quality of life, and urinary excretion of neuropeptides among postmenopausal women." *Menopause: Journal of the North American Menopause Society* 1995; 2(1): 3–12.
9. Blatt, M. H. G., Wiesbader, H., and Kupperman, H. S. "Vitamin E and climacteric syndrome." *Archives of Internal Medicine* 1953; 91: 792–796.
10. Kronenberg, F. "Hot flashes: Phenomenology, quality of life, and search for treatment options." *Experimental Gerontology* 1994; 29(3/4): 319–336.
11. Holm, L. E., Callmer, E., Hjalmar, M. L., Lidbrink, E., Nilsson, B., and Skoog, L. "Dietary habits and prognostic factors in breast cancer." *Journal of the National Cancer Institute* 1989; 81(16): 1218–1223.
12. Weed, Susun. Personal communication, July 1996.
13. Stoll, W. *Therapeutikon* 1987; 1: 23–31.
14. Lehmann-Willenbrock Riedal Zent. Bl. Gynakol 1988; 110: 611–618.
15. Dueker, E. M., Kopanski, L., Jarry, H., and Wuttke, W. "Effects of extracts from *Cimicifuga racemosa* on gonadotropin release in menopausal women and oophorectomized rats." *Planta Medica* 1991; 57: 420–424.
16. Todorov, S., Philianos, S., Petkov, V., Harvala, C., Zamifirova, R., and Olimpiou, H. "Experimental pharmacological study of three species from genus salvia." *Acta Physiologica Pharmacologica Bulgarica* 1984; 10(2): 13–20.
17. Li, W., Zhou, C. H., and Lu, Q. L. "Effects of Chinese materia medica in activating blood stimulating menstrual flow on endocrine function of ovary-uterus and its mechanisms." *Chung Kuo Chung Hsi I Chieh Ho Tsa Chih* 1992; 12(3): 165–168.
18. Usuki, S. "Effects of hachimijiogan, tokishakuyakusan, kei-shibukuryogan, ninjinto, and unkeito on estrogen and progesterone secretion in preovulatory follicles incubated in vitro." *American Journal of Chinese Medicine* 1991; 19(1): 65–71.
19. Ota, H., Fukushima, M., and Maki, M. "Stimulatory action of shakuyaku on aromatase activity in cultured rat follicles." *Nippon Sanka Fujinka Gakkai Zasshi* 1989; 41(5): 525–529.
20. Kato, T., and Okamoto, R. "Effect of shakuyaku-kanzo-to on serum estrogen levels and adrenal gland cells in ovariectomized rats." *Nippon Sanka Fujinka Gakkai Zasshi* 1992; 44(4): 433–439.
21. Epstein, M. T., Espiner, E. A., Donald, R. A., Hughes, H., Cowles, R. J., and Lun, S. "Licorice raises urinary cortisol in man." *Journal of Clinical Endocrinology Metabolism* 1978; 47(2): 397–400.
22. Walker, B. R., and Edwards, C. R. "Licorice-induced hypertension and syndromes of apparent mineralocorticoid excess." *Endocrinology Metabolism Clinics of North America* 1994; 23(2): 359–377.
23. Bernardi, M., D'Intino, P. E., Trevisani, F., Cantelli-Forti, G., Raggi, M. A., Turchetto, E., and Gasbarrini, G. "Effects of prolonged ingestion of graded doses of licorice by healthy volunteers." *Life Science* 1994; 55(11): 863–872.

24. Zhang, J. P., and Zhou, D. J. "Changes in leucocytic estrogen receptor levels in patients with climacteric syndrome and therapeutic effect of luiwei dihuang polls." *Chung Hsi I Chieh Ho Tsa Chih* 1991; 11(9): 521–523, 515.

25. Zhang, G. L. "Treatment of breast proliferation disease with modified xiao yao san and er chen decoction." *Chung Hsi I Chieh Ho Tsa Chih* 1991; 11(7): 400–402, 388.

26. Coope, J., Thomson, J. M., and Poller, L. "Effects of 'natural oestrogen' replacement therapy on menopausal symptoms and blood clotting." *British Medical Journal* 1975; 4: 139–143.

27. Lebherz, T. B., and French, L. "Nonhormonal treatment of the menopausal syndrome." *Obstetrics and Gynecology* 1969; 33: 795–799.

28. Clayden, J. R., and his group (Clayden, J. R., Bell, J. W., and Pollard, P.). "Menopausal flushing: Double-blind trial of a nonhormonal medication." *British Medical Journal* 1974; 1: 409–412.

29. Tulandi, T., Lal, S., and Kinch, R. A. "Effect of intravenous clonidine on menopausal flushing and luteinizing hormone secretion." *British Journal of Obstetrics and Gynaecology* 1983; 90: 854–857.

30. Jones, K. P., Ravnikar, V., and Schiff, I. "A preliminary evaluation of the effect of lofexidene on vasomotor flushes in postmenopausal women." *Maturitas* 1985; 7: 135–139.

31. Loprinzi, C. L., Michalak, J. C., Quella, S. K., O'Fallon, J. R., Hatfield, A. K., Nelimark, R. A., Dose, A. M., Fischer, T., Johnson, C., Klatt, N. E., et al. "Megestrol acetate for the prevention of hot flashes." *New England Journal of Medicine* 1994; 331(6): 347–352.

32. Rookus, M. A., and van Leeuwen, F. E. "Oral contraceptives and risk of breast cancer in women aged 20–54 years." *Lancet* 1994; 344(8926): 844–851.

33. Pethö, A. *Ärztl. Praxis* 1987; 47: 1551–1553.

34. Milewicz, A., Gejdel, E., Sworen, H., Sienkiewicz, K., Jedrzejak, J., Teucher, T., and Schmitz, "H. Vitex agnus castus-Extrakt zur Behandlung von Regeltempoanomalien infolge latenter Hyperprolaktinamie. Ergebnisse einer randomisierten Plazebo-kontrollierten Doppelblindstudie." *Arzneimittelforschung* 1993; 43(7): 752–756.

35. Sliutz, G., Speiser-Schultz, A. M., Spona, J., and Zeillinger, R. "Agnus castus extracts inhibit prolactin secretion of rat pituitary cells." *Hormone Metabolism Research* 1993; 25(5): 253–255.

36. O'Connor, H., and Magos, A. "Endometrial resection for the treatment of menorrhagia." *New England Journal of Medicine* 1996; 335: 151–156.

37. Carlson, K. J., Miller, B. A., and Fowler, F. J. "The Maine Women's Health Study: I. Outcomes of hysterectomy." *Obstetrics and Gynecology* 1994; 83: 556–565.

38. Tobachman, J. K., Tucker, M. A., Kase, R., et al. "Intra-abdominal carcinomatosis after prophylactic oophorectomy in ovarian cancer prone families." *Lancet* 1982; 11: 795–797.

39. Wilcox, G. "Oestrogenic effects of plant foods on postmenopausal women." *British Medical Journal* 1991; 301: 905–906.

40. Nachtigall, L. E. "Comparative study: Replens versus local estrogen in menopausal women." *Fertility and Sterility* 1994; 61(1): 178–180.

41. Punnonen, R., and Lukola, A. "Oestrogen-like effect of ginseng." *British Medical Journal* 1980; 281: 1110.

42. DiRaimondo, C. V., Roach, A. C., and Meador, C. K. "Gynecosmastia from exposure to vaginal estrogen cream." *New England Journal of Medicine* 1980; 302(9): 1089–1090.

43. Zhdanova, I. V., Wurtman, R. J., Lynch, H. J., Ives, J. R., Dollins, A. B., Morabito, C., Matheson, J. K., and Schomer, D. L. "Sleep inducing effects of low doses of melatonin ingested in the evening." *Clinical Pharmacology and Therapeutics* 1995; 57(5): 552–558.

44. Garfinkel, D., Laudon, M., Nof, D., and Zisapel, N. "Improvement of sleep quality in elderly people by controlled-release melatonin." *Lancet* 1995; 346(8974): 541–544.

45. Brown, E., and Walker, L. *Breezing Through the Change.* Berkeley, Calif.: Frog, p. 107. Also—Ito, D. *Natural Remedies for Menopause and Beyond.* New York: Random House, p. 143.
46. Weed, op. cit.
47. Petkov, V. D., Kehayov, R., Belcheva, S., Konstantinova, E., Petkov, V. V., Getova, D., and Markovska, V. "Memory effects of standardized extracts of Panax ginseng (G115), Gingko balboa (GK501), and their combination Gincosan (PHL-00701)." *Planta Medica* 1993; 59(2): 106–114.
48. Liberti, L. E., and Marderosian, A. D. "Evaluation of commercial ginseng products." *Journal of Pharmacology Science* 1978; 67: 1487–1489.
49. Michael, M. *The Healing Power of Herbs: The Enlightened Person's Guide to the Wonders of Medicinal Plants.* Rocklin, Calif.: Prima, 1995.
50. Semlitsch, H. V., Anderer, P., Saletu, B., Binder, G. A., and Decker, K. A. "Cognitive psychophysiology in nootropic drug research: Effects of Ginkgo biloba on event-related potentials (P300) in age-associated memory impairment." *Pharmacopsychiatry* 1995; 28(4): 134–142.
51. Nygaard, I. "Prevention of exercise incontinence with mechanical devices." *Journal of Reproductive Medicine* 1995; 40(2): 89–94.
52. Brown and Walker, op. cit.

Chapter 12   For Prevention:
First Look to Your Lifestyle!

1. Rose, D. P., Connolly, J. M., Rayburn, J., and Coleman, M. "Influence of diet containing eicosapentaenoic or docosahexaenoic acid on growth and metastasis of breast cancer cells in nude mice." *Journal of the National Cancer Institute* 1995; 87: 587–592.
2. Ornish, D. *Dr. Dean Ornish's Program for Reversing Heart Disease.* New York: Random House, 1990.
3. Feskanich, D., Willet, W. C., Stampfer, M. J., and Colditz G. A. "Protein consumption and bone fractures in women." *American Journal of Epidemiology* 1996; 143(5): 472–479.
4. Ellis, F. R., Holesh, S., and Ellis, J. W. "Incidence of osteoporosis in vegetarian and omnivorous women." *American Journal of Clinical Nutrition* 1972; 25: 555–558.
5. Marsh, A. G., Sanchez, T. V., Michelsen, O., Keiser. J., and Mayor, G. "Cortical bone density of adult lacto-ovo vegetarian and omnivorous women." *Journal of the American Dietetic Association* 1980; 76; 148–151.
6. Bennetts, H. W., Underwood, E. J., and Shier, F. L. "A specific breeding problem of sheep on subterranean clover pastures in Western Australia." *Australian Veterinarian Journal* 1946; 22: 2–129.
7. Findlay, J. K., Buckmaster, J. M., Chamley, W. A., Cummings, I. A., Hearnshaw, H., and Goding, J. R. "Release of luteinizing hormone by oestradiol 17 beta and gonadotrophin-releasing hormone in ewes affected with clover disease." *Neuroendocrinology* 1973; 11: 57–66.
8. Hughes, C. L. "Phytochemical mimicry of reproductive hormones and modulation of herbivore fertility by phytoestrogens." *Environmental Health Perspectives* 1988; 78: 171–175.
9. Anderson, J. W., Johnstone, B. M., and Cook-Newell, M. E. "Meta analysis of the effects of soy protein intake on serum lipids." *New England Journal of Medicine* 1995; 333: 276–282.
10. Barnes, S. Presentation at Menopause Conference: Advances in Hormone Replacement and Alternative Therapeutic Strategies. Philadelphia, Pa.: May 9–10, 1996.
11. Breslau, N. A., Brinkley, L., Hill, K. D., and Pak, C. Y. C. "Relationship of animal protein-rich diet to kidney stone formation and calcium metabolism." *Journal of Clinical Endocrinology Metabolism* 1988; 66: 140–146.

12. Naomi, O., Syuichi, A., Katumi, M., and Ikuko, E. "Evaluation of the effect of soybean milk and soybean milk peptide on bone metabolism in the rat model with ovariectomized osteoporosis." *Journal of Nutritional Sciences and Vitaminol* 1994; 40, 201–211.

13. Cassidy, A., Bingham, S., and Setchell, K. D. R. "Biological effects of a diet of soy protein rich in isoflavones on the menstrual cycle of premenopausal women." *American Journal of Clinical Nutrition* 1994; 60: 333–340.

14. Messina, M. J., Persky, V., Setchell, K. D. R., and Barnes, S. "Soy intake and cancer risk: A review of the in vitro and in vivo data." *Nutrition Cancer* 1994; 21: 113–131.

15. Lee, H. P., Gourley, L., Duffy, S. W., Esteve, J., Lee, J., and Day, N. E. "Dietary effects on breast cancer risk in Singapore." *Lancet* 1991; 337: 1197–1200.

16. Wang, C., and Kurzer, M. S. "Effects of isoflavones flavinoids and lignans on proliferation of estrogen-dependent and independent human breast cancer cells." *Proceedings of the American Association for Cancer Research* 1996; 37: 277.

17. Petrakis, N. L., Barnes, S., King, E. B., Lowenstein, J., Wiencke, J., Lee, M. M., Miike, R., Kirk, M., and Coward, L. "Stimulatory influence of soy protein isolate on breast secretion in pre- and postmenopausal women" [in Process Citation]. *Cancer Epidemiology Biomarkers and Prevention* 1996; 5(10): 785–794.

18. Setchell, K. D. R., Gosselin, S. J., Welsh, M. B., Johnston, J. O., Balistreri, W. F., Kramer, L. W., Dresser, B. L., and Tarr, M. J. "Dietary estrogens: A probable cause of infertility and liver disease in captive cheetahs." *Gastroenterology* 1987; 93: 225–233.

19. Liener, I. E. "Possible adverse effects of soybean anticarcinogens." *Journal of Nutrition* 1995; 125: 744S–750S.

20. Tew, B. Y., Xu, X., Wang, H. J., and Murphy, P. "A diet high in wheat fiber decreases the bioavailability of soybean isoflavones in a single meal fed to women." *Journal of Nutrition* 1996; 126: 871–877.

21. Seraino, S. "The effect of flaxseed supplementation on the initiation and promotional stages of mammary tumorgenesis." *Nutrition and Cancer* 1992; 17(2): 153–159.

22. Bierenbaum, M. L. "Reducing atherogenic risk in hyperlipemic humans with flaxseed supplementation: a preliminary report." *Journal of the American College of Nutrition* 1993; 12(5): 501–504.

23. Cumnane, S. C. "Nutritional attributes of traditional flaxseed in healthy young adults." *American Journal of Clinical Nutrition* 1993; 69(2): 443–453.

24. Messina, M. "The role of soy products in reducing risk of cancer." *Journal of the National Cancer Institute* 1991; 83(7): 541–545.

25. Shandler, N. *Estrogen: The Natural Way: Over 250 Easy and Delicious Recipes for Menopause.* New York: Villard, 1997.

26. Zheng, W., Doyle, T. J., Hong, C. P., Kushi, L. H., Sellers, T. A., and Folsom, A. R. "Tea consumption and cancer incidence in a prospective cohort study of postmenopausal women." *Proceedings of the Annual Meeting of the American Association for Cancer Research* 1995; 36: A1654 (meeting abstract).

27. Reid, I. R., Ames, R. W., Evans, M. C., Gamble, G. D., and Sharpe, S. J. "Effect of calcium supplementation on bone loss in postmenopausal women." *New England Journal of Medicine* 1993; 328(7): 460–464.

28. Prince, R. "The calcium controversy revisited: Implications of new data." *Medical Journal of Australia* 1993; 159: 404–407.

29. Manson, J. E., Willett, W. C., Stampfer, M. J., Colditz, G. A., Hunter, D. J., Hankinson, S. E., Hennekens, C. H., and Speizer, F. E. "Body weight and mortality among women." *New England Journal of Medicine* 1995; 333(11): 677–685.

30. Nishizawa, T., Akaoka, I., Nishida, Y., Kawaguchi, Y., and Hayashi, E. "Some factors related to obesity in the Japanese sumo wrestler." *American Journal of Clinical Nutrition* 1976; 29(10): 1167–1174.

31. Notelovitz, M., and Tonnessen, D. *Menopause and Midlife Health.* New York: St. Martin's, 1993.
32. Weed, S. *Menopausal Years: The Wise Woman Way.* Woodstock, N.Y.: Ash Tree, 1992.
33. Freudenheim, J. L., Marshall, J. R., Vena, J. E., Laughlin, R., Brasure, J. R., Swanson, M. K., Nemoto, T., and Graham, S. "Premenopausal breast cancer risk and intake of vegetables, fruits, and related nutrients." *Journal of the National Cancer Institute,* 1966; 88(6): 340–348.
34. Hennekens, C. H., Buring, J. E., Manson, J. E., Stampfer, M., Rosner, B., Cook, N. R., Belanger, C., LaMotte, F., Gaziano, J. M., Ridker, P. M., Willett, W., and Peto, R. "Lack of effect of long-term supplementation with beta carotene on the incidence of malignant neoplasms and cardiovascular disease." *New England Journal of Medicine* 1996; 334(18): 1145–1149.
35. Manson et al., op. cit.
36. Notelovitz and Tonnessen, op. cit.
37. Bernstein, L., Henderson, B. E., Hanisch, R., Sullivan-Halley, J., and Ross, R. K. "Physical exercise and reduced risk of breast cancer in young women." *Journal of the National Cancer Institute* 1994; 86(18): 1403–1408.
38. Notelovitz and Tonnessen, op. cit., p. 98.
39. Bravo, G. "Physical exercise benefits postmenopausal women." *Journal of the American Geriatric Society* 1996; 44: 756–762.
40. Blair, S. N., Kohl, H. W., Paffenbarger, R. S., Clark, D. G., Cooper, K. H., and Gibbons, L. W. "Physical fitness and all cause mortality: A prospective study of healthy men and women." *Journal of the American Medical Association* 1989; 262: 2395–2401.
41. Notelovitz and Tonnessen, op. cit.
42. Weed, op. cit.
43. Cousins, N. *Anatomy of an Illness.* New York: Bantam, 1979.
44. Benson, H. *Beyond the Relaxation Response.* New York: Berkeley, 1985.
45. Stolbach, Leo. Quoted in Love, S. *Dr. Susan Love's Breast Book.* Reading, Mass.: Addison-Wesley, 1995, pp. 438–439.
46. Benson, op. cit.
47. Jarte, J. L., Eifert, G. H., and Smith, R. "The effects of running and meditation on beta endorphin, corticotropin releasing hormone and cortisol in plasma and on mood." *Biological Psychology* 1995; 40(3): 251–265.
48. Smith, W. P., Compton, W. C., and West, W. B. "Meditation as an adjunct to a happiness enhancement program." *Journal of Clinical Psychology* 1995; 51(2): 269–273.
49. Fiore, N. *The Road Back to Health.* New York: Bantam, 1984.
50. Cousins, op. cit.
51. LeShan, L. *How to Meditate.* New York: Bantam, 1974, pp. 33, 39, 40.
52. Spiegel, D., Bloom, J. R., Kraemer, H. C., and Gottheil, E. "Effect of psychosocial treatment on survival of patients with metastatic breast cancer." *Lancet* 1989; 2(8668): 888.

Chapter 13   Alternatives: Acupuncture to Herbs

1. Omenn, G. S., Goodman, G. E., Thornquist, M. D., Balmes, J., Cullen, M. R., Glass, A., Keogh, J. P., Meyskens, F. L., Valanis, B., Williams, J. H., Barnhart, S., and Hammar, S. "Effects of a combination of beta carotene and vitamin A on lung cancer and cardiovascular disease." *New England Journal of Medicine* 1966; 334(18): 1150–1155.
2. Pennington, J. A. T. "Mineral content of foods and total diets: The selected minerals in foods survey." *Journal of the American Dietetic Association* 1986; 86(7): 876–891.
3. Sempos, C. T., et al. "A two year dietary survey of middle aged women: Repeated dietary records as a measure of usual intake." *Journal of the American Dietetic Association* 1984; 1008–1013.

4. Cumming, R. G. "Calcium intake and bone mass: A quantitative review of the evidence." *Calcified Tissue International* 1990; 47: 194–201.

5. Garland, C., Barrett-Connor, E., Rossof, A. H., Shekelle, R. B., Criqui, M. H., and Paul, O. "Dietary vitamin D and calcium and risk of colorectal cancer: A 19 year prospective study in men." *Lancet* 1985; February: 307–325.

6. Sowers, M. R., Wallace, R. B., and Lemke, J. H. "The association of intakes of vitamin D and calcium with blood pressure among women." *American Journal of Clinical Nutrition* 1985; 42: 135–142.

7. Weed, S. *The Menopausal Years: The Wise Woman Way.* Woodstock, N.Y.: Ash Tree, 1992.

8. Sojka, J. E., and Weaver, C. M. "Magnesium supplementation and osteoporosis." *Nutrition Reviews* 1995; 53(3): 71–80.

9. Abraham, G. E., and Grewal, H. "A total dietary program emphasizing magnesium instead of calcium." *Journal of Reproductive Medicine* 1990; 35: 503–507.

10. Koskinen, T., Pyykko, K., Kudo, R., Jokela, H., and Punnonen, R. "Serum selenium, vitamin A, vitamin E and cholesterol concentrations in Finnish and Japanese postmenopausal women." *International Journal for Vitamin and Nutrition Research* 1987; 57: 111–114.

11. Free-Graves, J., et al. "Manganese status of osteoporotics and age matched, healthy women." *FASEB Journal* 1990; 4: A777.

12. National Research Council. *Recommended dietary allowances.* Washington, D.C.: National Academy, 1989, p. 186.

13. Notelovitz, M., and Tonnessen, D. *Menopause and Midlife Health.* New York: St. Martin's, 1993, p. 86.

14. Krall, E. A., et al. "Effect of vitamin D intake on seasonal variations in parathyroid hormone secretion in postmenopausal women." *New England Journal of Medicine* 1989; 321: 1777–1783.

15. Sultenfuss, S. W., and Sultenfuss, T. J. *A Woman's Guide to Vitamins and Minerals.* Chicago: Contemporary, 1995.

16. Cargill, M. *Acupuncture: A Viable Medical Alternative.* Westport, Conn.: Praeger, 1994, p. 26.

17. Wolfe, H. L. *Menopause: A Second Spring.* Boulder, Colo.: Blue Poppy, 1995.

18. Dickens, P., Tai, Y. T., But, P. P., Tomlinson, B., Ng, H. K., and Yan, K. W. "Fatal accident aconitine poisoning following ingestion of Chinese herbal medicine: A report of two cases." *Forensic Science International* 1994; 67(1): 55–58.

19. Gertner, E., Marshall, P. S., Filandrinos, D., Potek, A. S., and Smith, T. M. "Complications resulting from the use of Chinese herbal medications containing undeclared prescription drugs." *Arthritis Rheumatism* 1995; 38(5): 614–617.

20. Chan, T. Y., Chan, A. Y., and Critchley, J. A. "Hospital admissions due to adverse reactions to Chinese herbal medicines." *Journal of Tropical Medicine Hygiene* 1992; 95(4): 296–298.

21. Yamamoto, M., Uemura, T., Nakama, S., Uemiya, M., and Kumagai, A. "Serum HDL-cholesterol-increasing and fatty liver improving actions of Panax ginseng in high cholesterol diet fed rats with clinical effect on hyperlipidemia in man." *American Journal of Chinese Medicine* 1983; 11(1–4): 96–101.

22. Bai, Y. R., and Wang, S. Z. "Hemodynamic study on nitroglycerin compared with salvia miltiotthiza chung kuo." *Chung Hsi I Chieh Ho Tsa Chih* 1994; 14(1): 24–25.

23. Jiu, L. J., Morikawa, N., Omi, N., and Ezawa, I. "The effect of tochu bark on bone metabolism in the rat model with ovariectomized osteoporosis." *Nutrition Science Vitaminol* 1994; 40(3): 261–273.

24. Chopra, D. *Perfect Health.* New York: Harmony, 1991.

25. Ibid.

26. Thakur, C. P., Thakur, B., Singh, S., Sinha, P. K., and Sinha, S. K. "The ayurvedic medicines haritaki, amala, and bahira reduce cholesterol induced atherosclerosis in rabbits." *International Journal of Cardiology* 1988; 21(2): 167–175.

27. Shaila, H. P., Udupa, A. L., and Udupa, S. L. "Preventative actions of terminalia belerica in experimentally induced atherosclerosis." *Journal of Cardiology* 1995; 49(2): 101–106.

28. Sharma, H. M., Hanna, A. N., Kauffman, E. M., and Newman, H. A. "Inhibition of human low density lipoprotein oxidation in vitro by maharishi ayur-veda herbal mixtures." *Pharmacology, Biochemistry, and Behavior* 1992; 43(4): 1175–1182.

29. Shanmugasundaram, E. R., Sundaram, P., Srinivas, K., Shanmugasundaram, K. R., and Shankara, J. R. "Double-blind crossover study of modified anna pavala sindhooram in patients with hyperlipidemia or ischemic heart disease." *Ethnopharmacology* 1991; 31(1): 85–99.

30. Zamarra, J. W., Schneider, R. H., Besseghini, I., Robinson, D. K., and Salerno, J. W. "Usefulness of the transcendental meditation program in the treatment of patients with coronary heart disease." *American Journal of Cardiology* 1996; 77(10): 867–870.

31. Schneider, R. H., Staggers, F., Alexander, C. N., Sheppard, W., Rainforth, M., Kondwani, K., Smith, S., and King, C. G. "A randomized controlled trial of stress reduction for hypertension in older African Americans." *Hypertension* 1995; 26(5): 820–827.

32. Collinge, W. *The American Holistic Health Association Complete Guide to Alternative Medicine.* New York: Warner, 1996.

Chapter 14   Drugs: Other Means of Prevention

1. Reginster, J. Y., Deroisy, R., Lecart, M. P., Sarlet, N., Zegels, B., Jupsin, I., de Longueville, M., and Franchimont, P. "A double-blind, placebo-controlled, dose-finding trial of intermittent nasal salmon calcitonin for prevention of postmenopausal lumbar spine bone loss." *American Journal of Medicine* 1995; 98: 452–458.

2. Rico, H., Revilla, M., Hernandez, E. R., Villa, L. F., and Alvarez de Buergo, M. "Total and regional bone mineral content and fracture rate in postmenopausal osteoporosis treated with salmon calcitonin: A prospective study." *Calcified Tissue International* 1995; 56: 181–185.

3. Lyritis, G. P., Tsakalakos, N., Magiasis, B., Karachalios, T., Yiatzides, A., and Tsekoura, M. "Analgesic effect of salmon calcitonin in osteoporotic vertebral fractures: A double-blind placebo-controlled clincal study." *Calcified Tissue International* 1991; 49: 369–372.

4. Landman, J. O., Hamdy, N. A., Pauwels, E. K., and Papapoulos, S. E. "Skeletal metabolism in patients with osteoporosis after discontinuation of long term treatment with oral pamidronate." *Journal of Clinical Endocrinology Metabolism* 1995; 8 (12): 3465–3468.

5. Liberman, U. A., Weiss, S. R., Broll, J., Minne, H. W., Quan, H., Bell, N. H., Rodriguez-Portales, J., Downs, R. W., Jr., Dequeker, J., Favus, M., et al. "Effect of oral alendronate on bone mineral density and the incidence of fractures in postmenopausal osteoporosis. The Alendronate Phase III Osteoporosis Treatment Study Group." *New England Journal of Medicine* 1995; 333: 1437–1443.

6. Shapiro, D. R., Thompson, D. E., Karpf, D. B., Santora, A. C., Lombardi, A., Hirsch, L. J., Seeman, E., Bell, N., Ortolani, S., Harris, S. T., and Ensrud, K. "Non-vertebral fracture incidence in patients treated with alendronate. Abstract." *American Society for Bone and Mineral Research*, October 17, 1995.

7. Black, D. "Alendronate prevents hip and other fractures in some osteoporosis patients." Presentation at 1996 World Conference on Osteoporosis, Amsterdam, May 1996.

8. Anonymous. "Warning about oesophagitis with Fosamax." *Lancet* 1996; 347: 959.

9. Riggs, B. L., O'Fallon, W. M., Lane, A., Hodgson, S. F., Wahner, H. W., Muhs, J., Chao, E., and Melton, L. J. "Clinical trial of fluoride therapy in postmenopausal osteoporotic women: Extended observations and additional analysis." *Journal of Bone and Mineral Research* 1994; 9: 265–275.

10. Pak, C. Y., Sakhaee, K., Adams-Huet, B., Piziak, V., Peterson, R. D., and Poindexter, J. R. "Treatment of postmenopausal osteoporosis with slow-release sodium fluoride. Final report of a randomized trial." *Annals of Internal Medicine* 1995; 123: 401–408.

11. Brandi, M. L. "New treatment strategies: Ipriflavone, strontium, vitamin D metabolites and analogs." *American Journal of Medicine* 1993; 95: 5A69S–5A74S.

12. Gotto, A. M., Jr. "Primary and secondary prevention of coronary artery disease." *Current Opinion Cardiology* 1992; 7: 553.

13. Bradford, R. H., Downtown, M., Chremos, A. N., et al. "Efficacy and tolerability of lovastatin in 3390 women with moderate hypercholesterolemia." *Annals of Internal Medicine* 1993; 118: 50.

14. "The Scandinavian Simvastatin Survival Study Group randomized trial of cholesterol lowering in 4444 patients with coronary heart disease. The Scandinavian Simvastatin Survival Study (4S)." *Lancet* 1994; 344: 1383.

15. Waters, D., Higginson, L., Gladstone, P., Boccuzzi, S. J., et al., for CCAIT Study Group. "Effects of cholesterol lowering on the progression of coronary atherosclerosis in women. *Canadian Atherosclerosis Intervention Trial (CCAIT) Substudy Circulation* 1995; 92: 2404.

16. Manson, J. E., Stampfer, M. J., Colditz, G. A., Willet, W. C., Rosner, B., Speizer, F. E., and Hennekens, C. H. "A prospective study of aspirin use and primary prevention of cardiovascular disease in women." *Journal of the American Medical Association* 1991; 266: 521–527.

Chapter 15 Hormones: The Menu of Options

1. Spicer, D., Pike, M. C., and Henderson, B. E. "The question of estrogen replacement therapy in patients with a prior diagnosis of breast cancer." *Oncology* 1990; 4(12): 49–59.

2. McDonnell, D. P., Clemm, D. L., Hermann, T., Goldman, M. E., and Pike, J. W. "Analysis of estrogen receptor function in vitro reveals three distinct classes of antiestrogens." *Molecular Endocrinology* 1995; 9: 659–669.

3. McDonnell, D. P., Clevenger, B., Dana, S. L., Santiso-Mere, D., Tzukerman, T., and Gleeson, M. A. "The mechanism of action of steroid hormones: A new twist to an old tale." *Journal of Clinical Pharmacology* 1993; 33: 1165–1172.

4. Clark, J. H., Paszko, Z., and Peck, E. J., Jr. "Nuclear binding and retention of the receptor estrogen complex: Relation to the agonistic and antagonistic properties of estriol." *Endocrinology* 1977; 100(1): 91–96.

5. Whittaker, P. G., Morgan, M. R., Dean, P. D., Cameron, E. H., and Lind, T. "Serum equilin, oestrone, and oestradiol levels in postmenopausal women receiving conjugated equine oestrogens ('Premarin')." *Lancet* 1980; 1(8158): 14–16.

6. Barrett-Connor, Elizabeth. Personal communication, 1996.

7. Ettinger, B., Genant, H. K., and Cann, C. E. "Postmenopausal bone loss is prevented by treatment with low-dosage estrogen with calcium." *Annals of Internal Medicine* 1987; 106: 40–45.

8. Ettinger, B., Golditch, I. M., and Friedman, G. "Gynecologic consequences of long-term unopposed estrogen replacement therapy." *Maturitas* 1988; 10: 271–282.

9. Lemon, H. M. "Antimammary carcinogenic activity of 17–alpha-ethinyl estiol." *Cancer* 1987; 60(12): 2873–2881.

10. Adlercreutz, H., Gorbach, S. L., Goldin, B. R., Woods, M. N., Dwyer, J. T., and Hamalainen, E. "Estrogen metabolism and excretion in Oriental and Caucasian women." *Journal of the National Cancer Institute* 1994; 86(14): 1076–1082.

11. Walter, S., and Jensen, H. K. "The effect of treatment with oestradiol and oestriol on fasting serum cholesterol and triglyceride levels in postmenopausal women." *British Journal of Obstetrics and Gynaecology* 1977; 84(11): 869–872.
12. Thorneycroft, I. "Practical aspects of hormone replacement therapy." *Progress in Cardiovascular Diseases* 1995; 38(3): 243–255.
13. Henderson, I. Craig. Personal communication, 1996.
14. Anonymous. "NSABP halts B-14 trial: No benefit seen beyond 5 years of tamoxifen use." *Journal of the National Cancer Institute* 1995; 87(24): 1829 (news).
15. Spicer, Pike, and Henderson, op. cit.
16. Early Breast Cancer Trialists Group (EBCTC). "Effects of adjuvant tamoxifen and of cytotoxic therapy on mortality in early breast cancer: An overview of 61 randomized trials among 28,896 women." *New England Journal of Medicine* 1988; 319: 1681.
17. Anonymous. "NSABP halts B-14 trial: No benefit seen beyond 5 years of tamoxifen use." *Journal of the National Cancer Institute* 1995; 87(4): 1829.
18. Ke, H. Z., Simmons, H. A., Pirie, C. M., Crawford, D. T., and Thompson, D. D. "Droloxifene, a new estrogen antagonist/agonist, prevents bone loss in ovariectomized rats." *Endocrinology* 1995; 136(6): 2435–2441.
19. Sato, M., Kim, J., Short, L. L., Slemenda, C. W., and Bryant, H. U. "Longitudinal and cross-sectional analysis of ralixofene effects on tibiae from ovariectomized aged rats." *Journal of Pharmacology and Experimental Therapeutics* 1995; 272(3): 1252–1259.
20. Going, J. J., Anderson, T. J., Battersby, S., et al. "Proliferative and secretory activity in human breast during natural and artificial menstrual cycles." *American Journal of Pathology* 1988; 130: 193–204.
21. Chang, K. J., Fournier, S., Lee, T. T., de Lignieres, B., and Linares-Cruz, G. "Influences of percutaneous administration of estradiol and progesterone on human breast epithelial cell cycle in vivo." *Fertility and Sterility* 1995; 63(4): 785–791.
22. Writing Group for the PEPI Trial. "Effects of estrogen or estrogen/progestin regimens on heart disease risk factors in postmenopausal women." *Journal of the American Medical Association* 1994; 273(3): 199–208.
23. Prior, J. C. "Progesterone as a bone-trophic hormone." *Endocrine Reviews* 1990; 11(2): 386–398.
24. Writing group for the PEPI trial, op. cit.
25. Ibid.
26. Marslew, U., Riis, B. J., and Christiansen, C. "Bleeding patterns during continuous combined estrogen-progestogen therapy." *American Journal of Obstetrics and Gynecology* 1991; 164: 1163–1168.
27. Hickok, L. R., Toomey, C., and Speroff, L. "A comparison of esterified estrogens with and without Methyltestosterone: Effects on endometrial histology and serum lipoproteins in postmenopausal women." *Obstetrics and Gynecology* 1993; 82: 919–924.
28. Colditz, G. A., Hankinson, S. E., Hunter, D. J., Willet, W. C., Manson, J. E., Stampfer, M. J., Hennekens, C., Roser, B., and Speizer, F. E. "The use of estrogens and progestins and the risk of breast cancer in postmenopausal women." *New England Journal of Medicine* 1995; 332: 1589–1593.
29. Rako, S. *The Hormone of Desire*. New York: Harmony, 1996.

Chapter 16   Decisions: What Should *I* Do?

1. Holzman, G. B., Ravitch, M. M., Metheny, W., Rothert, M. L., Holmes, M., and Hoppe, R. B. "Physicians' judgments about estrogen replacement therapy for menopausal women." *Obstetrics and Gynecology* 1984; 63: 303–311.
2. Notelovitz, M., and Tonnessen, D. *Menopause and Midlife Health*. New York: St. Martin's, 1993, p. 438.

3. Foundation for Informed Medical Decision Making. *Hormone Replacement Therapy.* A Shared Decision Making Program Videotape, 1995.

4. Grady, D., Rubin, S. M., Petitti, D. B., et al. "Hormone therapy to prevent disease and prolong life in postmenopausal women." *Annals of Internal Medicine* 1992; 117(12): 1016.

5. Ibid.

6. Bush, T. L., and Miller, V. T. "Effects of pharmacologic agents used during menopause: impact on lipids and lipoproteins." In Mishell, D. R., ed., *Menopause: Physiology and Pharmacology.* Chicago: Year Book Medical Publishers, 1987: 187–208.

7. Walsh, B. W., Schiff, I., Rosner, B., et al. "Effects of postmenopausal estrogen replacement on the concentrations and metabolism of plasma lipoproteins." *New England Journal of Medicine* 1991; 325: 1196–1204.

8. The Writing Group for the PEPI. "Effects of estrogen or estrogen/progestin regimens on heart disease risk factors in postmenopausal women." *Journal of the American Medical Association* 1995; 273: 199–208.

9. Love, R. R., Wiebe, D. A., Newcomb, P. A., Cameron, L., Levanthal, H., Jordan, V. C., Feyzi, J., and DeMets, D. L. "Effects of tamoxifen on cardiovascular risk factors in postmenopausal women." *Annals of Internal Medicine* 1991; 115(11): 860–4.

10. Oster, G., Borok, G. M., Mensin, J., Heyse, J. F., Epstein, R. S., Quinn, V., Benson, V., Dudl, R. J., and Epstein, A. M. "Cholesterol reduction intervention study (CRIS): a randomized trial to assess effectiveness and costs in clinical practice." *Archives of Internal Medicine* 1996; 156.

11. Schaefer, E. J., Lichtenstein, A. H., Lamon-Fava, S., Mcnamara, J. R., Schaefer, M. M., Rasmussen, H., and Ordovas, J. M. "Body weight and low density lipoprotein cholesterol changes after consumption of a low-fat ad Libitum diet." *Journal of the American Medical Association* 1995; 274: 1450–1455.

12. Anderson, J. W., Johnstone, B. M., and Cook-Newell, M. E. "Meta-analysis of the effects of soy protein intake on Serum Lipiserum lipids." *New England Journal of Medicine* 1995; 333: 276–82.

13. Boyden, T. W., Pamenter, R. W., Going, S. B., Lohman, T. G., Hall, M. C., Houtkooper, L. B., Bunt, J. C., Ritenbaugh, C., and Aickin, M. "Resistance exercise training is associated with decreases in serum low density lipoprotein cholesterol levels in premenopausal women." *Archives of Internal Medicine* 1993; 153(1): 97–100.

14. Felson, D. T., Zhang, Y., Hannan, M. T., Kiel, D. P., Wilson, P. W. F., and Anderson, J. J. "The effect of postmenopausal estrogen therapy on bone density in elderly women." *New England Journal of Medicine* 1993; 329: 1141–6.

15. Ettinger, B., Genant, H. K., and Cann, C. "Long-term estrogen replacement therapy prevents bone loss and fractures." *Annals of Internal Medicine* 1985; 102: 319–24.

16. Liberman, U. A., Weiss, S. R., Broll, J., Minne, H. W., Quan, H., Bell, N. H., Rodriguez-Portales, J., Downs, R. W., Jr., Dequeker, J., Favus, M., et al. "Effect of oral alendronate on bone mineral density and the incidence of fractures in postmenopausal osteoporosis." The Alendronate Phase III Osteoporosis Treatment Study Group. *New England Journal of Medicine* 1995; 333(22): 1437–43.

17. Nelson, M. E., Fisher, E. C., Dilmanian, F. A., Dallal, G. E., and Evans, W. J. "A 1-year walking program and increased dietary calcium in postmenopausal women: effects on bone." *American Journal of Clinical Nutrition* 1991; 53(5): 1304–11.

18. Caplan, G. A., Ward, J. A., and Lord, S. R. "The benefits of exercise in postmenopausal women." *Australian Journal of Public Health* 1993; 17(1): 23–6.

19. Agnusdei, D., Adami, S., Cervetti, R., Crepaldi, G., DiMunno, O., Fantasia, L., Isaia, G. C., Letizia, G., Ortolani, S., Passeri, M., et al. "Effects of ipriflavone on bone mass and calcium metabolism in postmenopausal osteoporosis." *Journal of Bone and Mineral Research* 1992; Suppl 1: S43–8.

20. Powles, T. J., Hickish, T. F., Kanis, J. A., and Ashley, S. "Tamoxifen preserves bone mineral density in postmenopausal women but causes loss of bone density in premenopausal women" (Meeting Abstract). *Proceedings Annual Meeting of American Society of Clinical Oncology* 1995; 14: SA344.

21. Blair, S. N., Kohl, H. W., Paffenbarger, R. S., Clark, D. G., Cooper, K. H., and Gibbons, L. W. "Physical fitness and all-cause mortality: A prospective study of healthy men and women." *Journal of the American Medical Association* 1989; 262: 2395–2401.

22. Ettinger, B., Friedman, G. D., Bush, T., and Quesenberry, C. P. "Reduced mortality associated with long-term postmenopausal estrogen therapy." *Obstetrics and Gynecology* 1996; 87: 6–12.

23. Blair, S. N., Kohl, H. W., Paffenbarger, R. S., et al., op. cit.

24. Ibid.

25. Ulrich, C. M., Georgiou, C. C., Snow-Harter, C. M., and Gillis, D. E. "Bone mineral density in mother-daughter pairs: Relations to lifetime exercise, lifetime milk consumption, and calcium supplements." *American Journal Clinical Nutrition* 1996; 63(1): 72–79.

26. Cauley, J. A., Lucas, F. L., Kuller, L. H., Vogt, M. T., Browner, W. S., and Cummings, S. R., for the Study of Osteoporotic Fractures Research Group. "Bone mineral density and risk of breast cancer in older women: the study of osteoporotic fractures." *Journal of the American Medical Association* 1996; 276: 1404–1408.

Index

copper, 228
corn oil, 193
coronary care unit (CCU), 106
corpus luteum, 6
cortisone, 86
coumarin, 166
Council of Acupuncturist Schools and Colleges, 156
Cousins, Norman, 218, 220
cranberry juice, 187
crash diets, 203
creativity, menopause and, 222
Crenshaw, Theresa L., 18
"crone's year," 217
cross-sectional studies, 63, 64, 83
crush fractures, 81
cyclical therapy, continuous therapy vs., 269–71
Cycrin, 254
cynicism, as risk factor for heart disease, 103

daily charts, 278
D and C (dilation and curettage), 32, 47, 174, 175
dandelion (*Taraxacum oficiniale*), 166
dang qui shao yao san, 153, 166, 167
dan shen (Salvia miltiorrhiza), 155, 165, 235
DCIS (ductal carcinoma *in situ*), 114
DDT, 117
decision making, 275–300
   questionnaires for, 281–83, 292–96
   for symptoms, 283–85
   values in, 276–81
deoxyacteine, 165
depression, menopausal-related, 49–50
DES, 61, 118, 260, 279
DEXA (dual-energy X-ray absorptiometry), 81
diabetes, 103–4, 129, 259
diadzein, 196, 197
Didronel (etidronate), 242
diet, 192–207
   bone formation in, 76–77
   calcium in, 201–2
   cancer prevention and, 205
   crash, 203
   eating habits and, 206–7
   fat in, 102, 153, 192–93, 204, 205–6
   flaxseed in, 199–201
   fluid intake in, 201
   high soy-protein, 111, 205
   late-night meals and, 203–4
   meat-based, 138
   mood swings and, 183
dilantin, 298
dilation and curettage (D&C), 32, 47, 174, 175
diosgenin, 172

doctors:
   Chinese, 151, 155–56, 235
   and tapering off of hormones, 299–300
   values of, 277–79
dolomite, 226
dong quai (Angelica sinensis), 165–66, 179, 183, 184, 223
Doress-Worters, Paula B., 26
double-blind, 67
dowager's hump, 74, 81
Dr. Dean Ornish's Program for Reversing Heart Disease (Ornish), 193
dried raw soybeans, 198
Droloxifene, 265
drug companies, xv
   as driving force for medicalization of menopause, 24–31
   hormone replacement therapy marketed by, 25–27
   media exploitation by, 33–35
   "natural" hormones marketed by, 251–52
drugs:
   delivery systems of, 252–55
   see also hormone replacement therapy; non-hormonal drugs; *specific drugs*
dual-energy X-ray absorptiometry (DEXA), 81
ductal carcinoma *in situ* (DCIS), 114
Duda, Rosemary, 148
dysuria, 57

edamame, 198
eggs, 5
elder flower (*Sambucus* species), 166
embolic stroke, 137
endocrinology, reproductive, 8
endometrial ablation, 174
endometrial biopsies, 32, 47, 110, 175, 271
endometrial cancer, 28, 47, 126–33, 271
   prevention and, 288
   realities of, 126–29, *127, 128*
   risk factors for, 129–33
endometrial hyperplasia, 47, 127–28, 175, 259, 271
endometriosis, 11, 143, 176
endometrium, 5, 173, 261
endothelium, 99
England, 24, 31
epinephrine, 216
equilin, 136
equilin sulfate, 257
Equisetum arvense (horsetail), 232–33
er chen tang, 154
ergotamine, 168
ERT, *see* estrogen
Estinyl, 260
Estrace, 180, 253, 255, 260
Estraderm, 253, 261

ABOUT THE AUTHORS

SUSAN M. LOVE, M.D., is an author, teacher, surgeon, researcher, and activist. She is the author of many books and articles, including *Atlas of Surgical Techniques* and *Dr. Susan Love's Breast Book*, which has been called "the bible" for women with breast cancer. In 1996, after twenty years of direct patient care, Dr. Love left clinical practice to devote more time to her basic research as an adjunct associate professor of clinical surgery at UCLA and director of the Santa Barbara Breast Cancer Research Institute. In addition, as a result of her growing interest in women's health, she is starting an independent think tank that will be a conscience for the nation on women's health issues and will study ways to improve the health care of women in the managed care environment. She lives in Southern California with her life partner, Helen Cooksey, their eight-year-old daughter, Katie, Brownie the dog, and Cream the cat.

If you are interested in supporting her work, you can reach her at P.O. Box 846, Pacific Palisades, CA 90272.

KAREN LINDSEY is the coauthor of *Dr. Susan Love's Breast Book*. She is the author of *Friends as Family* and *Divorced, Beheaded, Survived: A Feminist Reinterpretation of the Wives of Henry VIII*. She teaches writing at Emerson College and women's studies at the University of Massachusetts in Boston.

ABOUT THE TYPE

This book was set in Photina, a typeface designed by
José Mendoza in 1971. It is a very elegant design
with high legibility, and its close character fit has
made it a popular choice for use in quality magazines and art gallery publications.